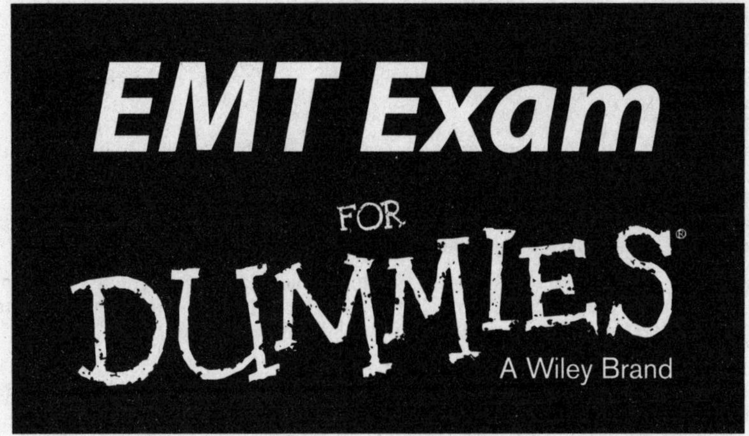

by Art Hsieh, MA, NREMT-P

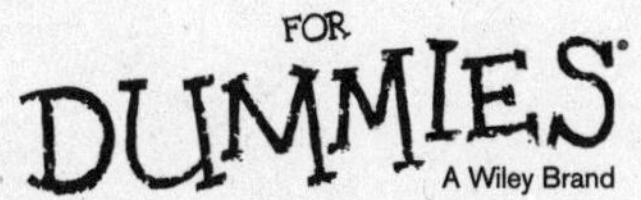

EMT Exam For Dummies®

Published by: **John Wiley & Sons, Inc.,** 111 River Street, Hoboken, NJ 07030-5774, www.wiley.com

For general information on our other products and services, please contact our Customer Care Department within the U.S. at 877-762-2974, outside the U.S. at 317-572-3993, or fax 317-572-4002. For technical support, please visit www.wiley.com/techsupport.

Wiley publishes in a variety of print and electronic formats and by print-on-demand. Some material included with standard print versions of this book may not be included in e-books or in print-on-demand. If this book refers to media such as a CD or DVD that is not included in the version you purchased, you may download this material at http://booksupport.wiley.com. For more information about Wiley products, visit www.wiley.com.

Library of Congress Control Number: 2014930403

ISBN 978-1-118-76817-4 (pbk); ISBN 978-1-118-81396-6 (ebk); ISBN 978-1-118-81402-4 (ebk)

Manufactured in the United States of America

10 9 8 7 6 5 4 3 2 1

Contents at a Glance

Table of Contents

Introduction

The emergency medical services (EMS) profession is a noble one. People don't become rich by being EMS providers, and many gladly volunteer their time and resources providing the service to their community.

As an EMS professional of more than 30 years, I welcome you to our world with open arms. I hope that you'll find as much satisfaction and enjoyment in providing emergency care and compassion as I have!

Although the amount of time it takes to become an emergency medical technician (EMT) may be relatively small, your responsibilities are huge. In the prehospital setting, the decisions you make in providing basic care to a critically sick or injured person may make a huge difference in whether the patient has a good outcome, recovers with difficulty, or, in the worst case, dies. Mastering the information in your EMT course and being able to apply it with accuracy and efficiency are of the utmost importance.

The fact that you're reading this book means one of two things: Either you have completed an EMT course and you're getting ready to take the National Registry of Emergency Medical Technicians (NREMT) examination, or you're interested in learning about the role of the EMT in the healthcare setting. My goals in writing this book are to address both of these areas — to improve your test-taking skills and provide an overview of EMS and of the EMT.

About This Book

EMT Exam For Dummies contains a lot of information in a well-organized format, logically laid out and in relatively few chapters. Features include the following:

- **This is not a rehash of your textbook.** Each chapter summarizes key findings of the many conditions you'll come across as a practicing EMT. You don't have to read this book from cover to cover; you can dip into any section, chapter, or part you need. You already have a textbook; why add another?
- **Practice questions are written in the NREMT format.** The questions may seem more challenging at first; they're written to test your ability to reason and make decisions, not your ability to remember simple facts.
- **Practice exams evaluate your overall knowledge.** There are three practice exams, two in this book and one other online at `learn.dummies.com`. Each one is designed to test your overall knowledge base of the EMT.
- **I let you in on tricks of the trade.** Who wouldn't want to know about little tricks and shortcuts to help make life easier as an EMT? You find them in their own chapters at the end of this book.
- **You get some "nice to know" information.** In a few places, I provide a behind-the-scenes look to better explain a principle or process. I denote this information either with the Technical Stuff icon or in a shaded box called a *sidebar;* feel free to skip this material if you're short on time.

- **It's a Dummies book.** When I was asked to write this book, I was honored to do so. I have several of these books on my personal shelf, and I wrote this book in a similar way — making it easy to read and understand, and keeping all the fluff to a minimum. I try to keep it light, but medicine is a serious business and some jokes are simply inappropriate.
- **Medical terminology appears throughout.** While most of the book is written in a conversational, easy-to-understand style, medical terms are used. An EMT is a healthcare professional and is expected to speak and understand the "language" of medicine at a foundational level. *Italics* indicate terms that are defined in the text; **boldface** highlights key words in bulleted lists or the main parts of numbered steps.
- **Web addresses may break.** Within this book, you may note that some web addresses break across two lines of text. If you're reading this book in print and want to visit one of these web pages, simply key in the web address exactly as it's noted in the text, pretending as though the line break doesn't exist. If you're reading this as an e-book, you've got it easy — just click the web address to be taken directly to the web page.

Foolish Assumptions

In writing this book, I made a few assumptions about you:

- **You're getting ready to take the NREMT EMT exam.** In fact, you may have taken it one or more times before. I assume that you've completed the vast majority of an EMT course and have been taught according to a standard curriculum.
- **You have a textbook.** This book isn't meant to be a mini-textbook. It emphasizes only the essential elements you need to know to pass the exam. Your course textbook serves as your reference — use its index pages, found in the back of the book, to find key terms or concepts that you find unfamiliar.
- **You're pressed for time.** I've tried my best to be direct. I want you to get the most out of this book in the least amount of time. Don't read this book like a novel. Use the sections you need to become better at the exam.
- **You're open to suggestions.** After all, you bought this book because you want extra help. I provide a variety of suggestions and explain some of the more difficult concepts a little differently in order to give you more tools to better master the material.

If you aren't about to take the exam, that's fine! If you're at the beginning or in the middle of an EMT course, the suggestions about studying and answering the practice questions in each chapter will strengthen your core knowledge. And if you're just thinking about taking an EMT class, you may find the information illuminating and perhaps helpful in solidifying your decision.

Icons Used in This Book

Icons are the small drawings found in the margins of this book. I use several icons to call your attention to key points:

This icon highlights points that you should keep in mind while taking the exam or taking care of a patient.

This icon points to a bit of information that helps make a key concept or exam process easier to understand or perform.

Watch out! If you see this icon, pay attention to the information provided. It describes situations that can get you into a lot of trouble on the exam — and with the care of your patients.

This is "nice to know" information that explains some ideas or processes in more detail but isn't 100 percent necessary to remember. You can skip these paragraphs if you're pressed for time.

Examples are sample questions that highlight specific concepts or procedures. Explanations are provided immediately after the answers. By the way, there are also additional practice questions at the end of each chapter in Part III.

Beyond the Book

EMT Exam For Dummies has three full practice exams located online at learn.dummies.com. All you have to do to access them is register by following these simple steps:

1. **Find your PIN code.**
   - **Print-book users:** If you purchased a hard copy of this book, turn to the front of this book to find your PIN.
   - **E-book users:** If you purchased this book as an e-book, you can get your PIN by registering your e-book at www.dummies.com/go/getaccess. Simply select your book from the drop-down menu, fill in your personal information, and then answer the security question to verify your purchase. You'll then receive an e-mail with your PIN.
2. **Go to http://learn.dummies.com.**
3. **Enter your PIN.**
4. **Follow the instructions to create an account and establish your own login information.**

Now you're ready to go! You can come back to the online program as often as you want — simply log on with the username and password you created during your initial login. No need to enter the PIN a second time.

If you have trouble with your PIN or can't find it, contact Wiley Product Technical Support at 877-762-2974 or go to http://support.wiley.com.

Use the exams to check your study practice; for example, you may want to take the two in this book first, review Part III, and then take the third exam online. You'll also find 200 flashcards at learn.dummies.com.

But wait — that's not all! Check out the free Cheat Sheet at www.dummies.com/cheatsheet/emtexam for details on EMT certification, features of the EMT exam, and tips for preparing and taking the exam. At www.dummies.com/extras/emtexam, discover free articles on computer adaptive testing, the process for distinguishing medical complaints, and common medical abbreviations.

Where to Go from Here

You can go to any chapter from here. Like other *Dummies* books, this one is not designed to be read from the first page to the last page. If you haven't started an EMT course and are interested in finding out more, I suggest you start with Chapter 1. If you're currently in a course, you may want to start with Chapter 6, as it provides study tips and ideas that you can use right away. If you're starting your review in preparation for the NREMT EMT exam, begin with Chapter 3, which introduces the exam process.

If you feel that you aren't a good test-taker, consider reading Part II before you begin your review. If you want to jump right in with content review, I suggest you take the preassessment in Chapter 8 before reviewing Chapters 9 through 14. Chapters 15 and 17 have full-length practice exams; Chapters 16 and 18 provide answers and explanations.

While this book contains lots of good information, it's not the end-all and be-all. Your textbook and class notes will serve as additional reference material while you work your way through this book. Doing quick searches on the web will provide additional resources. And don't forget your classmates — you spent (or will spend) a significant amount of time with them and probably have study buddies you should stay in touch with, just in case.

Part I
Making Sense of the EMT Exam

getting started with the EMT exam

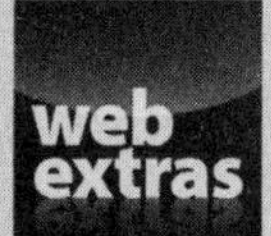

Visit www.dummies.com for great (and free!) Dummies content online.

In this part . . .

- Discover what an emergency medical technician (EMT) does and where an EMT works. (Essentially, an EMT provides basic emergency care, such as oxygen administration, spinal immobilization, and splinting; EMTs typically work in ambulances, but they're also deployed as part of wilderness and search and rescue teams.)
- Read about the education you need to certify as an EMT. Not only is there the textbook information to acquire, but there are skills to master as well as time you'll spend with actual patients while you're in training.
- Get the scoop on the National Registry of Emergency Medical Technicians (NREMT) exam. You may have heard that the exam is really hard. There's a reason for that, but it's not what you think!

Chapter 1

Becoming an Emergency Medical Technician

In This Chapter

- Knowing what an EMT does
- Becoming a certified EMT
- Renewing your EMT certification

Welcome to the world of emergency medical services, or EMS! This is a noble profession. The training is challenging, the work unpredictable, and you won't become rich performing the job. But you will have the privilege of helping people when they need it the most — when doing the right thing at the right time may very well save a life. Even in instances when the job isn't that dramatic, the simple care, comfort, and words of reassurance you provide may be all someone needs to feel better.

This chapter gives you the basics on what EMTs do, how to become one, and how to maintain your certification.

Understanding What Being an EMT Means

An emergency medical technician, or EMT, provides a basic level of emergency and non-urgent patient care. Some EMTs are paid for their work, while others volunteer their time, especially in more rural parts of the United States. In most states, the EMT is the minimum level of training required to provide ambulance transportation or care for the patient in the ambulance. The following sections explain what EMTs do, where they work, and the value of EMT training.

Note: The profession is transitioning from using the older term EMT-Basic (EMT-B) to simply EMT. This book uses the term EMT, but you can assume that the two terms are interchangeable.

What does an EMT do?

The EMT is one component of an EMS system, which may use other trained prehospital professionals to care for patients as well. The four general levels of EMS providers in the United States are

- **Emergency medical responder (EMR):** 48–60 hours of training. An EMR provides minimum, basic first aid. Lifeguards, police officers, and some firefighters are often required to have this certification.

- **Emergency medical technician (EMT):** 120–180 hours of training. This level serves as the foundation for higher certification levels. An EMT provides basic emergency care, such as oxygen administration, spinal immobilization, and splinting. Many states require this certification as a minimum to work as a staff member on an emergency ambulance. Many firefighters and police officers also earn EMT certification so that they can perform basic emergency care as part of their duties.
- **Advanced emergency medical technician (AEMT):** 160–300 hours of training beyond EMT. This training can vary quite widely from one state to the next. In addition to the skill set of the EMT, AEMTs may perform intravenous therapy, administer a limited set of medications, and manage a patient's airway at a higher level than an EMT.
- **Paramedic:** 1,100 hours or more of training beyond EMT. In addition to the skill set of the AEMT, the paramedic receives more information about human anatomy and physiology, the pathophysiology of disease, and trauma, and can administer a greater array of emergency medications. Paramedics can insert endotracheal tubes to help patients breathe and perform various types of electrical therapy to help heart rhythm disturbances.

In the majority of states, you have to be certified first as an EMT before taking on additional training to become an AEMT or paramedic. All EMS providers function under medical direction; usually a physician oversees the clinical practice of each level of responder.

An EMT does a patient assessment, which includes taking the patient's history and vital signs, and performing a physical examination. The care an EMT provides includes oxygen administration, artificial ventilation, cardiopulmonary resuscitation (CPR), splinting of broken bones, and immobilization for spinal injuries. EMTs are trained to assist patients with specific types of emergency medication that are prescribed for them, such as nitroglycerin for chest pain, an inhaler for breathing difficulties, and an epinephrine autoinjector (EpiPen) for *anaphylaxis,* a severe, life-threatening allergic reaction. Some states permit EMTs to do more procedures, such as monitor oxygen levels in the blood *(oximetry),* test blood glucose levels *(glucometry),* and administer certain emergency drugs.

Because the practice of the EMT isn't consistent throughout all states, the test questions don't evaluate your knowledge of things like glucometry. The questions assume only that you were taught to the foundational level as determined by the EMS National Scope of Practice, which is a federal document that describes what each level of EMS provider is permitted to perform. You can see this document at `www.ems.gov/education/EMSScope.pdf`.

Where do EMTs work?

EMTs traditionally work in ambulances, caring for and transporting patients from one location to the next: from a hospital bed to the person's home, from an emergency care scene to a hospital, or even from one hospital to another.

In emergency response systems, an EMT may work alongside another EMT, or partner with a more advanced level provider such as an AEMT or paramedic. Firefighters and police officers who are EMT-certified may respond to an emergency call and arrive sooner than the ambulance that may be farther away.

You often find EMTs working as part of an emergency-department team or working at a clinic. It's not unusual for the EMT to receive additional training in skills such as *phlebotomy* (blood draws) or recording a patient's *electrocardiogram* (tracing of the heart's electrical activity).

Wilderness and search-and-rescue teams often deploy EMTs because their skill set is ideal for providing care in remote areas. As in the hospital or clinic setting, EMTs may receive more training to better handle these conditions.

Can you use EMT training for other purposes?

Many students become EMTs to help prepare them for a career in the healthcare field. The information is valuable and serves as a foundation to build upon. EMTs go on to become AEMTs, paramedics, nurses, physician assistants, doctors, or other allied health professionals.

Even if you're not planning to further your education or pursue a career as an EMT, the training you receive is invaluable. Learning to stay calm, manage a scene, and provide basic care in a medical emergency makes you a more valued member of society.

Walking through the Steps of Becoming an EMT

As you find out in the following sections, you need to complete a few steps before you can apply your skills and knowledge as an EMT. ***Note:*** Because emergency medical services are regulated at the state level, these steps can vary from one state to the next. Always check your state's EMS website for the details.

Finding and completing a class

EMT classes are conducted by a wide variety of institutions. Your local community college may offer the class for college credit. Hospitals may also provide the training. The local EMS agency or fire department may offer the course, especially if it's to help train volunteers. Private organizations provide the training as well.

Searching online usually yields a list of classes closest to you. You can also check your state's office of EMS to see whether it offers a listing of approved training programs. If you feel adventurous, try visiting your local EMS or fire station and introduce yourself to the EMTs on duty. Ask whether they have any suggestions or recommendations on where to take a course.

After you find a class that meets your needs, you complete your training program. This means passing all the tests your instructor provides, including all the practical examinations. Seems obvious, but you really can't proceed to the next step without completing this one. Chapter 2 provides the scoop on finding a class and meeting its requirements.

Passing the National Registry Exam

A desire to pass the National Registry Exam may be the main reason you have this book. The National Registry of Emergency Medical Technicians (NREMT) is a nongovernmental organization that serves as the national EMS certification organization. The computer-based NREMT examination has been exhaustively evaluated for its ability to measure your EMT knowledge. Part of the NREMT examination is a practical exam, often given by your training program. Passing the NREMT exam means that you have a level of understanding that experts call "entry-level competent." You discover more about the exam in Chapter 3.

Note: Although most states require you to pass the NREMT exam, not all do. States that don't mandate the NREMT exam usually require you to complete a state-level examination. You can check the NREMT website (`www.nremt.org/nremt/about/stateReciprocityMap.asp`) to see whether your state requires the NREMT exam.

Finishing the process

Passing the NREMT exam doesn't authorize you to function as an EMT. That responsibility resides with your state. You typically present your NREMT credentials to the state EMS office, complete an application, and pay a fee to become state-certified. Because EMTs enter people's homes and businesses as part of the job, as well as solicit personal information about patients, many states require that you submit to a criminal background check.

To work as an EMT, an employer may require you to pass a medical examination and/or pass a test regarding the operation of an ambulance. You should check with these agencies to see what they require.

Maintaining Your EMT Certification

All states require you to renew your EMT certificate periodically. The time frame varies from one part of the country to the next, but many states have a two-year interval. Some states require you to use the NREMT renewal process to recertify. Other states have their own renewal process. You should consult your state EMS office for exact details.

If your state requires you to follow the NREMT renewal process, you need to do one of the following every two years:

- **Take a refresher course plus continuing education classes:** This option requires you to complete a combination of an approved, 24-hour EMT refresher course and an additional 48 hours of ongoing continuing education classes.
  - **EMT refresher class:** The refresher class is exactly that — a course designed to refresh your original knowledge base and, in some cases, verify your skill competency. It's designed to renew baseline knowledge that you may not have used or may have forgotten over your certification period. A written test is usually given at the end of the class to confirm that you possess the appropriate baseline knowledge and skill set for EMT practice (sometimes a practical test is also given).
  - **Continuing education classes:** Receiving your NREMT card doesn't signal the end of your training; in fact, it's really the beginning! Medicine is a continuously evolving science and art. New discoveries occur every day, and eventually some make it into the world of prehospital medicine.

    Continuing education classes help increase your body of EMT knowledge. They can be traditional, in-classroom courses; online courses; or a combination of the two, called a *hybrid.* Regardless of how the instruction is delivered, continuing education courses keep you up to speed in the world of prehospital medicine.

  Refresher and continuing education classes are offered by a variety of organizations, such as EMS agencies, fire departments, community colleges, and private education providers. You can search the web for organizations near you. Also, several providers provide online continuing education; you need to check whether the courses they teach are accepted in your state.

- **Retake the NREMT exam:** This option gives you the ability to renew your registration by retaking the initial exam. This is a good choice if your state requires fewer continuing education hours than the NREMT renewal process, and you'd prefer to take only the minimum number of hours necessary to maintain your certification. You can find additional information at the NREMT website (`www.nremt.org`).

A valid CPR card is also necessary. In addition, you must be working as an EMS professional and have your skills verified by your agency's training program director, director of operations, or physician medical director. Complete information can be found at `www.nremt.org/nremt/about/reg_basic_history.asp#EMT_Recertification`.

States that don't require the NREMT renewal process have their own recertification process. Check with your state's EMS office for details. A listing of state EMS offices can be found at `www.nremt.org/nremt/about/emt_cand_state_offices.asp`.

Chapter 2

Taking an EMT Course and Registering for the EMT Exam

In This Chapter

- Taking and passing an EMT course
- Signing up for the big test

It's time to take that first step — undergoing the training you need to qualify to take the NREMT examination. Depending on where you live, finding a program that best fits your needs may be a bit confusing. Determining where to take the training is an individual choice. You may be a 19-year-old student taking the course for credit or a 45-year-old working professional looking to volunteer in your local community.

Regardless of your particular needs, some common thoughts and tips about locating and completing an EMT course apply. This chapter walks you through the process and then explains how to register for the EMT exam.

Enrolling in and Completing an EMT Course

You need to find and complete a course that prepares you properly, not just for the exam but also for real-world conditions. The following sections explain how to find and succeed in an EMT course.

Finding a course that fits your needs

You have several options for finding an EMT course in your neck of the woods:

- Perhaps the easiest way to find a course is to perform a web search. Entering "EMT training" and the name of your town, city, or county in your browser of choice often brings up programs that are available in your area. Easy!
- Every state has an office of EMS, which may provide a list of training organizations that are approved or authorized to provide EMT training. Do an online search for the name of your state plus "EMS office."
- EMT programs may advertise in the local community. For example, volunteer fire or EMS departments may conduct EMT training at little or no cost to students in an effort to attract new volunteers to the organization. You may find additional information on their websites, in local newspapers, or at community centers.
- You may get a recommendation via word-of-mouth. Take a field trip down to the EMS or fire department to see whether the staff can recommend a particular training program.

Before you sign up for the first course you come across, carefully consider what the course needs to have to maximize your chances of success:

- Distance matters, of course. A training program that's close by is easier to attend. If you have other priorities in life, such as work or family, a local program makes it simpler to travel between locations.
- Cost is a consideration. Some courses require additional expenses beyond the tuition. These may include books, lab fees, uniforms, and medical equipment. Many programs offer the practical portion of the NREMT exam as part of their curriculum. Make sure you find out about all the costs upfront so you can budget ahead of time; this way, you won't stress about a "sudden" cost that you didn't anticipate. Also keep in mind that there may be additional costs beyond your training program, such as paying for the NREMT exam and your certification application.
- What about the time commitment? Some courses meet weekends only, whereas others meet during the week. Day and evening options exist as well. Compare EMT course schedules to your own schedule for work and/or school, and see what matches up best. If you can't find a course that fits your schedule exactly, consider what you can move around in your personal schedule. The bottom line is that you can't miss too many class sessions — there is a lot to cover, and the program probably has a minimum attendance policy.
- An increasing number of EMT courses are provided online. This option may be great for folks who have little time to attend a traditional face-to-face class or who work odd hours that conflict with class schedules. However, the majority require some type of hands-on labwork as part of the class; make sure you know exactly what the time commitments are. ***Note:*** Not everyone is cut out for an online class; you must be a highly motivated student who's capable of independent learning in order to maximize your chance of success.
- Being a good consumer of education can help you select the right course. Your state EMS office may have public data regarding how well graduates of various courses perform on the NREMT or state examination. You can also call the training organizations you're considering and ask what their NREMT passing rates are, as well as their attrition rate (the percentage of students who don't complete the training).

Being prepared for the course

If you haven't been to a classroom in a while, the prospect of formal learning may intimidate you. Don't worry — EMT education is very interactive and interesting, and it'll be what you make of it. Be prepared to have fun and be challenged! On one hand, you get to discover how to do things such as administer oxygen, immobilize patients using long backboards, perform CPR, operate an automated external defibrillator (AED), and manage chaotic emergency scenes. On the other hand, you have to get a handle on basic anatomy and physiology, plus a few complex concepts related to serious medical conditions such as shock, anaphylaxis, and diabetes.

A good rule of thumb is to set aside one to two hours of study time for each hour of instruction. For example, if the course meets six hours a week, plan to spend another six to twelve hours either reading, studying in groups, or practicing skills.

Create a study schedule that's realistic and maximizes your learning. Maybe you can only spend an hour a day or two hours every other day studying. That's fine, as long as you commit to focusing on your learning during those time periods. It's better to be totally focused for one hour than to sit in front of your books for three hours while being distracted by the television, telephone, or social media.

Figure 2-1 shows an example of a class/study/life schedule.

Sunday	*Monday*	*Tuesday*	*Wednesday*	*Thursday*	*Friday*	*Saturday*
Morning: Church	Morning: Work	Morning: Work	Morning: Work	Morning: Work	Morning: Work	*Morning: 8 a.m.–1 p.m. Class lab*
Afternoon: 1–5 p.m. Study previous week's materials	Afternoon: Work	Afternoon: Work	Afternoon: Work	Afternoon: Work	Afternoon: Work	Afternoon: 2–5 p.m. Study group
Evening: 7–9 p.m. Read this week's chapters	Evening: 7–10 p.m. Prep for weekly quiz	*Evening: 6–10 p.m. Class*	Evening: 7–10 p.m. Prep for Thursday class	*Evening: 6–10 p.m. Class*	Evening: 5–6 p.m. Prep for Saturday lab	Evening: Relax!

Figure 2-1: A sample class/study/life schedule.

In this sample, 16 hours of study time are set aside for 13 hours of classroom instruction. Free time is also set aside each day, as well as an evening off, to allow your brain to rest and recharge. Your schedule will probably be different, but the point is the same: Creating a schedule can help you stay on track and avoid falling behind in your studies.

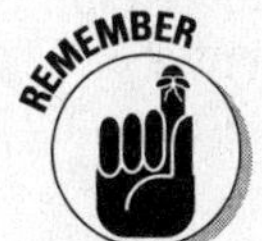

After you make your schedule, follow it religiously. Consider it as important as being on time for work, having dinner, or going to bed. You may need to give up some time with family and friends, or even reduce your work hours while attending the course. Whatever your sacrifice, know that it will be short-lived!

Create a positive study environment. Have a place in your home where you can minimize outside distractions. Have a good task light to read with and a table with a comfortable but supportive chair. (Beds and couches are more conducive to napping than studying.)

If you can't make the space at home, look for other places where you can study. The campus or public library is one place. A nearby coffee shop is a favorite spot for many students, but you'll want to know whether the shop charges for Internet access or requires minimum purchases for "parking" to study.

Speaking of Internet access, many courses use online resources to supplement what's taught in the classroom. If that's true of the course you're taking, you'll need to have reliable access to the web. A tablet may be adequate, but a smartphone may be too small to view the videos or readings that may be required. Check with the instructor before the course begins regarding the technology requirements.

Understand how you learn! For example, you may not be a strong textbook reader, but instead, you may pick up a lot of information from listening to someone talk about the subject matter. You may benefit from recording the instructor's lectures and playing them back when you're in the car or at home. Several different learning-style assessments are free to use online. One example can be found at `www.edutopia.org/multiple-intelligences-learning-styles-quiz`.

Meeting the course requirements

Besides the classroom portion, most EMT courses also have a clinical component, where you may observe on an ambulance or fire engine, in an emergency department, or in a combination of locations. You may need to provide proof of vaccinations and immunizations in order to participate in clinical "ride-alongs."

These clinical hours are important. You'll see real patients and perhaps have the opportunity to practice your skills under the watchful eye of an experienced EMS provider. It's crucial that you don't miss these sessions; your instructor will certainly consider these hours to be just as important as your classroom sessions.

EMT courses typically have a series of exams and practical skills tests that you have to successfully pass. The exams may be done in the classroom, using pencil and paper; others may be done through a website; and others may even be done outside the classroom. Check with the instructor at the beginning of the course as to the requirements for completion. The course syllabus should contain that information, along with other requirements and guidelines for the course.

The final exam is a comprehensive test that evaluates your overall knowledge of the course. Usually this is a test created by the instructor; it's not the NREMT or state exam. Passing the final exam doesn't certify you as an EMT; only the state's process of using either the NREMT or its own exam can perform that function. However, you have to successfully pass the course in order to qualify for the certification exam.

If your state requires the NREMT exam as part of the certification process (and it probably does if you're reading this book!), the practical skills exam portion is likely to be conducted in your course. The hands-on portion tests your ability to perform the skills listed in Chapter 3.

Getting the most out of your instructors

The majority of EMT instructors are interested in your success as a student. That said, you are your own best advocate when it comes to your learning. Introduce yourself to the instructor on the first day of the course. Ask questions that are appropriate to the subject being taught. If you're challenged by a specific concept or skill, don't hesitate to ask for clarification or additional information. Most instructors appreciate enthusiasm and a desire to learn.

Many instructors are also EMS providers, actively working in the field. Besides the instruction they provide, instructors can also help you gain employment, from passing along information about job opportunities to providing interview tips and recommendations about your performance as a student. When the opportunity arises, take the time to find out more about your instructor's background and see whether he or she may be able to provide job placement assistance.

Signing Up for the EMT Exam

After you complete your training, you're ready to focus on passing the certification exam. First, determine whether your state has its own examination process. Chances are, your instructor knows this and may have already provided you with information on how to register for the state exam.

If you're taking the NREMT exam, you must fulfill the following minimum requirements:

- Be 18 years of age or older
- Successfully complete an EMT training program that meets or exceeds the National EMS Education Standards for the EMT
- Complete that course within two years of taking the exam
- Have a current CPR certificate at the healthcare-provider level
- Successfully pass a state-approved practical examination (your final practical test)

If your state requires the NREMT examination (and if you're reading this book, I assume it does), you'll need to set up a testing account, which is easy to do. Begin by going to the website at `www.nremt.org`. Toward the upper left of the home page, click on the link "Create New Account" (Figure 2-2 shows you the exact location). Fill out the requested information. You're requesting to use your new login as a "nationally certified EMS professional."

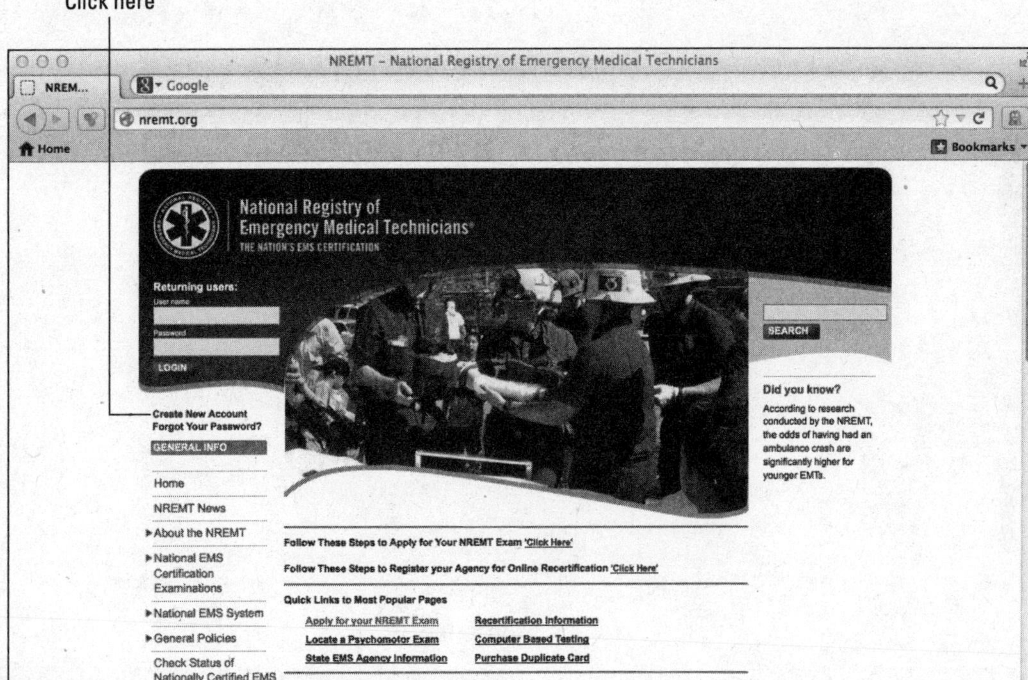

Figure 2-2: Create a new account on the NREMT website.

Courtesy of the National Registry of Emergency Medical Technicians

After you complete the first page, you'll be required to respond to statements related to licensing action and felony statements. *Do not hide* any criminal convictions that you may have. Like most states, the NREMT has certain criteria for who they allow to take the exam. Although very serious convictions may keep some people from taking the exam, most incidences are evaluated on a case-by-case basis. The fastest, easiest way to be barred from taking the exam is to try to hide any past criminal record.

After you submit your information, an account will be created. Your training program will be notified through the website that you have registered an account, and the course director will be asked to verify that you have successfully completed your training and have a current CPR healthcare-provider-level card.

Once that's done, your account will show that you're ready to register for an examination. You'll pay the exam fee of $70 via the website, or follow the instructions to print a money order tracking slip for mailing your money order to the NREMT.

After your application has been verified and approved, and you've paid your fee, your NREMT account will show that you've received an authorization to test (ATT), allowing you to determine the date and location of the exam you want to take. This step takes you to the Pearson VUE website (`www.vue.com`), which allows you to schedule your exam. Chapter 3 provides more information.

Chapter 3

Getting to Know the EMT Exam

In This Chapter

- Walking through the cognitive exam
- Discovering what's on the practical portion

One of the greatest confidence killers is the fear of the unknown. The NREMT exam is one such point of stress. A lot of rumors are out there about how difficult it is and how it's nearly impossible to pass the first time. Frankly, those rumors simply aren't true. I'm not suggesting that the test is super easy — it's not. The exam is designed to evaluate whether you have an entry-level knowledge base appropriate to the certification. If you do, the test, although difficult, is straightforward.

This chapter provides you more information about how the exam is constructed and delivered. Keep this information in mind as you prepare yourself for the test.

Checking Out the Cognitive Exam

Reading this section carefully is like pulling the curtain back on the booth in *The Wizard of Oz.* Knowing what's tested on the exam, how it's presented, and how it evaluates your performance can help you to not only better prepare for the exam, but also approach the exam with confidence.

The cognitive exam is what most students call the "written exam." It covers all the information you spent a few months learning in class. However, the exam isn't just about remembering facts and figures; it's more about how to apply that information to "real life" situations.

You take the cognitive portion of the EMT exam on a computer at a testing center. Doing so allows for greater accuracy in determining your level of comprehension of the material. You find out more about *computer adaptive testing* later in this chapter.

In addition, you have to pass a hands-on portion called the *practical exam* (sometimes called the *psychomotor exam*). I discuss the practical exam later in this chapter.

Breaking down the exam

The NREMT EMT exam is broken down into the five content areas listed in Table 3-1. The breakdown of the percentage of questions for each content area varies slightly. Within each area, 85 percent of the questions are geared toward adult patients and 15 percent toward pediatric patients.

Table 3-1 NREMT EMT Exam Content Areas

Content Area	*Percentage of Exam Content*
Airway, Respiration, and Ventilation	17–21%
Cardiology and Resuscitation	16–20%
Medical and Obstetrics/Gynecology	27–31%
Trauma	19–23%
EMS Operations	12–16%

These five areas may not correspond directly to how your class covered the information or the chapters in your textbook. However, the following sections give you a general idea of how the information is broken down on the test.

Airway, respiration, and ventilation

The airway, respiration, and ventilation category covers the following topics (for a more-detailed review, see Chapter 9):

- Airway management
- Respiratory emergencies
- Primary assessment
- Human anatomy and physiology related to the airway and breathing

Cardiology and resuscitation

The following three topics are integral to the cardiology and resuscitation portion of the test (for the lowdown on these topics, turn to Chapter 10):

- Anatomy and physiology related to cardiology and the vascular system
- Cardiac arrest
- Shock

Medical and obstetrics/gynecology

Medical, obstetrics, and gynecology are combined into one broad category (see Chapter 11 for more information). Following are the topics you should be versed in for this portion of the test:

- Neurologic emergencies
- Gastrointestinal emergencies
- Urological emergencies
- Endocrine emergencies
- Hematologic emergencies
- Immunologic emergencies
- Infectious diseases
- Toxicology
- Psychiatric emergencies
- Gynecologic emergencies

- Obstetrics and neonatal care
- Nontraumatic musculoskeletal disorders
- Anatomy and physiology related to each system listed
- Secondary assessment related to medical patients
- Reassessment of trauma patients

Trauma

Trauma-related topics that you need to be familiar with include the following (check out Chapter 12 for the specifics):

- Bleeding
- Chest trauma
- Abdominal and genitourinary trauma
- Orthopedic trauma
- Soft tissue trauma
- Head, facial, neck trauma
- Spine trauma
- Environmental emergencies
- Multisystem trauma
- Anatomy and physiology related to each system listed
- Secondary assessment related to trauma patients
- Reassessment of trauma patients

EMS operations

The EMS operations portion of the test goes beyond patient care to address such issues as medical legal standards, emergency vehicle operation, environmental hazards, and incident management. Topics to bone up on for this portion of the test include the following (head to Chapter 14 for more details):

- EMS systems
- EMT safety and wellness
- Communications and documentation
- Therapeutic communications
- Medical legal concepts and ethics
- Ambulance operations
- Incident management
- Multiple casualty incidents
- Hazardous materials
- Terrorism and disasters

Within each of these areas, about 15 percent of the questions are based on pediatric patients (see Chapter 13), and the remaining 85 percent focus on adult and geriatric patients.

Getting a grip on computer adaptive testing

Unlike a traditional paper and pencil examination, the number of questions on the NREMT EMT exam varies, roughly from 70 to 120 items per exam attempt. The actual number of questions you see depends on how well or how poorly you're performing. How does that happen?

The NREMT EMT exam is a computer adaptive test (CAT). While you're taking the exam, the computer you take it on constantly evaluates how you respond to each question and makes adjustments to the level of difficulty of each subsequent exam item accordingly. In other words, the NREMT exam isn't a one-size-fits-all paper exam! CAT is considered much more accurate in verifying knowledge. It also makes the test appear very challenging. You find out more about CAT in Chapter 5.

However, the exam isn't impossible to pass. According to the NREMT 2012 Annual Report, the national average first-time pass rate in 2012 was 72 percent. Some states reported first-time pass rates as high as 84 percent.

The test questions aren't vague or confusing. They're written in a way that mimics realistic decision-making. In real life, you don't always have all the information you want, but you still need to make decisions about your patient's care. Also, sometimes there's more than one right approach, but only one of them is the best. This concept is important and is covered in more detail in Chapter 4.

You have an almost three out of four chance of passing the exam on your first attempt. If you've been diligent in your studies and reasoned your way through the different course exams, you should be in good shape.

Scoring the exam and getting your results

After you complete the exam, your test results are transmitted to the NREMT, which verifies that all necessary steps have been completed.

The NREMT uses a different method than you may expect in scoring your exam. Rather than having a simple pass/fail process, which you may be used to with paper exams, the nature of a computer adaptive test results in a more complex scoring process. Your performance on each exam item is evaluated to be above or below the given standard. Over time, the computer recognizes that your overall performance in that section is either above or below the standard. Once it does, it moves on to the next section. This means that there is no minimum number of questions that you must answer correctly; it depends on your performance.

However, how the computer scores the exam isn't necessarily how it may order the questions themselves. In fact, the order of the questions may seem very random at times — you may first see an airway, respiration, and ventilation question, followed by a trauma question, then a medical question, then back to airway, respiration, and ventilation. Don't worry about the order — just focus on the question in front of you.

You not only have to perform above the overall exam standard, but you must also do so in each of the five sections listed in Table 3-1. Passing each section proves that your breadth of knowledge is enough to allow you to practice.

Your results are posted in your account on www.nremt.org (see Chapter 2 for details on setting up an account). Although the NREMT states that it can take one to two business days, sometimes your result may appear as early as the same day you took the exam. If you passed, go ahead and perform a happy dance — you deserve it! On the other hand, if you didn't pass, you're told how you performed in each content area so that you can prepare for your next attempt. You have an opportunity to retake the exam two more times, for a total of three attempts. (Flip to Chapter 7 for more information on what to do if you don't pass the exam the first time around.)

Completing the Practical Exam Portion

Before you can take the cognitive exam (described earlier in this chapter), your training program director must verify your ability to perform the following procedures competently:

- Patient assessment/management of a trauma patient
- Patient assessment/management of a medical patient
- Cardiac arrest management/automated external defibrillator (AED)
- Bag-valve-mask ventilation of an apneic patient
- Spinal immobilization (for both seated and supine patients)
- Long bone fracture immobilization
- Joint dislocation immobilization
- Traction splinting
- Bleeding control/shock management
- Upper airway adjuncts and suction
- Mouth-to-mouth ventilation with supplemental oxygen
- Supplemental oxygen administration to a breathing patient

Your course instructor verifies your skills either throughout the program or at the end of your training; it varies from one program to the next.

You also need to successfully complete a practical (or psychomotor) skills examination. This is usually provided in the form of a final practical exam at the end of your course. The state EMS office determines which exact skills are tested; your instructor will tell you what will be evaluated on the final practical exam.

Find out how your final practical exam will be conducted at the beginning of your course. This way, you'll know what to pay attention to in your training.

Your results are submitted to the NREMT by your EMT program director after you complete the testing. Once this information is entered into your account and you pay your testing fee, you'll be cleared to sign up for the cognitive exam.

Part II

Test-Taking Tips and Strategies

Five Ways to Improve Your Study Habits

- Set the stage for optimal studying by creating an environment free of distractions.
- Develop and stick to a study schedule that is realistic and keeps you on track for success.
- Don't reread the entire textbook! Use the practice exams in this book and online to guide your studies and focus on areas of weakness.
- Study with buddies. They can be your "outside voice" to keep you honest about your knowledge.
- Using tools like flashcards, talking aloud during studying, and finding other explanations about difficult topics can help improve your retention.

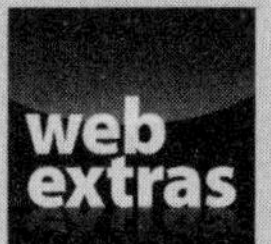

Dig deeper into computer adaptive testing for the EMT exam in an article at `www.dummies.com/extras/emtexam`.

In this part . . .

- Break down the different parts of a multiple-choice test item so you have a better understanding of how to answer it.
- Know how computer adaptive testing (CAT) evaluates your knowledge so you can be prepared for the stress that you may feel during the EMT exam.
- Find out how to study more effectively and learn more in less time. Studying is a skill!
- Discover that it takes more than just book knowledge to pass the EMT exam. Attitude and a healthy body give you the capacity to handle the fear and stress of taking a high-stakes exam.

Chapter 4

The Anatomy of the Multiple-Choice Question

In This Chapter

- Picking out the parts that make up a multiple-choice test item
- Using deduction when choosing an answer

Life is full of questions such as the following:

- "Why is the sky blue?"
- "Is there life after death?"
- "An adult male is unresponsive on the floor of a restaurant. Patrons report the patient was having lunch when he suddenly grabbed his throat and collapsed. He is cyanotic, with agonal breaths. What should you do next?"

While the first two questions may require a meteorology or theological degree to answer, as an EMT you should be able to respond correctly to the last one. After all, it seems pretty straightforward. But what if these were your choices?

(A) Perform abdominal thrusts.

(B) Perform chest compressions.

(C) Roll him onto his side.

(D) Ventilate with a pocket mask.

At first glance, many of the answers look good — that is, more than one of the answers seem to be right. But a closer examination reveals that one answer is better than the others (see the later section "Aiming for the best answer" for the lowdown). And that's how the NREMT exam is set up: It contains multiple-choice questions that check your ability to make accurate decisions, given a set amount of information. You'll see questions that are as fairly straightforward as this one — that is, if your knowledge base and your reasoning ability are good enough. It's worth looking at just how the NREMT exam questions are created and how to deduce the correct answer; you get the scoop in this chapter.

Looking at the Parts

A multiple-choice question, or item, is made of several parts: the stem, distractors, and the correct answer. Each part plays a specific role.

The stem

The *stem* is the "question" part of the item. It's the first part that sets up the situation for you to respond to, providing only the information necessary for you to answer the item correctly. The stem ends in the form of a question, for example, "What should you do next?" or asks you to complete a statement, such as "You suspect the underlying condition to be. . . ."

This chapter's introduction gives you an example of a stem: "An adult male is unresponsive on the floor of a restaurant. Patrons report the patient was having lunch when he suddenly grabbed his throat and collapsed. He is cyanotic, with agonal breaths. What should you do next?"

Distractors and the answer

The choices that are provided after the stem come in two flavors, answers and distractors. The *answer* is the best choice, given the stem. A *distractor* is exactly that — it's designed to draw your attention away from the answer. The following sections explain the differences between good distractors and the best answer.

Noting the importance of high-quality distractors

Where a multiple-choice question shines is in the quality of the distractors. Good distractors look like they could be right answers. In fact, they often are; however, in such cases the stem asks for the *best* answer, not the *right* one. This means that you really have to choose which "right" answer is the best one.

On the other hand, bad distractors are obviously incorrect. Bad distractors don't test your knowledge base or your ability to reason. Here's a simple example.

You look up and see a small animal with wings flying overhead. As it does, you can hear it make a "quack quack quack" sound. You suspect it is

(A) a cow.

(B) a dog.

(C) a duck.

(D) a brick.

Unless you've been partaking in some sort of mind-altering substance, you immediately recognize that Choices (A), (B), and (D) aren't even remotely described by the stem. This question really doesn't evaluate knowledge — the distractors are so off the mark that Choice (C) is the only possible answer.

What if the choices were these instead?

(A) an American Black Duck.

(B) a Tufted Duck.

(C) a Ruddy Duck.

(D) a Steller's Eider.

Unless you're a duck aficionado, this question is much more difficult to answer. All the distractors are of the duck variety. Three of the choices include the word "duck." You'd need to know something about ducks to answer this question correctly. (And in case you want to really know, it's the American Black Duck; the others don't quack. For example, the Tufted

Duck makes a "kar kar" sound, and the Ruddy Duck makes a low belching sound — quite rude, those Ruddy Ducks. But you get what I mean: You need to know this information to answer the question.)

Aiming for the best answer

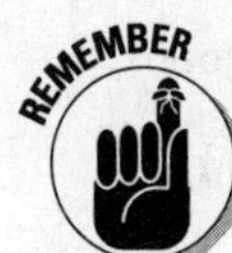

The NREMT exam asks you to select the *best* answer from the choices. Don't mistake "best" with "right." On the exam, more than one of the distractors may be right. The more right answers you have to select from, the harder the question is to answer.

The following example is the EMS question from the beginning of this chapter. Take another look.

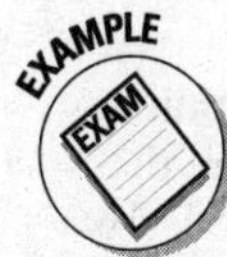

An adult male is unresponsive on the floor of a restaurant. Patrons report the patient was having lunch when he suddenly grabbed his throat and collapsed. He is cyanotic, with agonal breaths. What should you do next?

(A) Perform abdominal thrusts.

(B) Perform chest compressions.

(C) Roll him onto his side.

(D) Ventilate with a pocket mask.

Given the situation described in the scenario, most of these answers are correct. But, the stem is asking for what to do *next*. Here are some factors you need to consider:

- Cyanosis with agonal breathing makes you conclude that the patient is in cardiac arrest, which requires chest compressions, Choice (B), as soon as possible.
- You need to recognize that abdominal thrusts, Choice (A), are performed only if a patient is conscious and obstructed, not when he's unconscious.
- Ventilation, Choice (D), comes after chest compressions.
- Rolling the patient onto his side, Choice (C), won't change the state of the patient.

So, although Choices (B) and (D) are both appropriate in cardiac arrest, the *best* choice is (B).

You may be thinking, "Wait! There's no information about whether the patient has a pulse. How do I know that he's in cardiac arrest?" The step of checking for a carotid pulse isn't a choice. You need to know that agonal respirations set in at the beginning of cardiac arrest.

Answering NREMT exam items is similar to the real-life decision-making you'll do in the field. Based on limited findings and your knowledge base, you'll need to make some conclusions about the patient and then use those to decide what to do about the situation.

Breaking Down a Question Step by Step

Using a step-by-step approach is a reliable, effective way to analyze and answer a multiple-choice question. Having a consistent approach can also take a bit of fear or nervousness out of taking the NREMT.

Looking at the stem and answering it

After you read a test item, you may be very tempted to look at the answers and choose the one that seems correct. This strategy may work in many cases, but it can also work against you, *if more than one answer appears correct.* Many of the NREMT exam items are challenging for exactly this reason.

A stem should be written well enough so that you should be able to answer it without looking at the responses. Doing so gets you to slow down and consider *exactly* what the question is asking. You may have to draw certain conclusions about the patient's status or condition, based on the information provided in the stem, *before* answering the question.

After you have the answer in your head, compare it to the four choices that are presented. If you're spot on, the best answer should immediately be apparent. If none of the choices appear to match what you thought the answer should be, move to the next step (in the following section).

Take a look at the following example. First, read the stem and tell yourself what you think the answer is.

A 62-year-old female is experiencing chest pain that began at rest. She describes the pain as "sharp," and points to the right side of her chest when you ask her to locate where the discomfort is. Her heart rate is 90, her blood pressure is 130/70, and her respiratory rate is 16 and nonlabored. Her oxygen saturation level is 97 percent. You should

(A) administer high-flow oxygen using a nonrebreather mask.

(B) transport immediately.

(C) question her further about the chief complaint.

(D) place her in a supine position.

Based only on the information provided — before you even look at the answer choices — you should understand that the patient is not in a serious or critical state that requires a major intervention to airway, breathing, or circulation. Given that her oxygen saturation level is normal, supplemental oxygen isn't indicated either. Although you can say that the discomfort doesn't appear to be cardiac in nature, you still need to investigate further.

With this information in mind, you're ready to consider the answer choices. Choice (A) isn't indicated because her saturation level is normal and she's not in respiratory distress. Choice (B) is not correct; none of the information given indicates that she needs to be rushed to an emergency department. Her blood pressure is normal and there are no signs of shock, making Choice (D) incorrect. The leaves Choice (C) as the best answer; you want to know more about the chief complaint.

NREMT exam items rarely test you on simple "recall" performance. The test assumes that you possess basic knowledge contained within the EMT curriculum. The questions build upon your knowledge and test your ability to use it in a scenario or to deduce certain conclusions about a patient.

Eliminating what's not right

Begin by discarding answers that are clearly incorrect. On the NREMT exam, answers that are obviously wrong may not appear often, but when they do, make the most of it and get rid of them. It's better to make an educated guess when you have three possibilities rather than four!

If you're not lucky enough to remove an obvious incorrect answer, read each choice carefully. Consider whether what you read has some relationship to the stem and make a mental judgment as to how likely that answer is to be the best one. You may grade the choice as "very unlikely," "maybe," or "very likely." Repeat this process for each choice. When you're done, sort the responses according to how likely they are to be the best answer. The one that comes to the top of your list is likely your best answer. (If you're having trouble deciding between choices, follow the advice in the next section.)

A 20-year-old female was struck in the chest with a bat during a fight. She complains of chest pain and trouble breathing. There is tenderness when you palpate the left anterior chest wall, in the area of T3 and T4. Lung sounds are clear and equal on inspiration. She is alert and is breathing 20 times per minute. Her pulse rate is 90. Which of the following injuries is most likely?

(A) Tension pneumothorax

(B) Rib fractures

(C) Pneumothorax

(D) Pulmonary contusion

Given the mechanism of injury, any of the choices could be correct. However, you would expect to see additional findings in the stem for most of the responses. For example, you'd expect to see tachycardia, hypotension, altered mental status, and jugular venous distension for Choice (A), which makes it very unlikely. While Choice (C) is possible, you'd expect a faster breathing rate and/or a difference in lung sounds on the affected side, making this choice less likely. You'd also expect tachypnea with Choice (D). This line of thinking leaves Choice (B) as the most likely answer.

The following are common mistakes test-writers make that good test-takers recognize, sometimes unconsciously. However, the writers of the NREMT exam work really hard to eliminate these issues; as a result, the vast majority of the test items really test your knowledge and not your test-taking abilities.

- If the answer contains absolute words, such as *never* and *always,* it's not likely to be correct. Virtually no situations are so clear-cut.
- If the answer doesn't grammatically key into the stem, it's probably not right.
- The correct choice may be the longest one. That's because the test-writer provides an explanation or extra details to make it the best answer.
- Sometimes a word or phrase appears in the stem and is repeated within an answer. If so, it may point to the correct response.

Remember that these are not hard and fast rules. For example, the test-writer may intentionally put the same word in both the stem and in a wrong answer, just to mislead you.

Choosing which answer is best

Using the approach in the preceding section usually eliminates two or three choices from the mix. If you end up having to select between two options, try these tips:

- Reread the stem once more just to make sure that you didn't miss any subtle clues.
- Sometimes the best answer is the longest one or the one that has the most specificity. This is not likely to happen with the NREMT exam because they check for such item-writing "errors," but you never know.
- A test item may ask you a sequencing question — what you should do *next,* for example. If you're trying to choose between two answers, look to see whether there's an order to how things should happen. For example, does Choice (A) happen before Choice (B)?

- You can apply a "true-false" test to the answer choices. Reread the stem with each answer and ask yourself whether it sounds true or false. Your intuition is your subconscious mind speaking to you. You may have learned the information, but it may not be coming to the surface. Rereading the stem and answer together may allow your subconscious to match a learned nugget that you're unable to recall at the moment. If more than one answer rings true, check to see whether there's a sequencing component.
- Sometimes two of the four choices are opposites of each other. If so, there's a good chance that one of them is correct.

A 19-year-old male has been shot in the chest. He has an open wound to the left anterior chest wall that is oozing blood. He responds incomprehensibly to verbal stimulus. His respiration rate is 8, with shallow breathing. His pulse rate is 110, and his skin is cool, pale, and diaphoretic. What should you do first?

(A) Insert an oropharyngeal airway.

(B) Ventilate with a bag-valve mask (BVM).

(C) Apply gauze to the open chest wound.

(D) Administer high-flow oxygen with a nonrebreather mask.

You might want to select Choice (D) because it's the longest answer, and it certainly seems that the patient requires oxygen. However, his breathing rate is slow, and his tidal volume is shallow. These facts point more to Choice (B) as a better answer. While he is altered, he does respond to a verbal stimulus, which may mean he has a gag reflex. This consideration makes Choice (A) less of a good answer. If Choice (C) were to apply an occlusive dressing to the chest wound, that would make it a very good answer. But applying gauze alone makes this a poor choice as air could still pass through the wound.

If you follow these tips, you're making an educated guess on questions to which the answer isn't clear. This tactic is very different from performing a WAG — a wild-&#!ed guess. WAGs are simply playing the odds and hoping that you end up choosing the best answer. Educated guessing is really applying the skill of deduction, which increases your chances of being correct.

Chapter 5

Checking Out Computer Adaptive Testing

In This Chapter

- Getting a handle on computer adaptive testing
- Acclimating to CAT

You may be worrying about taking your NREMT exam on a computer. You shouldn't be. While it's true that the computerized version isn't just a digitized paper examination, you shouldn't fear it. After you review the basic elements of a computer adaptive test (CAT), which are described in this chapter, you'll have a better understanding of how the computer will test your knowledge and capabilities.

Understanding How Computer Adaptive Testing Works

Once upon a time, tests could be provided only on paper. You used a quaint little device called a pen (or its rough cousin, the pencil) to make marks on the paper in response to questions. Your teacher then had to correct the test by hand, checking each response you provided against a key.

Then came a major advance in technology. It was called a Scantron, and it used fancy pieces of paper that were filled with bubbles that you penciled in with your response. State of the art!

However, despite that change, the tests were still basically unchanged — they were one-size-fits-all evaluation tools. The teacher had to estimate the *cut score,* the minimum score you had to get in order to pass the test. Most of the time, it was 70 percent, an arbitrary number.

Over the years, an experienced teacher could evaluate how well the test determined who had enough information to pass the test and who didn't. She might change the cut score, adjusting it upward if the test had a lot of easy questions or setting it lower if a lot of the questions were hard. Nevertheless, for the most part, the tests were still uniform in what they tested.

Then came computer adaptive testing (CAT), which replaces the paper test with one that actually evaluates your specific level of understanding. How? Based on how you answer a question (right or wrong), the test adjusts, or adapts, and sends you an appropriate question accordingly. Over time, the test figures out whether you have the minimum level of knowledge needed to accomplish a task — in this case, to practice as an EMT. Confused? Read on.

How does CAT adapt?

Approaching the CAT is a little like jumping a high bar. The bar is set at a certain height, and you need a certain amount of speed and skill to make it over the first time. If you do, the next time you jump, the bar may be set higher. On the other hand, if you don't make the first jump, the bar may be adjusted a little lower before you try again.

A CAT exam begins like the first high bar setting. You see a couple of multiple-choice questions, in a content area like EMS operations, that have been judged to be of medium or medium-easy difficulty. Say that you're Mr. or Ms. Smarty Pants, and you answer these questions correctly. The computer records the information and sets a more difficult question in front of you. You, being as smart as you are, answer that question correctly too. The computer records that result and adds it to the previous results.

It then continues to give you increasingly difficult questions to answer until statistically you've proven you know your stuff in this area. The computer then switches to another content area, say medical and obstetrics/gynecology, and begins the process all over again.

If you correctly and consistently answer a majority of questions that are above a set minimum standard, the test abruptly stops, and you're done. If you're really prepared and knowledgeable about all things EMT, you may only have to answer as few as 70 questions for the computer to decide that you're ready to go.

If this happens to you, you may think, "Wow, I must have passed since the test shut off after 70 questions." But that's not necessarily the case.

Imagine the same scenario, but this time, say you miss the first couple questions of medium difficulty. The computer records this, just as before. But now it shows you a question that's easier. You end up missing that one too. The computer records your result and adds it to the others.

If you continue to miss similarly easy questions, eventually you demonstrate that you don't know the material. The computer switches to the next content area and repeats the same process, until you've demonstrated that you're *not* ready to go. This may *also* take as few as 70 questions.

The result? If your test shuts off after 70 or so questions, you either did really great or really poorly. And to add insult to injury, you may not know how you did. Think about it: Because the test adapts the difficulty of each question to *your* level of ability, *every* question will appear to be difficult. In fact, many EMT students report how uncertain they feel about how they did after an NREMT exam.

The two preceding scenarios represent the extremes. The fact is, most people need to answer somewhere between 70 and 120 questions before the computer decides statistically that they're either at or above the standard or below it. For example, say you do just fabulous on the EMS operations section, but when it comes to medical and obstetrics/gynecology, you flub a question that's considered medium in difficulty. The computer then asks you a similar question at a lower level of difficulty. You answer that question correctly. The computer then asks a more difficult question related to the same topic and continues to do so until you show that you are at or above the standard. Then it moves on to the next section.

As a result of a few ups and downs, you have to answer more questions to show that you have enough understanding compared to someone who has a better level of comprehension. The number of questions you have to answer doesn't matter though; as long as you meet or exceed the standard in all sections, you pass the exam. That's what matters, which reminds me of a joke:

What do you call someone who graduates from an EMT program at the bottom of the class?

An EMT.

In other words, passing the NREMT exam means that your understanding of being an EMT is enough for you to be a safe, beginning practitioner.

Educators utilize a concept known as classical test theory to create a paper-based exam. *Classical test theory* basically says that by asking a few well-constructed and well-chosen questions about a particular topic area, your performance on those questions can predict how well you'd do if you were asked every possible question about the same topic. Writing good test questions and choosing the right ones to ask is challenging. A computer adaptive test, on the other hand, uses item response theory as a basis for choosing its questions. *Item response theory* says that how well you do on a question is based upon how good your knowledge base is and how difficult the question is. CAT, combined with item response theory, delivers a much more targeted exam process that's highly accurate in determining your readiness level.

Who judges the questions' difficulty, anyway?

You may be wondering: "Who judges the questions' level of difficulty on a CAT exam?" The answer: You do. No, really — new questions are introduced into every test. Your performance on these "test" test questions doesn't count toward your final score. However, it is recorded by the computer, along with hundreds of other students' attempts. Over time, the test question is answered correctly by a certain percentage of students, which equals a difficulty level of easy, medium, or hard. After the level of difficulty is determined, the question is released into the pool of questions and called up by the computer when needed.

By the way, unlike the questions that may have been written by your instructor or taken from a test bank, NREMT exam questions are written by teams of EMS experts from around the country. Creating a question that meets certain criteria takes weeks to months and costs about a thousand dollars. The NREMT test bank contains thousands of questions, for each level of provider. You're very unlikely to see the same question on two different exams.

What makes CAT better?

NREMT switched to CAT in 2007. What are the benefits of using CAT rather than paper tests? CAT has earned a reputation for being

- **Sophisticated:** The CAT is more sophisticated than a traditional paper-based exam; it really becomes your test, giving you questions based on your performance on the previous ones.
- **Short and sweet:** In general, CAT exams are shorter than paper exams. And because they're administered electronically, the good folks at the NREMT get your results very quickly, which means you get to find out how you did very quickly — sometimes on the same day.
- **Safe:** CAT exams are also easier to secure. Paper exams can be copied or stolen. As you find out in Chapter 7, stealing questions from the computer exam is virtually impossible.
- **Sound:** CAT exam results are considered more accurate and reliable in determining competency than paper exams. Because traditional paper exams are one-size-fits-all, they're pretty generic when it comes to determining competency across all students. CAT exams can really drill down on *your* knowledge base and get a real sense of how deep your comprehension level really is.

Adapting to Computer Adaptive Testing

If you've never taken a test on a computer before, you may expect it to be intimidating. However, a CAT such as the NREMT EMT exam is designed to be user-friendly. You use a mouse to click through the different screens and select answers. And at the beginning of the exam, there are even sample screens for you to practice on before you begin the actual test.

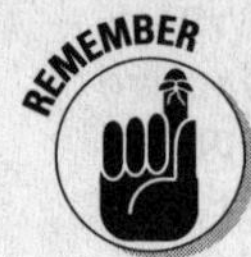

Keep these three key points in mind when it comes to taking a computer adaptive test:

- Your NREMT exam will feel difficult, no matter how well you perform. It's designed to be that way, so don't panic if you feel like a total failure at the end of the exam. Losing your confidence can lead to uncertainty, and you may very well begin second-guessing yourself on your answers. You find out more about this topic in Chapter 7.
- How long it takes you to complete the exam depends on how well prepared you are to take the exam. The more questions you answer correctly, the sooner the test will end.
- The importance of being prepared cannot be overstated. You want to complete the minimum number of questions necessary to pass; the questions you see will hone in on your level of knowledge and preparedness. Turn your attention to Chapter 6, designed to maximize your studying habits so you can be as prepared as possible.

Chapter 6

Preparing for the Exam

In This Chapter

- Developing your study routine — and sticking to it
- Getting the most from your study time
- Making additional plans for success

You've spent well over a hundred hours in the classroom discovering what it takes to be an EMT. You've probably spent at least another hundred hours outside of the classroom, studying and practicing. It makes sense that spending a few more hours preparing for the NREMT exam is appropriate.

But what should you study? There's so much information to cover. You could reread the textbook and all of your notes, but that approach may be too time-consuming. Indeed, a study released by the NREMT in 2008 shows that you should try to take the exam within 26 days after your last class date. After that, the longer you wait, the higher the likelihood of performing poorly on the exam.

Having only a couple of weeks to prepare for the exam may not seem like enough time, but as you find out in this chapter, with proper planning and discipline, you can maximize your study efforts and be more than ready for the exam. Being prepared has the added benefit of increasing your confidence level, which is almost as important. You want to go into the exam feeling prepared to pass.

If you stick to your study schedule, stay focused while studying, and maintain a healthy routine, you'll be in great shape for the exam. In Chapter 7, you find out how to do your best during the exam.

Gearing Up to Study

Studying for a major exam such as the NREMT can be daunting. Because it can feel overwhelming, you may be tempted to put it off for as long as possible. Anxiety builds, and before long, panic sets in and you end up cramming the last couple of days before the exam.

Don't procrastinate! Studies repeatedly show that cramming does little to prepare you for an exam. It's far better to take a few minutes to plan your studies — when you'll study and where it'll happen. Following a study plan takes more discipline, but it's definitely worth it.

Setting the stage

Create a space that promotes learning — not just the physical space but the mental space as well. Contrary to popular belief, most people don't multitask very well. Your brain needs to focus intently as it figures out how all that information you're feeding it fits together. Your goal is to clear all the clutter that can get in the way of a great study session.

Ideally, you want to find a space that affords you privacy and a little solitude. This space is *not* your bedroom or a super comfy couch. Studying is an active process; you don't want to be so comfortable that you drift off or fall asleep! A sturdy chair supports your body, and a table or desk allows you to keep things like your books and notes handy. Have a good task lamp for when lighting is dim; reading in poor light doesn't necessarily make you go blind, but your eyes have to work harder, which can be distracting.

On the other hand, you may not be lucky enough to have a designated space to study at home. Places like a library may have quiet areas that promote a better study environment. A coffee shop may be too noisy and distracting, depending on the time of day. Keep track of when these spaces are open and when they may be less busy.

Have your study materials available to you. You don't want to sit down to study, only to find out you're missing your books or your notes. Keep everything you need in one place, whether on a table or in a backpack. This way, everything is available to you when you're ready to go to work.

Distractions can be disastrous. You may feel you need to have the television running in the background. Posting a Facebook status like "Studying for my exam while my friends are partying" may be fun. Listening to music through your earphones may be entertaining. But in the meantime, you're not focused on the real task at hand — studying. So, as difficult as it may be, turn everything off — except your brain. Being off the grid and studying for an hour is likely to be far more effective than being distracted every couple of minutes for a few hours. Don't worry; the world will still be there when you plug back in.

Staying on schedule

Studying is a task, and it takes priority over other tasks as you get ready for the NREMT exam. Give it its due! Start by taking a minute to consider just how much time you have to spend studying. The answer is different for everyone. Work and family commitments, along with sleeping, eating, and going to the bathroom, limit the amount of serious study time that's available.

Don't assume that you'll be able to study at work — it's too distracting. And don't try studying if it's your turn to take care of the kids. Keep in mind that you want to have the time and space to study effectively. Trying to fit it in somewhere is frustrating and unpredictable.

Be realistic in scheduling your time. You may think that you have superhuman abilities and can study for hours on end. That's not likely. Just as you did during your EMT course, make the schedule work for you. Map out a new timetable, similar to the one in Chapter 2, that accommodates your work and life schedule. Keeping your study intervals to an hour or two at a time is more realistic. This strategy makes scheduling study time easier and reduces your frustrations when life gets in the way. If you need more time than that, consider studying twice a day, maybe once in the morning and again at night. The bottom line: Make it work for you!

How much time overall should you spend preparing for the NREMT exam? It depends. As I mention earlier in this chapter, the sooner you attempt the exam after graduation, the greater the likelihood of passing. I recommend that you try to take the exam within two or three weeks. That will give you enough time to review any weak areas that you may have in your EMT knowledge. You can use the preassessment test in Chapter 8 to evaluate yourself and determine what areas to study first.

After you set a schedule, stick to it closely. Maintaining a schedule makes studying a habit. Your brain will anticipate when it's time to focus on your EMT studies. However, don't be too strict with yourself. If something happens and you can't stick to your schedule, simply find another time slot and study then.

Making the Most Out of Studying

After you create the space and the time to study, make the most of it. Making every minute count during your study session maximizes your potential to pass the exam; it's also very satisfying to know that you've done the best you possibly can.

Using objectives

Textbooks are not written like novels; you don't read one from beginning to end. A textbook is designed to be more of a reference. You read only the sections that you need to read to gain comprehension or understanding. But how do you know which sections to look at?

Textbook authors base what they write about on *objectives*. An objective is a statement that describes some idea or principle that you should have learned from the course. For example, your EMT textbook might have an objective regarding bleeding that looks like this one:

Differentiate between arterial, venous, and capillary bleeding.

This objective focuses on how arterial bleeding tends to look bright red and spurts from a wound, whereas venous bleeding tends to be dark red in color and flows steadily. Finally, capillary bleeding tends to be minor and oozes from a wound.

Each of your textbook chapters has a list of objectives somewhere in it, usually at the beginning. In addition, your course syllabus should have a list of learning objectives. You should be able to elaborate on each one with some specificity, meaning with some detail.

You'll definitely come across objectives that you won't be able to answer with confidence or with detail. That's normal. An EMT course covers a lot of objectives, and you aren't expected to get them all at once. If you aren't able to explain an objective while you're studying, look it up in your textbook or your notes. Some textbooks conveniently list the chapter pages that relate to each objective. If that's not the case, you may have to skim through the chapter to find the paragraphs related to the objective.

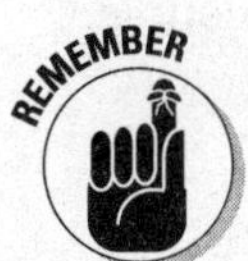

Simply reading a chapter from beginning to end, without knowing exactly what you're supposed to get out of it, may not be the most effective way of solidifying your understanding. Studying by objective can help you focus on the materials and may make information easier to organize in your head. You'll concentrate on what you don't know, rather than what you do know.

Another way to focus on less-familiar concepts is to take an assessment exam. Chapter 8 has a short exam that can help you understand where your strengths and weaknesses are. Take the test without assistance and don't flip the pages to see the answers. When you score yourself, pay attention to the questions that gave you problems; review the chapters in this book that correlate to those questions.

Studying with buddies

Studying with classmates can be helpful. You can quiz each other on topics and get better explanations for some concepts that are confusing. "Teaching" concepts to another person is a great way to solidify your own understanding as well!

The trick is to have the group session be effective. Gossiping about other students or griping about things in general can be all too easy. It's best if you set a time limit that everyone agrees upon and stick to a few specific topics. For example, three or four students can review cardiology in detail in about 60 to 90 minutes. Go through the objectives (see the preceding section) and have each person explain one in a minute or two. If one person can't explain an objective to the satisfaction of others, have the next person try to explain it.

Trying a few tips for retaining info

Everyone learns differently and at different rates. There are a few ways to retain information and improve comprehension. Here are a few tips that have helped other students; consider trying a couple to see whether they help you:

- **Use flashcards:** During your studies, you may come across a fact or concept that you have difficulty remembering or understanding. On one side of an index card, write the name of the point you want to remember; then, write down the related information on the other side of the card. For example, you might write "Rule of Nines" on one side and the percentage of body surface area for each area of the body on the other side. (Flip to Chapter 13 for more about this rule.) Flashcards are great in that you can pull them out anytime and use them to quiz yourself.

  Check out digital flashcards to help you prep for the EMT exam at `learn.dummies.com`; see the Introduction for details on accessing them.

- **Think aloud:** If some concepts are difficult for you to remember, record yourself reading aloud the relevant section of the textbook. Although hearing your own voice may feel strange, listening to the explanation may help you retain the information better if you're an auditory learner. If that's too weird, just repeat a sentence or two aloud several times in a row.

- **Surf the web:** Sometimes the explanations provided in your textbook don't work well for you. Search key terms from the paragraph using your favorite Internet browser to see whether someone else does a better job explaining the concept.

If you're reading this part before you begin your EMT course, try these study habits while you're in class. This way, you'll build up good study habits and tricks all during the course.

Giving your brain a break

When study time is over, step away. Your brain needs time to process the information you just worked on. Close your books, take a deep breath, and go do something else. If your schedule has you studying for a couple of hours at a time, simply taking a break for a few minutes after the first hour and thinking about something else will give your brain a rest. You may find yourself more refreshed, more alert, and able to focus better during the next hour.

When you're not studying, don't stress about it. Have fun. Focus on work, play with your kids, make dinner, hang out with your friends — your brain will continue to process the information while you're doing something else. You may find yourself feeling more refreshed the next time you sit down to study.

Practicing for the practical exam

In addition to your cognitive exam (taken on a computer), you need to successfully complete a hands-on practical (or psychomotor) skills examination, usually in the form of a final practical exam at the end of your course. Your state EMS office determines the exact skills that are tested; your instructor will tell you what will be evaluated. Here are a few pointers for succeeding on your practical exam, no matter what's covered (see Chapter 3 for more about this exam):

- Know which skills you'll be tested on early; if possible, find out from the instructor at the beginning of the course.
- Practice early and often. Many of the skills an EMT performs aren't intuitive or simple; skills such as splinting or spinal immobilization have many steps. Your brain memorizes facts and figures to help with answering written questions; your body memorizes each physical movement of a skill in order to put it together in a fluid motion.
- Practice with friends. Having a classmate watch you perform a skill provides you with better feedback on how well you performed. Make sure your classmate has a skill sheet to look at while you perform and check off what you did and didn't do correctly.
- As you get better at a skill, test yourself under the same conditions as the actual test. For example, there may be a time limit to the skill — use the same limit as you perform your final practice runs to make sure you can get it done in time.

Picking Out Other Pointers for Success

Franklin Roosevelt once said, "The only thing we have to fear is fear itself." Many students come to fear the exam, having heard rumors about how difficult it is and how after the test is over, you don't know how it went. Put those concerns aside and approach the exam like any other challenge — plan for it, work for it, and go for it.

Having the right mindset

The design of the NREMT exam makes it feel difficult no matter how prepared you are. Computer adaptive testing (CAT; see Chapter 5) adjusts the level of difficulty for each question based on your performance on the previous one. The more you answer correctly, the harder the questions become until you reach a level that's above the minimum standard. So, don't stress about what you've heard. Be aware that the test will feel difficult. If your study habits are solid and you dedicate your efforts toward passing the exam, you'll do just fine. Confidence quells any fear you may have about not remembering all the information.

But what happens if you don't do well on exam day? You simply retake the exam. Even the NREMT recognizes that anyone can have an "off" day. In fact, you can retake the exam up to six times before you're required to retake an EMT course. So, don't panic if you don't pass the first time — you can try again after doing some additional preparation. (Flip to Chapter 7 for more information on retaking the exam.)

Making a few final plans before exam day

The NREMT exam is like a sports game, such as baseball or football. Sure, you can just play in a pickup game and have great fun. But if you're competing in a league, placing first takes practice, preparation, and determination. So it is for the exam. You want to be at your best on "game day"!

- **Pick an optimal time to take the exam.** You know yourself best — pick a time that you know you'll be most awake, alert, and ready to test. Most testing centers have appointments that begin first thing in the morning, in the evening, and on weekends. Choose the best time slot for you; then clear your schedule of other tasks that day so you're sure to make your appointment.
- **Get enough rest.** Scientific studies have made it clear that a well-rested brain is needed to think through exam questions. Please, don't try to cram your studies into the last 24 hours. Doing so isn't likely to help and will just make you tired.
- **Don't sacrifice exercise.** Physical exercise can help clear the brain of cobwebs and reduce the stress built up within the body. Go for a run or take a time-out at the gym — your brain and body will thank you.

Chapter 7

Doing Your Best During the Exam

In This Chapter

- Understanding what happens at the testing center
- Maintaining focus and a positive attitude
- Taking action after you get your results

The day has arrived. Weeks of preparation have led up to the big event — your NREMT exam. It's time to step up to the plate and knock it out of the park! Just like baseball, though, now isn't the time to forget everything you've done prior to game day. Knowing what to do during the exam will help keep you focused on the task at hand and your confidence high.

Knowing What to Expect in a Nutshell

The NREMT administers its computer adaptive testing (CAT) exams through Pearson VUE Testing Centers. Pearson VUE conducts testing for a wide variety of licenses and certifications across the world in a secure, comfortable environment. When your application to take the exam is approved by the NREMT, you're given a list of testing centers and their locations. You can take the test anywhere in the country, but most folks find the one closest to their home or workplace.

When you arrive at the testing center, you're asked to provide two forms of government identification and validate your identity with an electronic palm print. You're instructed to place all of your personal belongings in a locker; you're not permitted to carry anything into the testing room. You're given a small dry erase board and pen that you can use to make notes.

Other people are likely to be there with you to take different exams. At the appointed time, a proctor escorts everyone into the room and you're directed to take a seat at a cubicle. In front of you is a computer. The proctor logs you into the computer and tells you when to begin the exam.

When the exam begins, you start by reviewing some basic information about the exam, such as the penalty for cheating and when your test results will become available. After that, the first question appears on the screen. Only one question at a time is shown to you. Once you answer that question, you're shown another one. You aren't able to return to the previous question. This allows the computer to decide where your abilities lie and provide you an appropriately difficult question (see Chapter 5 for details on how this adaptive testing works).

A timer is on the screen at all times. It tells you how much time is remaining on the test. It doesn't flash or otherwise signal how much time you have left; make sure you check it every few questions to stay on time. Don't worry too much, though; you'll likely finish the exam before the timer runs out. Overall, you have two and a half hours to complete the exam.

The NREMT provides accommodations for certain types of reading disabilities on a case-by-case basis. If approved, additional time will be provided to you so you can adequately review each question. You need to provide this information to the NREMT well before your exam date; most people provide the documentation when they first apply to take the exam.

If you need to take a break for any reason during the exam, you can signal the room proctor. The proctor then temporarily signs you out of your test and escorts you out of the room. When you return, you need to be escorted back into the room and logged back into the computer you were working on. The time continues to run while all of this is happening.

When the computer has enough information to determine whether you pass or fail, the program immediately shuts off. A note appears on the screen indicating that the test is over. Don't be anxious — it's designed to do this. When you are done, you're escorted out of the room. You can then collect your personal belongings, bid the staff a fond farewell, and leave. That's it!

Staying Focused and Positive During the Exam

While you're actually taking the exam, you need to stay focused and positive. It's okay to feel nervous, a little scared even. But those testing jitters should go away as you chip away at each question. After all, you have prepared yourself well for this moment. Following are some tips to help you keep your cool and do your best when you're taking the exam.

Answering one question at a time

Each question is presented by itself during the exam. Once you submit your answer to a question, you can't look at it again. Therefore, take each question as it comes. Consider what the question stem is asking and see whether you can answer it without looking at the responses. If you feel that you have a solid answer, check it against the responses provided. If none of them match up precisely, reread the stem to see whether you may have missed or misinterpreted part of it. Read all the responses, keeping in mind that just because a response is *right* doesn't mean it's *best.* Check out the tips in Chapter 4 to optimize your ability to choose the most correct response.

Try not to guess — the odds of choosing the best answer are against you. Silently reread the question and each response together. Choose the sentence that sounds most correct. If you have absolutely no clue what the answer is, choose one and move on to the next question.

If later in the exam you see a question that's related to a previous question and you realize you may have answered the earlier question incorrectly, don't panic. It serves no purpose other than to distract you from answering the question that's in front of you right now. Forget about the previous question and go about answering the current one.

I know this sounds all zen-like and all, but I do mean it: Be one with the exam. If you feel the stress building within you, stop for a moment; close your eyes; and take a slow, deep breath. You are doing the best that you can, and nothing can keep that from happening. The questions are designed to feel difficult, as I explain in Chapter 6. So be in the moment during the exam. It's just you and the test question in front of you. Understand what is being asked, consider the responses, choose your best answer, and move on to the next question.

Maintaining a positive attitude

Any successful person will tell you that having a positive attitude plays a large part in that success. Sports players spend time making mental images about winning. Special military units like the Rangers or SEALS go out on missions with the assumption that they will achieve the goal. Likewise, if you have practiced and studied with diligence, you should absolutely believe that you will be successful, even if you weren't on previous attempts.

The worst thing you can do to yourself during the exam is to lose confidence. If you aren't sure what the question is asking or none of the answers seems to apply, step back for a moment (mentally — your proctor may get anxious if you literally step out of your cubicle). Use all of your test-taking strategies to reason out the best answer. And remember — you don't need to get every question correct in order to pass the exam.

When the computer screen shuts off, you're done — figuratively and literally. When you leave the testing center, relax. You have my permission to take some time for yourself and feel good. You just took an exam that is challenging, and passing it really means you've proven that you have the education to perform the job.

Getting Your Results and Moving Ahead

Your results are posted in your account on `www.nremt.org` on the same day as your exam or shortly thereafter. (Chapter 2 has details on setting up an account; Chapter 3 explains how the exam is scored.) How you move forward depends on whether you passed:

- **If you passed:** The NREMT will mail you your registration card and paperwork explaining the renewal process that you'll need to undertake in two years. You won't receive any other information about how well you did on the exam.
- **If you didn't pass:** You'll get a report that details how you did on each section of the exam. The NREMT uses the statements "above passing," "near passing," and "below passing" to indicate your performance. "Above passing" and "below passing" are self-explanatory. The term "near passing" is a bit vague but doesn't imply satisfactory performance. You can assume that you didn't do especially well in that area.

Whether you pass or fail in your attempt, NREMT doesn't provide any specific information about how you did on specific exam questions. Remember that the exam evaluates your knowledge base and ability to think about all things EMT. Your exam selected questions from a very large test bank as it evaluated your performance during the testing. It's extremely unlikely that you'll see the same exact question on your next attempt. In other words, knowing the answer to a specific question is of no benefit.

Although I'm confident that your best effort was good enough to pass the exam on the first try, it wouldn't be fair to you if I didn't address this question: What if you *didn't* pass? Not passing the first time isn't unusual; NREMT's own research says that one out of every four students has to retake the exam two or more times. The good news is that the vast majority of students who have to do this pass on the second attempt. There are probably a couple of reasons why this happens:

- Taking the test once provides better insight regarding how the questions are asked.
- Failed students get a brief report telling them which section(s) they didn't perform well enough in. That information allows them to focus their studies before retaking the exam, often with better results.

Having to take the exam a second time can be depressing. Don't let it be. Take a deep breath, relax, and look at the exam results. Focus your studying on the sections that you did poorly on first. Then spend some time reviewing the sections that you passed, just to keep that information fresh. Retake the practice exams and evaluate your performance. Rebuild your confidence and go take the exam with the assumption that you will pass.

What happens if you don't pass the second time? Well, you get a third attempt. If you fail that one, you have to engage in at least 24 hours of remedial training and provide documentation of that remediation to the NREMT before scheduling your fourth attempt. The remedial training may be provided by your program; check with your course instructor for details.

At the end of your remediation, the instructor should provide you with a letter stating that you successfully completed 24 hours of remedial training. You submit that to the NREMT when you register for the exam.

In total, you have six opportunities to pass the exam. If you fail the sixth time, you must complete another EMT course before you can apply again.

Part III

Assessing What You Know and Reviewing Essential Information

An Overview of Body Systems, Structures, and Functions

System	*Major Organs and Structures*	*Main Functions*
Nervous	Brain, spinal cord, nerves	Fast, short-acting control system Conscious thought
Gastrointestinal	Mouth, teeth, esophagus, stomach, small and large intestines, liver, gallbladder, pancreas, appendix, rectum, anus	Digestion — break down food and absorb nutrients Absorb water Excrete unused food components and unwanted solid waste products
Immune	Thymus, bone marrow	Protection from foreign substances and organisms, such as allergens and infections
Endocrine	Pancreas, ovaries, testes	Slow, long-acting control system
Hematologic	Red blood cells (erythrocytes), white blood cells (leukocytes), platelets, plasma	Carry oxygen and nutrients to cells and remove carbon dioxide and waste
Urinary	Kidneys, ureters, bladder, urethra	Regulate water balance Excrete unwanted liquid wastes
Reproductive	Male: Testes, urethra, penis Female: Ovaries, uterus, fallopian tubes, vagina, mammary glands	Reproduction (sperm production for males; egg development, ovulation, and pregnancy for females) Secondary sex characteristics (deeper voice, greater muscle growth for males; breast development, higher voice for females)

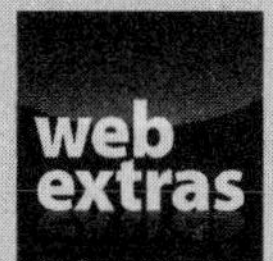

Discover how to differentiate the medical complaint in a free article at `www.dummies.com/extras/emtexam`.

In this part . . .

- Take a preassessment to see which exam topics you should focus on first as you study.
- Get the scoop on the key conditions and findings you need to know for the EMT exam. The information in this part is separated in the same way as the NREMT divides its exam, which can help you focus on weaker areas. The main topics are the airway, cardiology, medical fundamentals, trauma, and EMS operations, with a special chapter dedicated to pediatrics. Keep your notes and textbook handy in case you need greater detail while you review each chapter.

Chapter 8

Taking a Preassessment with Answers and Explanations

In This Chapter

- Walking through practice exam questions
- Getting the answer explanations
- Jumping into further study

One way to understand how prepared you are to take the NREMT exam is to perform a preassessment — take a practice exam to see where you stand, right now. You may find out that you're doing just fine and that all you need is a little tune-up on just a couple of areas. If so, that's great! On the other hand, you may realize that you need to review a few areas and study them further. The preassessment can help you focus first on the areas that you need to study the most. Later, you can review the areas you're more familiar with.

Keep in mind that test-taking is a skill that you can improve with practice. However, your base knowledge must be good enough to allow you to analyze a question for its information.

Going through the Preassessment Questions

Try to go through this first set of questions without looking up the answers. It's important for you to get a good sense of what you know — and what you don't. An honest appraisal helps you identify your areas of weakness. Then, you can focus your precious study time on what matters most and do any last-minute "cleanup" on topic areas that you know well.

If you can, try to answer the questions all in one sitting. Doing so helps get your brain in "game mode." Chapters 15 and 17 contain much longer practice exams; the 60 questions in this chapter will likely take 40 minutes to an hour to complete.

When you study each question, take a moment to consider how confident you are in your chosen answer. If you don't feel very confident about your choice, you may want to make a notation to that effect in the margin next to the question. When you check the answer later, you can find out whether your self-appraisal was accurate.

Finally, leave no question unanswered. Even if you're not confident and can only venture a guess, go ahead. Sometimes your subconscious brain has information that you're not fully aware of; besides, you don't want to leave any question unanswered during your actual EMT exam.

1. You determine that your unconscious patient has an inadequate airway. You insert an oropharyngeal airway. The patient vomits. You should first

   (A) place the patient into a prone position.

   (B) remove the airway.

   (C) suction the airway until it's clear.

   (D) place the patient in a sitting position.

2. Your patient is supine in bed, unresponsive to verbal stimulus and having difficulty breathing. You note that the patient's lips, face, and fingers are cyanotic and that there's pink, frothy sputum in the mouth and nose. You should first

   (A) suction the mouth and nose.

   (B) place the patient into a sitting position with feet dangling.

   (C) begin bag-valve-mask ventilations.

   (D) apply a jaw thrust.

3. A 7-month-old infant presents limp and unresponsive in his mother's arms. You note no air exchange and a weak, slow brachial pulse. The mother reports that the infant was playing with toys in a crib when he suddenly turned blue and stopped breathing. You should

   (A) administer five abdominal thrusts.

   (B) suction the mouth.

   (C) administer five back blows and five chest thrusts.

   (D) begin chest compressions.

4. A 16-year-old female says she is short of breath. She is alert and is speaking seven to eight words in between breaths. She has hives on her chest and arms, and her skin is pale. You should

   (A) ventilate the patient with a bag-valve mask.

   (B) insert a nasopharyngeal airway.

   (C) administer supplemental oxygen.

   (D) apply continuous positive airway pressure (CPAP).

5. An unconscious 25-year-old female has pale, cool, and diaphoretic skin. Her respiratory rate is 6 times a minute. You cannot hear lung sounds with a stethoscope. Your next step is to

   (A) administer abdominal thrusts.

   (B) administer high-flow oxygen.

   (C) ventilate with a bag-valve mask.

   (D) turn the patient onto her side.

6. A 4-year-old child is having breathing difficulty. He isn't responding to your commands, he has cyanosis around his lips and fingers, and he's drooling from his mouth. His parents report the patient has a high fever and didn't want to lie down to rest. What should you do?

   (A) Administer oxygen via blow-by mask.

   (B) Ventilate using a bag-valve mask.

   (C) Apply a nasal cannula and oxygen at 6 LPM.

   (D) Administer a combination of back blows and abdominal thrusts.

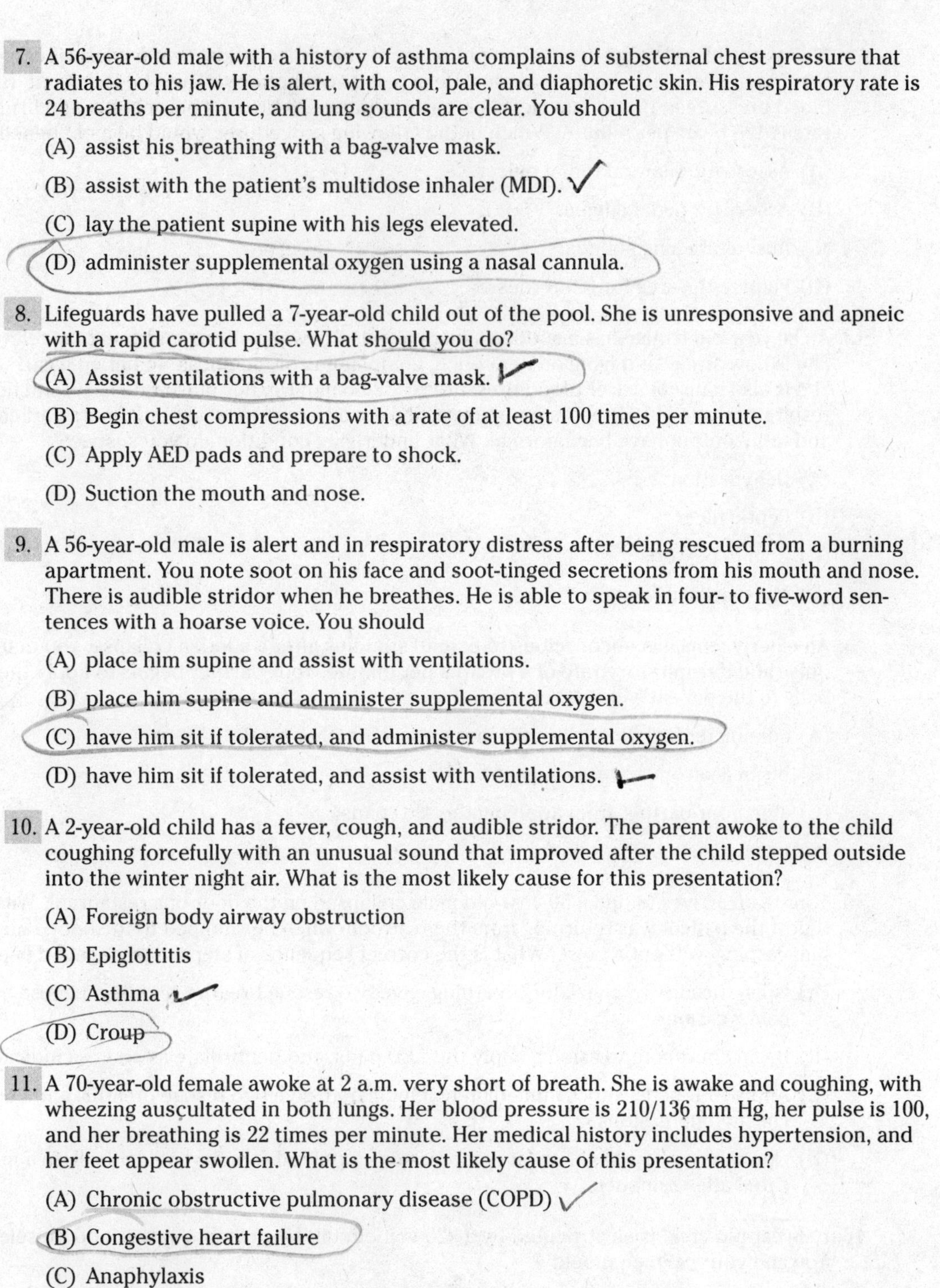

7. A 56-year-old male with a history of asthma complains of substernal chest pressure that radiates to his jaw. He is alert, with cool, pale, and diaphoretic skin. His respiratory rate is 24 breaths per minute, and lung sounds are clear. You should

(A) assist his breathing with a bag-valve mask.

(B) assist with the patient's multidose inhaler (MDI).

(C) lay the patient supine with his legs elevated.

(D) administer supplemental oxygen using a nasal cannula.

8. Lifeguards have pulled a 7-year-old child out of the pool. She is unresponsive and apneic with a rapid carotid pulse. What should you do?

(A) Assist ventilations with a bag-valve mask.

(B) Begin chest compressions with a rate of at least 100 times per minute.

(C) Apply AED pads and prepare to shock.

(D) Suction the mouth and nose.

9. A 56-year-old male is alert and in respiratory distress after being rescued from a burning apartment. You note soot on his face and soot-tinged secretions from his mouth and nose. There is audible stridor when he breathes. He is able to speak in four- to five-word sentences with a hoarse voice. You should

(A) place him supine and assist with ventilations.

(B) place him supine and administer supplemental oxygen.

(C) have him sit if tolerated, and administer supplemental oxygen.

(D) have him sit if tolerated, and assist with ventilations.

10. A 2-year-old child has a fever, cough, and audible stridor. The parent awoke to the child coughing forcefully with an unusual sound that improved after the child stepped outside into the winter night air. What is the most likely cause for this presentation?

(A) Foreign body airway obstruction

(B) Epiglottitis

(C) Asthma

(D) Croup

11. A 70-year-old female awoke at 2 a.m. very short of breath. She is awake and coughing, with wheezing auscultated in both lungs. Her blood pressure is 210/136 mm Hg, her pulse is 100, and her breathing is 22 times per minute. Her medical history includes hypertension, and her feet appear swollen. What is the most likely cause of this presentation?

(A) Chronic obstructive pulmonary disease (COPD)

(B) Congestive heart failure

(C) Anaphylaxis

(D) Pulmonary embolus

12. A 47-year-old male experiences a rapid onset of chest discomfort that he describes as "stabbing" in between his shoulder blades. He is pale and diaphoretic, and he feels faint. His blood pressure is 102/64 mm Hg, his breathing rate is 20 breaths per minute, and his heart rate is 120 beats per minute. Which of the following procedures would be most beneficial?

    (A) Assess for bilateral radial pulses.

    (B) Assess for pedal edema.

    (C) Auscultate lung sounds.

    (D) Palpate the area for tenderness.

13. An 80-year-old female has a sudden syncopal episode while sitting and watching television. She is now awake and lying on her couch, complaining of "achiness" in her epigastric region. She is also nauseous. Her blood pressure is 132/86 mm Hg, her pulse rate is 60, and her respiratory rate is 16 breaths per minute. She ate a normal meal about 2 hours earlier. Bowel and urine output have been normal. What underlying condition do you suspect?

    (A) Dehydration

    (B) Peptic ulcer

    (C) Angina pectoris

    (D) Myocardial infarction

14. An elderly female is unconscious to painful stimulus after a sudden collapse. You detect a pulse and a respiratory rate of 4 breaths per minute. Your partner begins to apply the AED pads to the patient's chest. You should

    (A) administer high-flow oxygen using a nonrebreather mask.

    (B) begin a secondary assessment.

    (C) stop your partner from applying the AED pads.

    (D) begin chest compressions.

15. Your team arrives to find a 50-year-old male collapsed on the floor of a restaurant. Witnesses report the patient was returning from the restroom when he slumped to the floor. You find him gasping, without a pulse. What is the correct sequence of steps in managing this patient?

    (A) Open the airway, check for breathing, give two rescue breaths, and begin chest compressions.

    (B) Begin chest compressions, apply the AED pads, and defibrillate as soon as indicated.

    (C) Apply AED pads, shock immediately if indicated, give two rescue breaths, and begin chest compressions.

    (D) Open the airway, begin chest compressions, apply AED pads, and defibrillate if indicated after 2 minutes.

16. A 2-year-old child is electrocuted by a 220-volt circuit. He presents apneic and pulseless. You and your partner should

    (A) perform compressions and ventilations at a ratio of 30:2.

    (B) perform compressions at a rate of at least 100 per minute and at a depth of 1 inch.

    (C) perform compressions and ventilations at a ratio of 15:2.

    (D) apply AED pads and defibrillate immediately if indicated; then begin compressions.

17. A 78-year-old female has a sudden episode of confusion and dizziness. Family reports the patient can speak clearly but her words "don't make sense." She has a history of hypertension and Type 2 diabetes. Her skin is pink, warm, and dry. Her blood pressure is 146/86 mm Hg. You suspect that the patient is experiencing

(A) a stroke.

(B) diabetic ketoacidosis.

(C) insulin shock.

(D) a hypertensive emergency.

18. After 2 minutes of CPR, you analyze a patient's rhythm using your AED. A shock is indicated. What should you do next?

(A) Check for a carotid pulse; if no pulse, defibrillate.

(B) Defibrillate and then check for a carotid pulse.

(C) Defibrillate and then administer chest compressions.

(D) Analyze again to confirm rhythm; then defibrillate.

19. A 65-year-old male presents with chest pressure and difficulty breathing. His blood pressure is 86/50 mm Hg, he has a pulse rate of 110, and he's breathing 24 times per minute. You can hear crackles in both lung fields during auscultation. You should

(A) sit the patient upright to improve his breathing ability.

(B) assist his ventilations with a bag-valve mask.

(C) provide supplemental oxygen.

(D) assist the patient with his prescribed nitroglycerin.

20. The purpose of the automated external defibrillator is to reverse which of the following cardiac rhythm disturbances?

(A) Ventricular standstill

(B) Ventricular fibrillation

(C) Asystole

(D) Sinus rhythm without a pulse

21. A driver has been struck on the driver's side door by a second motor vehicle moving at a high rate of speed. He is awake, confused, and breathing fast. There's profuse bleeding from a large laceration to his left forearm. You can palpate a weak, fast carotid pulse only. What should you do next?

(A) Control the bleeding.

(B) Administer high-flow oxygen.

(C) Assist his ventilations with a bag-valve mask.

(D) Rapidly extricate him from the vehicle.

22. A patient has been assaulted with a metal bar. You see bruises to the left side of his head, the left lateral chest wall, and the right upper quadrant of his abdomen. His blood pressure is 98/68 mm Hg, he has a heart rate of 136 beats per minute, and he has a respiratory rate of 26 breaths per minute with equal, clear lung sounds. His skin is cool, diaphoretic, and pale. Which injury would most likely cause his presentation?

(A) Hemothorax

(B) Brain injury

(C) Ruptured spleen

(D) Lacerated liver

23. A 19-year-old male has been shot. A small, round wound is located in the right anterior chest wall. The patient is coughing up blood and has difficulty breathing. Lung sounds are absent over the right side. His blood pressure is 146/84 mm Hg, and he has a heart rate of 98 and a respiratory rate of 24 breaths per minute. You should

(A) place the patient in a supine position, with legs elevated.

(B) assist ventilations with a bag-valve mask.

(C) seal the wound with an occlusive dressing.

(D) place the patient on his left side.

24. In a head-on collision, a poorly restrained 18-month-old child became loose from his car seat, causing him to strike the back of the front passenger seat. He presents supine on the car floor, tachypneic and with cyanotic, cool skin. He doesn't cry, and he grunts when he breathes. Lung sounds are diminished over the left side, and you note crepitus of the rib cage over that side. You should

(A) immobilize the patient on a pediatric backboard and lay him on the affected side.

(B) assist ventilations with a pediatric bag-valve mask.

(C) administer high-flow oxygen via a pediatric nonrebreather mask.

(D) administer low-flow oxygen via a pediatric nasal cannula.

25. A 45-year-old female has abdominal pain after being assaulted by her boyfriend. Her left upper quadrant is tender to palpation, and you observe bruising to the area. Her blood pressure is 136/84 mm Hg, and she has a heart rate of 86 and a respiratory rate of 16 breaths per minute. She is alert, anxious, and upset. What should you do?

(A) Place her supine on the gurney, administer high-flow oxygen, and transport to a trauma center.

(B) Determine the full extent of her relationship with the assailant.

(C) Place the patient in a position of comfort and transport her to her hospital of choice.

(D) Advise the patient to see her primary physician for pain management.

26. A 9-year-old child fell off his skateboard. He presents awake, crying, and cradling his left arm. The elbow is bent at an unusual angle. The child can't feel his hand, and you observe that the fingers appear white with prolonged capillary refill. You should

(A) splint the elbow in the position of deformity.

(B) apply gentle manual traction in line with the limb.

(C) carefully flex the injured arm and secure it with padded board splints.

(D) make two attempts to restore distal circulation by manipulating the elbow.

27. A 35-year-old man has severed his left hand with an electric saw. There is minimal bleeding from the distal arm. Which of the following describes the most appropriate care?

(A) Use direct pressure to control bleeding; wrap the severed hand in plastic and place on ice.

(B) Use a tourniquet to control bleeding; wrap the severed hand in plastic and place on ice.

(C) Use a pressure point and elevation to control bleeding; wrap the severed hand with cool, wet towels.

(D) Use direct pressure to control bleeding; place the severed hand into an ice bath.

28. You find a 75-year-old male lying unresponsive in bed. Family reports that the patient was last seen two days ago in a normal state. He takes thyroid medication and a blood thinner. His pulse rate is 60, his blood pressure is 210/104 mm Hg, and he has a respiratory rate of 8 breaths per minute. Lung sounds are clear, and there's bruising to the left side of his head and to his abdomen. Which is the most likely cause of the patient's presentation?

(A) Acute alcohol poisoning

(B) Subdural hematoma

(C) Acute ischemic stroke

(D) Internal hemorrhage

29. A 10-year-old female was struck by a motor vehicle while riding her bicycle. She is unresponsive to painful stimulus, is breathing shallowly at 10 times per minute, and has a pulse rate of 68 per minute. You note her pupils are unequal and notice an obvious deformity to the right humerus and right femur. Her abdomen is firm. Her helmet is damaged on the right side. Your priority of care is to

(A) ventilate the patient with a bag-valve mask and oxygen, immobilize the patient with a cervical collar and backboard, splint the femur with a traction splint, and begin transport.

(B) immobilize the patient with a cervical collar and backboard, administer oxygen with a nonrebreather mask, begin transport, and splint the femur with a traction splint.

(C) ventilate the patient with a bag-valve mask and oxygen, immobilize the patient with a cervical collar and backboard, begin transport, and splint the femur and humerus if time permits.

(D) ventilate the patient with a bag-valve mask and oxygen, place the patient on a gurney, begin transport, and splint the femur and humerus if time permits.

30. A patient has been struck over the head during an assault. He responds to pain by moaning only. His arms are slightly flexed which increases with a sternal rub. His eyes remain closed throughout your exam. How would he score on the Glasgow Coma Scale?

(A) 6

(B) 8

(C) 9

(D) 10

31. An 87-year-old female presents in a nursing home bed with a rapid onset of confusion, screaming, and altered mental status. Staff reports that the patient is normally quiet and keeps to herself. She has a history of hypertension, atrial fibrillation, Type 2 diabetes, and glaucoma. Her pulse rate is 90, her blood pressure is 200/104 mm Hg, and she's breathing at 20 breaths per minute. Her skin is pale, warm, and dry. You suspect that she's experiencing

(A) acute hypoglycemia.

(B) acute hyperglycemia.

(C) a stroke.

(D) a psychotic episode.

32. A mother is holding her 14-month-old son. She reports the patient was getting ready to fall asleep when his body stiffened for a few seconds and then began to "jerk" rhythmically for about a minute. The child had been running a high fever and has had normal urine output and bowel movements. The child is awake and is crying loudly and clinging to his mother. You should

(A) cool the child with wet towels.

(B) transport the child and parent to the hospital.

(C) have the mother bottle-feed the child.

(D) administer a baby aspirin to the child.

33. A 65-year-old female has been experiencing vomiting and loose stools for 72 hours. She is confused, and her skin feels cool and diaphoretic. You can detect carotid pulses only. You should

(A) perform a detailed physical exam.

(B) elevate her legs and reassess.

(C) have her drink fluids.

(D) prepare for immediate transport.

34. A 27-year-old male complains of itching and coughing after a meal. You observe hives on the patient's face and arms. His blood pressure is 160/92 mm Hg, his pulse rate is 90, and he's breathing 22 times per minute. Lung sounds are clear bilaterally; the patient is alert, anxious, and agitated. What should you do next?

(A) Assist the patient in administering his prescribed epinephrine autoinjector.

(B) Administer an oral dose of diphenhydramine (Benadryl).

(C) Administer syrup of ipecac.

(D) Prepare for transport.

35. Your patient presents with difficulty breathing and feeling faint. He had returned from the dentist's office, where he'd taken a dose of antibiotics after a surgical procedure. You can auscultate wheezes in both lungs; his pulse rate is 120, and his blood pressure is 88/50 mm Hg. You should

(A) contact the dentist to determine the type of antibiotics.

(B) help the patient sit up to help his breathing.

(C) help administer the patient's prescribed epinephrine autoinjector.

(D) administer continuous positive airway pressure (CPAP).

36. A 74-year-old female presents in her bed, unresponsive to painful stimulus. Family reports the patient has had flu-like symptoms for a week but has refused to see a doctor. Her pulse is 110 and regular, her blood pressure is 70 by palpation, and her respirations are 28 and shallow. Her skin is cool, cyanotic around her lips, and dry. Which of the following best describes your treatment?

(A) Assist ventilations with a bag-valve mask and oxygen; keep the patient supine.

(B) Administer high-flow oxygen with a nonrebreather mask; place the patient in a sitting position.

(C) Expose the patient to promote cooling; assist ventilations with a bag-valve mask and high-flow oxygen.

(D) Administer low-flow oxygen with a nasal cannula; place the patient in recovery position.

37. A 7-year-old child has been coughing and vomiting for the past 6 hours. He presents very tired, not reacting to your presence, and saying, "My head hurts." His skin feels very warm to the touch. What should you do next?

(A) Transport immediately.

(B) Don protective eyeglasses and a mask.

(C) Place the child in a cool water and alcohol bath.

(D) Have the patient drink several glasses of water.

38. A 53-year-old female presents lying on her couch. She responds to verbal stimulus by moaning. Her husband reports she has been feeling "weak" for the past three days, sleeping on the couch. Her pulse is 104, her blood pressure is 106/82 mm Hg, and her breathing rate is 18 per minute, with deep breaths. Her skin is warm, flushed, and dry. She has a history of Type 2 diabetes and hypertension. You should

(A) administer oral glucose.

(B) assist ventilations with a bag-valve mask.

(C) assist the husband with administering the patient's diabetic medications.

(D) prepare the patient for immediate transport.

39. A 70-year-old man is sitting in his kitchen, confused but cooperative. His wife reports that this episode began about an hour ago. He is a diabetic who takes insulin daily. He also has a history of hypertension. His skin feels cool and diaphoretic and looks pale. His blood pressure is 110/70 mm Hg, his pulse rate is 96, and his respiratory rate is 20 breaths per minute. He moves his arms equally and speaks clearly. Which of the following conditions best fits the patient's presentation?

(A) Hyperglycemia

(B) Stroke

(C) Hypoglycemia

(D) Transient ischemic attack (TIA)

40. A 35-year-old male says that there are people "out to get him." He asks if you hear the voices, too. You should

(A) focus on reality, such as people in the room.

(B) agree with what the patient hears.

(C) forcefully tell him that voices are not real.

(D) restrain the patient.

41. Parents report their 3-year-old child may have ingested two or three tablets of a grandparent's antihypertensive medication about 45 minutes earlier. The child appears alert, clings to a parent, and appears frightened. You should

(A) administer activated charcoal.

(B) administer syrup of ipecac.

(C) contact poison control.

(D) have the child drink milk.

42. You respond to a report of a "person down" in an apartment. On arrival, you find several members of a family complaining of headaches and nausea, and another person is unresponsive in bed. You should first

(A) begin resuscitation of the unresponsive person.

(B) retreat out of the apartment.

(C) administer oxygen to patients with headaches.

(D) call for additional resources.

43. A 32-year-old male is found unresponsive on the floor of his apartment. There are no signs of trauma. His blood pressure is 168/108 mm Hg, his heart rate is 50 beats per minute and bounding, and he is breathing 9 times per minute and irregularly. You note a medical alert bracelet that states he has hemophilia. You should first

(A) administer high-flow oxygen via a nonrebreather mask.

(B) transport immediately.

(C) perform a detailed physical exam to detect possible injuries.

(D) assist his ventilations with a bag-valve mask with high-flow oxygen.

44. A patient is having difficulty breathing at a dialysis center. A nurse reports that the patient had not yet begun her dialysis session when she became short of breath. The patient is alert and using accessory muscles to breathe. You auscultate crackles in both lung fields. Her blood pressure is 170/112 mm Hg, and her heart rate is 90 beats per minute and irregular. She is breathing 22 times a minute. Her skin is pale, warm, and diaphoretic. You should

(A) sit her up and administer oxygen via a nonrebreather mask.

(B) lay her supine and administer oxygen via a nonrebreather mask.

(C) place her in a semi-Fowler's position and assist ventilations with a bag-valve mask and oxygen.

(D) sit her up and assist her ventilations with a bag-valve mask and oxygen.

45. A 57-year-old female was robbed, badly beaten, and sexually assaulted. Your priority in treatment is to

(A) preserve evidence of the sexual assault.

(B) determine baseline vital signs.

(C) identify traumatic injuries.

(D) get a detailed description of the attack.

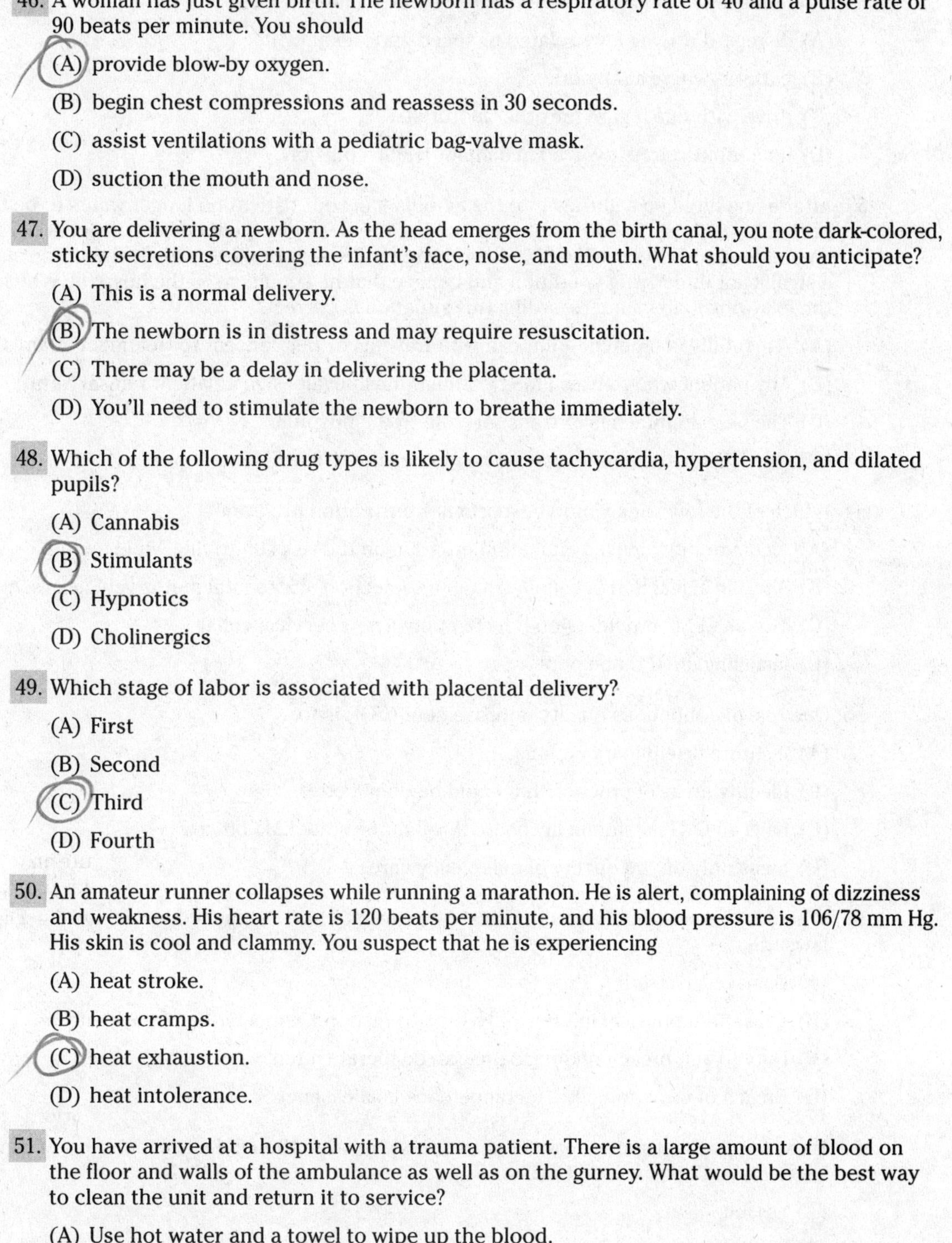

46. A woman has just given birth. The newborn has a respiratory rate of 40 and a pulse rate of 90 beats per minute. You should

(A) provide blow-by oxygen.

(B) begin chest compressions and reassess in 30 seconds.

(C) assist ventilations with a pediatric bag-valve mask.

(D) suction the mouth and nose.

47. You are delivering a newborn. As the head emerges from the birth canal, you note dark-colored, sticky secretions covering the infant's face, nose, and mouth. What should you anticipate?

(A) This is a normal delivery.

(B) The newborn is in distress and may require resuscitation.

(C) There may be a delay in delivering the placenta.

(D) You'll need to stimulate the newborn to breathe immediately.

48. Which of the following drug types is likely to cause tachycardia, hypertension, and dilated pupils?

(A) Cannabis

(B) Stimulants

(C) Hypnotics

(D) Cholinergics

49. Which stage of labor is associated with placental delivery?

(A) First

(B) Second

(C) Third

(D) Fourth

50. An amateur runner collapses while running a marathon. He is alert, complaining of dizziness and weakness. His heart rate is 120 beats per minute, and his blood pressure is 106/78 mm Hg. His skin is cool and clammy. You suspect that he is experiencing

(A) heat stroke.

(B) heat cramps.

(C) heat exhaustion.

(D) heat intolerance.

51. You have arrived at a hospital with a trauma patient. There is a large amount of blood on the floor and walls of the ambulance as well as on the gurney. What would be the best way to clean the unit and return it to service?

(A) Use hot water and a towel to wipe up the blood.

(B) Spray 1:10 bleach and water solution to contaminated areas and wipe with a towel or mop.

(C) Allow the blood to dry and then use a broom to brush it away.

(D) Heat-sterilize the ambulance.

52. Operating an ambulance in an emergency mode allows you to

(A) disregard driving laws related to speed and signal lights.

(B) park anywhere at any time.

(C) drive with due regard for other motorists.

(D) not stop if you're involved in a minor traffic collision.

53. After being lifted on a gurney into the ambulance, your patient no longer wants to be transported to the hospital. He is alert, appears not to be under the influence of alcohol or drugs, and understands the ramifications of refusing transport. However, you feel that the man has a significant underlying condition and believe that he should go to the hospital. Which of the following statements regarding this situation is correct?

(A) A mentally competent adult can withdraw his or her consent to treatment at any time.

(B) Any patient who refuses EMS treatment must legally sign a patient refusal form.

(C) The best approach is to transport him to the hospital.

(D) Once inside the ambulance, he cannot legally refuse EMS transport.

54. Which of the following would be a primary prevention program?

(A) A community-focused education program on the risks of driving while texting

(B) A traffic signal that is installed at an intersection after a fatal motor vehicle crash

(C) Training EMS providers on how to apply a new cervical collar

(D) Installing an AED at a pool

55. One role of continuous quality improvement (CQI) is to

(A) institute disciplinary actions.

(B) identify areas of practice that could be done better.

(C) have all EMTs maintain licensure through the state EMS office.

(D) focus only on the quality of emergency care.

56. What four general legal elements must be proven to have happened in a medical negligence lawsuit?

(A) Damages, causation, duty to act, breach of duty

(B) Causation, physical injuries only, duty to respond, expectation of payment

(C) Duty to act, breach of duty, damages, deliberate intent

(D) Breach of duty, damages, incompetence, malfeasance

57. If you forcibly transport a patient against his will, even though he is capable of refusing your services, you may be found guilty of

(A) assault.

(B) battery.

(C) false imprisonment.

(D) defamation.

58. Although laws may vary from state to state, EMTs in all states must report which of the following circumstances to proper authorities?

(A) Elder abuse

(B) Drug use

(C) Domestic violence

(D) Child abuse and neglect

59. People react differently toward death and dying. However, common stages of grieving include

(A) denial, bargaining, depression.

(B) acceptance, anger, euphoria.

(C) anger, suicidal thoughts, bargaining.

(D) excitement, acceptance, delirium.

60. Hepatitis B is an example of which type of communicable disease?

(A) Airborne

(B) Bloodborne

(C) Foodborne

(D) Vectorborne

Looking at the Preassessment Answers and Figuring Out How to Proceed

When you're done, look at the answers to see how you did. You may be tempted to rationalize that you really did know the answer, but set that thought aside for a moment. Knowing the actual answer is like having 20/20 hindsight; the answer seems so obvious. Yet you had a reason for answering the question the way you did; you may have misunderstood the question or missed a vital piece of information.

As you score your answers, record the topic sections for each of the questions you answered incorrectly. Here's the breakdown of topic sections and question numbers:

- Questions 1–10 cover Airway, Respiration, and Ventilation.
- Questions 11–20 cover Cardiology and Resuscitation.
- Questions 21–30 cover Trauma.
- Questions 31–50 cover Medical and Obstetrics/Gynecology.
- Questions 51–60 cover EMS Operations.

If you like, you can use the following table to record your results.

Topic Section	*Number Correct (Enter Hash Marks)*	*Total Number of Questions in Section*	*% Correct*
Airway, Respiration, and Ventilation		10	
Cardiology and Resuscitation		10	
Trauma		10	
Medical and Obstetrics/ Gynecology		20	
EMS Operations		10	

Record the number of questions you got right for each section, and then divide each number by the total number of questions in each section. Multiply your result by 100; that number is your percent score for that section. For example, suppose you got eight questions right in the Airway, Respiration, and Ventilation section; there are ten questions in that section. Eight divided by ten is 0.8; multiply that number by 100 to get 80 (80%).

You may find out that you did more poorly in some sections than others; study the chapter of this book that covers the section you scored most poorly on first. When you finish that, focus on the next-worst section; repeat the process until you've reviewed all the sections.

One final note: You'll see questions related to children throughout the NREMT exam. However, pediatric emergency care is different enough from adult care that it has its own chapter in this book. Refer to Chapter 13 if you have any questions about providing emergency care for children.

1. **B.** It's most likely that the oropharyngeal airway triggered the patient's gag reflex. Removing it will stop the reflex. Turning the patient face down, Choice (A), or upright, Choice (D), won't help maintain a patent airway. Suctioning the airway, Choice (C), will be helpful, but not until the airway has been removed.
2. **A.** You need to ensure that the patient's airway is patent, so clearing the airway of any potential obstructions comes first. You may need to ventilate the patient, Choice (C), but the question doesn't give you enough information to make that decision. Without knowing the blood pressure, putting the patient into a sitting position, Choice (B), may be dangerous. None of the information in the question suggests a trauma mechanism, so a jaw thrust, Choice (D), would be inappropriate.
3. **D.** A likely scenario for this presentation is a foreign body airway obstruction. Given the patient's age, abdominal thrusts, Choice (A), are inappropriate. Back blows and chest thrusts, Choice (C), would be indicated if the patient were still awake. There's no indication that the obstruction is in the mouth, so you wouldn't suction the mouth, as Choice (B) suggests.
4. **C.** The patient is alert and responding appropriately, which indicates respiratory distress and not respiratory failure. This makes bag-valve-mask use, Choice (A), and a nasopharyngeal airway, Choice (B), inappropriate. You have no information about lung sounds, and she has a near normal speaking rate, so CPAP, Choice (D), is not indicated.
5. **C.** The patient's respiratory effort is too slow to support adequate ventilations, so you need to assist with a bag-valve mask. High-flow oxygen alone, Choice (B), isn't helpful without adequate rate and tidal volume. There's no information to suggest that she's experiencing a foreign body airway obstruction, so you wouldn't administer abdominal thrusts, as Choice (A) suggests. If her ventilations were adequate, the recovery position, Choice (D), would be helpful; this isn't the case.
6. **B.** This child appears to have signs of an upper airway disorder, possibly due to epiglottitis. You can deduce that his ventilations are inadequate due to his mental status and skin signs. Therefore, supplemental oxygen alone, Choices (A) and (C), isn't adequate. There are no signs of a foreign body airway obstruction, so back blows and abdominal thrusts, Choice (D), aren't appropriate.

7. **D.** This patient appears to have adequate breathing, based on his rate and lung sounds. Therefore, you don't need to assist with ventilations, ruling out Choice (A). The complaint sounds more related to a cardiac condition than to asthma, making Choice (B), assisting with a multidose inhaler, less likely. The patient should be placed in a position of comfort, which is more likely to be sitting than lying, Choice (C).

8. **A.** The patient is in respiratory arrest. Her heart rate is fast, making chest compressions, Choice (B), unnecessary at this point and contradicting the use of the AED, Choice (C). There's no indication of secretions or water in the upper airway, so suctioning, Choice (D), isn't needed.

9. **C.** Stridor and a hoarse voice indicate some type of air restriction in the upper airway. Having the patient in a sitting position is most likely to promote optimal airway patency; laying the patient supine, as Choices (A) and (B) suggest, would most likely make the air restriction worse. The patient is alert and responding appropriately; assisting ventilations, Choice (D), at this point may cause more harm than good if the patient becomes agitated.

10. **D.** The description best fits an upper airway disorder; however, asthma, Choice (C), is a lower airway condition. Epiglottitis, Choice (B), and a foreign body airway obstruction, Choice (A), don't respond to changes in humidity or ambient temperature.

11. **B.** Her very high blood pressure and swollen legs make COPD, Choice (A), a less likely cause of the wheezing. There are no indications of an excessive immune reaction such as anaphylaxis, Choice (C). A pulmonary embolus, Choice (D), rarely causes unusual lung sounds like wheezing; if it does, the wheezing is usually well localized in one small region of a lung.

12. **A.** Although the description and location of the pain may reflect a myocardial infarction, you'd more strongly suspect an aortic aneurysm or dissection. If the wall of the aorta near where it exits the left ventricle weakens and begins to bulge (aneurysm) or separate (dissection), blood flow to the head and arms may be compromised. Uneven pulses can quickly point to the presence of this life-threatening condition, so you need to assess for bilateral radial pulses, Choice (A). Although you'll perform the procedures noted in Choices (B), (C), and (D) — assessing for pedal edema, auscultating lung sounds, and palpating the area for tenderness — as part of your assessment, they aren't likely to produce more definitive information.

13. **D.** Older patients and females often experience heart attacks differently from adult men. For example, chest discomfort may be absent. Having a sudden fainting episode while sitting still indicates a sudden pressure change within the Cardiology and Resuscitation system, most likely the heart in this case. A normal urine output reduces the likelihood of dehydration, Choice (A). Peptic ulcers, Choice (B), aren't likely to cause syncope, and angina, Choice (C), is usually brought on by a predictable level of exertion and resolves with rest.

14. **C.** The AED may detect a shockable rhythm such as ventricular tachycardia that's still generating a pulse; however, the AED doesn't know that and will try to shock the patient. The patient has a pulse and therefore doesn't require chest compressions, Choice (D). However, she requires ventilation with a bag-valve mask, not just supplemental oxygen, as Choice (A) indicates. You'll perform a secondary assessment, Choice (B), but not at this point in the scenario.

15. **B.** The research points to early and effective chest compressions as a major contributor to positive outcomes in cardiac arrest. Any delay in administering chest compressions, as is the case in Choices (A) and (C), results in worse outcomes. Current research supports defibrillating the patient in ventricular fibrillation as soon as possible, not waiting 2 minutes, as Choice (D) suggests.

16. **C.** Unlike adult cardiac arrest, pediatric cardiac arrest is usually the result of respiratory failure and arrest rather than a primary cardiac event. The American Heart Association continues to recommend administering five cycles of CPR before applying the AED, contrary to Choice (D). Two-person CPR is considered to be superior to one-person CPR; with two rescuers available, delivering more ventilation is possible with a ratio of 15 compressions to two breaths, not 30:2, as Choice (A) indicates. Chest compressions in a child between 1 year old and puberty should be at least one-third the depth of the chest, which is closer to 2 inches than 1, ruling out Choice (B).

17. **A.** Although the patient has a history of diabetes, she doesn't show the clinical signs associated with changes in blood sugar levels. Blood sugar so high that it results in diabetic ketoacidosis, Choice (B), takes days to weeks. Very low blood sugar causes the patient to become pale, cool, and diaphoretic — signs that are similar to a patient experiencing shock; that's why the term "insulin shock," Choice (C), is used to describe hypoglycemia. Blood pressure so high that it causes a hypertensive emergency, Choice (D), is usually greater than 180/120 mm Hg; although this patient's pressure is higher than normal, it is still within the range of simple hypertension.

18. **C.** In treating cardiac arrest, you shouldn't delay chest compressions for any period of time; the immediate response helps maintain adequate blood flow to the heart muscle. This means that Choices (A) and (B) aren't appropriate; Choice (D) isn't indicated because, by design, AEDs are very accurate in detecting ventricular fibrillation or ventricular tachycardia.

19. **C.** This patient's blood pressure is too low to support nitroglycerin use, Choice (D). Having the patient sit up, Choice (A), with such a low blood pressure may cause his pressure to fall even further, cutting off blood flow to the heart and brain. There's no information to suggest that the patient is in respiratory failure to indicate Choice (B).

20. **B.** In ventricular fibrillation, Choice (B), an AED provides a brief power-spike of electricity to a heart, which causes all the cells to stop fibrillating at once. If the heart is ready, it will then begin to contract normally. A heart in asystole, Choice (C), won't respond to a defibrillation shock. A heart that has an organized electrical rhythm, Choice (D), but doesn't contract has what's known as pulseless electrical activity (PEA). An AED by design won't defibrillate this rhythm. Ventricular standstill, Choice (A), is when the atrial may be conducting energy but the ventricles are not responding. This, too, fails to respond to a defibrillation shock.

21. **A.** In trauma, every blood cell counts. We depend on red blood cells to carry as much oxygen as possible. No doubt you'll need to provide oxygen, as Choices (B) and (C) suggest, but both of those procedures take time to begin, and the patient continues to bleed in the meantime. You shouldn't delay definitive treatment with extrication, Choice (D).

22. **D.** The patient has signs of shock: hypotension, tachycardia, and poor skin signs. With no external signs of bleeding, you must assume that he's bleeding internally. Clear lung sounds rule out a hemothorax, Choice (A). It's unlikely that massive bleeding that could cause shock would occur inside the skull, as Choice (B) suggests. The spleen, Choice (C), is located in the far upper-left quadrant of the abdomen; there's no indication of an injury there.

23. **C.** Based on the description, the patient's right lung has been compromised, likely by a pneumothorax. Being supine, Choice (A), or on his side, Choice (D), will likely worsen his breathing, and there's no indication that the patient is in shock. Likewise, there's no indication that the patient is in respiratory failure, so you wouldn't assist ventilations, Choice (B).

24. **B.** The crepitus, diminished lung sounds, and mechanism of injury (MOI) point to the presence of at least several broken ribs, if not a full flail segment. Regardless, the patient's skin signs and respiratory effort indicate impending respiratory failure. Administering supplemental oxygen, Choices (C) and (D), won't help if the patient isn't ventilating adequately. You'll likely immobilize the child's spine but not until later in the process; laying the patient on his side, Choice (A) likely won't help and may make care during transport more difficult.

25. **C.** There are no signs to indicate that the patient has an internal hemorrhage from the assault, so treating for shock and transporting to a trauma center, Choice (A), aren't necessary. Your focus is on identifying and managing the injuries, not determining the full extent of the relationship, Choice (B). At this point, EMS providers are not permitted to refuse transportation to a patient, as Choice (D) implies.

26. **B.** You need to reduce the dislocation if the arteries supplying blood to the distal arm and the associated nerve bundle are being impinged by the injury. Splinting the elbow in its position, Choice (A), likely won't improve circulation, nor will flexing the elbow, Choice (C), assuming you can do so. Excessive manipulation of the elbow, Choice (D), may cause more damage and should be avoided.

27. **A.** Given the amount of bleeding described, a tourniquet, Choice (B), isn't necessary. Direct pressure and elevation, Choice (C), hasn't been demonstrated to be effective, and it isn't necessary in this situation. The severed hand is best preserved when kept dry and as cold as possible, without freezing. This contradicts the use of an ice bath, Choice (D).

28. **B.** None of the information points to acute alcohol use, Choice (A). He could be experiencing a stroke, Choice (C), but the injury to the head points more toward a trauma-related event. Although bleeding in the abdomen, Choice (D), is possible, you'd expect shock signs rather than severe hypertension.

29. **C.** This patient has experienced multiple injuries and is critically injured. Although she has signs of possible internal bleeding to the abdomen, her slower heart rate and poor respiratory rate point more toward a brain injury. Beginning controlled ventilations is imperative; simply providing supplemental oxygen, Choice (B), won't accomplish this. The spine has to be protected from further harm, making Choice (D) incorrect. The femur and humerus injury, although significant, can be splinted during transport; you shouldn't do this before you transport, as Choice (A) indicates, thereby delaying care at the hospital. In fact, unless you have an adequate number of rescuers to assist, applying a traction splint while en route may be impractical.

30. **A.** In the Glasgow Coma Scale, no eye opening = 1, incomprehensible sounds = 2, and abnormal flexion = 3, for a total of 6. A score of less than 8 is very serious.

31. **C.** Don't be misled by the setting — you must first suspect a medical cause of acute altered mental status rather than a psychotic episode, Choice (D). In hyperglycemia, Choice (B), the patient tends to be less responsive and more lethargic than what the question describes. Low blood sugar, Choice (A), usually presents signs similar to shock — cool, clammy skin and a fast pulse rate but not hypertension.

32. **B.** Although the child could have suffered a seizure as a result of the fever, the seizure could also be due to something more serious, such as meningitis. Exposing the child's skin to let the body cool slowly may be helpful, but rapidly cooling with towels, Choice (A), may be too drastic. There's no indication of dehydration, so any feeding, as Choice (C) suggests, should be withheld until the child is evaluated by a pediatrician. Aspirin and children don't mix, and EMTs aren't authorized to dispense aspirin, ruling out Choice (D).

33. **D.** Your primary assessment indicates the patient has inadequate circulation, probably due to severe dehydration. Elevating the legs, Choice (B), hasn't been shown to be helpful in restoring blood pressure. Taking time to perform a detailed physical exam, Choice (A), is inappropriate in this situation because the patient is showing signs of shock and requires immediate transport. She can't have anything by mouth at this point as Choice (C) suggests; if she vomits, she could have further problems with a now-compromised airway.

34. **D.** The patient is not exhibiting signs of anaphylaxis, so epinephrine, Choice (A), isn't indicated. As an EMT, you aren't authorized to administer diphenhydramine, Choice (B). Inducing vomiting with syrup of ipecac, Choice (C), is unlikely to help reduce the allergic reaction, because the allergen is already in the patient's bloodstream.

35. **C.** This patient is experiencing anaphylaxis that's causing his bronchioles to constrict and his arteries to dilate excessively. An epinephrine autoinjector, Choice (C), will buy the patient some time by temporarily reversing the reaction. With such a low blood pressure, having the patient sit up, Choice (B), is dangerous. CPAP, Choice (D), may actually lower the blood pressure even further as it creates pressure on the great vessels in the chest, restricting blood flow. Finding out more information about the antibiotic, Choice (A), may be helpful, but it won't change the course of treatment.

36. **A.** This patient appears to be in septic shock. She isn't maintaining her own ventilations, making supplemental oxygen, Choices (B) and (D), ineffective. You should preserve the patient's body temperature in shock instead of cooling her any further as Choice (C) indicates; if the patient begins to shiver, she will waste precious energy stores that can be used to maintain perfusion.

37. **B.** You suspect the patient has signs of meningitis, a very contagious infectious disease, especially through airborne droplets. To reduce cross-contamination, you need to isolate yourself — and the patient — before transport, Choice (A). Using alcohol as part of a bath, Choice (C), isn't considered a standard practice in alleviating fever. The patient should have nothing by mouth, contrary to Choice (D), until he's evaluated more fully at a hospital emergency department.

38. **D.** You suspect that the patient is experiencing hyperglycemia. The patient is not alert enough to administer oral glucose, Choice (A). Her breathing rate and depth appear adequate, so no further assistance is necessary, eliminating Choice (B). As an EMT, you are only permitted to assist someone with specific prescribed medications such as nitroglycerin, an inhaler, or an epinephrine autoinjector, ruling out Choice (C).

39. **C.** You suspect that the patient's blood sugar level is lower than normal, giving him signs of insulin shock. Hyperglycemia, Choice (A), produces more of a normal or flush skin and takes days to weeks to develop. The fact that he has good movement of his arms and speaks clearly reduces the likelihood of either a stroke, Choice (B), or a TIA, Choice (D).

40. **A.** For patients who appear to be delusional, don't go along with them, Choice (B), or make a big deal, Choice (C). You may consider restraining the patient, Choice (D), if he becomes aggressive, but at this point, you have no reason to do so.

41. **C.** Poison control will have information on how to treat the specific medication ingestion and will also be able to tell how serious the situation is. Having the child ingest anything further at this point, as Choices (A) and (D) indicate, may not be helpful, and it may cause further problems such as compromising the airway during forced vomiting, the result of Choice (B).

42. **B.** Multiple persons sickened inside a closed space should immediately clue you in to a major safety issue, carbon monoxide in this case. Although you may perform some care on-scene as Choices (A) and (C) indicate, you must wait until the scene is safe for you to enter. You'll likely call for additional resources, Choice (D), but only after ensuring your own safety.

43. **D.** His breathing effort is inadequate; simple supplemental oxygenation, Choice (A), wouldn't be enough. Immediate transport is warranted, but you have to manage problems with airway, breathing, and circulation before extrication and transport, Choice (B). A detailed physical exam, Choice (C), should be conducted but only after transportation has begun, because the exam can prolong on-scene time.

44. **A.** The patient could be fluid overloaded from her renal failure, causing pulmonary edema. Her blood pressure is high enough to support her in the sitting position, which will help improve her breathing ability. Laying her in semi-Fowler's position, Choice (C), or flat, Choice (B), will worsen her breathing ability. She isn't in respiratory failure (she's alert and not breathing faster than 30 or less than 10), so a bag-valve mask, Choice (D), is unnecessary at this stage.

45. **C.** Although preserving a crime scene, Choice (A), is important, it's a secondary concern to managing any major injuries sustained during the attack. Taking a set of vital signs, Choice (B), is also important, but that occurs after the primary assessment, as does soliciting a history of the event, Choice (D).

46. **A.** The newborn's respiratory rate is adequate, but the heart rate is below normal, so assisting ventilations as Choice (C) suggests isn't appropriate; however, if the heart rate remains low after supplemental oxygen is provided, it may become necessary. The heart rate is above 80, which is considered to be the cutoff for chest compressions, Choice (B). Suctioning, Choice (D), should have occurred before the vital signs were assessed because creating and maintaining airway patency is critical.

47. **B.** The dark secretions are *meconium,* the newborn's fecal matter. Meconium isn't normal as Choice (A) suggests; it's a sign that the infant is in distress. There's no relation between the presence of meconium and the timing of placenta delivery, Choice (C). You *don't* want to stimulate breathing, Choice (D), until you can suction as much of the meconium as possible out of the mouth and nares.

48. **B.** Stimulants, Choice (B), activate the sympathetic branch of the autonomic nervous system (ANS), causing the body to have a "flight or fight" reaction. Heart rate increases, blood pressure rises, and the pupils dilate. Marijuana, Choice (A), causes feelings of euphoria and drowsiness; it doesn't affect the ANS directly. Hypnotics, Choice (C), are sedatives that depress the ANS, which may result in respiratory depression. Cholinergics, Choice (D), stimulate the parasympathetic branch of the ANS, causing bradycardia, hypotension, increased salivation, mucous production, nausea, and vomiting.

49. **C.** The first stage of labor, Choice (A), is the dilation of the cervix, which allows the soon-to-be newborn to pass out of the uterus and be delivered during the second stage, Choice (B). The placenta is delivered afterward, during the third stage, Choice (C). There is no fourth stage of labor, Choice (D).

50. **C.** When the body experiences strenuous activity, it begins to heat up. It cools itself through several mechanisms, including secreting sweat — *diaphoresis* — and allowing it to evaporate. If that fluid is not replaced, the body becomes dehydrated and leads to heat exhaustion, Choice (C), as it did for this runner. Heat stroke, Choice (A), occurs when cooling mechanisms fail and body temperature rises to a dangerously high level. Victims of heat stroke, Choice (A), tend to have dry, hot skin and worsening altered mental status. Heat cramps, Choice (B), are muscle spasms, possibly caused by localized electrolyte imbalances due to excessive sweating. Heat intolerance, Choice (D), is more of a chronic issue than a sudden, emergent problem.

51. **B.** Using hot water alone, Choice (A), may not disinfect surfaces contaminated with bloodborne pathogens. Allowing the blood to dry, Choice (C), takes much too long and keeps the unit out of service. You can't find a heat-sterilizer unit, as Choice (D) suggests, that's big enough to handle an ambulance!

52. **C.** Even while driving with lights and siren, you're responsible for not only your personal safety but also the safety of those around you. In other words, you're required to take the driving environment into consideration before driving faster than the posted speed limit or proceeding through a controlled intersection without stopping, Choice (A). Unless you're at a scene of an emergency, you're required to follow all laws regarding parking, contrary to Choice (B). If you're involved in even a minor crash, Choice (D), you must stop at the incident and cancel your response.

53. **A.** Although having a patient sign a form, Choice (B), each and every time he refuses treatment is optimal, it doesn't always happen. In such cases, have a reliable witness such as a law enforcement officer or family member sign a statement stating that you tried to have the patient sign but were unable to. You can't transport a competent adult patient against his will, ruling out Choice (C). A patient can accept treatment without having to consent to transport, contrary to Choice (D).

54. **A.** A *primary prevention program* aims to reduce the likelihood of a negative event happening. Installing a traffic signal after a fatal crash, Choice (B), is a bit like closing the barn door after the horses are gone. Training EMS providers on using cervical collars, Choice (C), doesn't prevent the incidence of cervical collar use. While installing an AED at a pool, Choice (D), may be helpful in a cardiac arrest after a drowning, it doesn't prevent the drowning from occurring.

55. **B.** The intent of continuous quality improvement (CQI) is to identify both strengths and weaknesses of an organization's practice, and develop processes that improve both. CQI incorporates clinical, operational, and administrative practices, not just emergency care, as Choice (D) states. Quality assurance is more focused on ensuring practices adhere to a certain standard, such as licensing, Choice (C). While disciplinary procedures, Choice (A), may arise from CQI review, they're not a responsibility.

56. **A.** Negligence is a civil action in which four legal elements must be proven to have occurred. The EMT must have had a duty to act (and by implication, act within acceptable guidelines). The EMT must have subsequently breached, or failed to perform that act (or have performed in an unacceptable manner). There must be an injury that occurred during the time of treatment, but it's not limited to physical injuries alone as Choice (B) indicates. Finally, there must be a relationship between the breach of duty and the injury itself. This is *causation*. Deliberate intent, as noted in Choice (C), must be proven in a gross negligence lawsuit. Malfeasance, a component of Choice (D), also relates to deliberate intent.

57. **C.** You cannot treat or transport a patient who refuses your services when he is legally able to make his own decisions. Threatening someone with bodily harm is assault, Choice (A). Battery, Choice (B), is the unlawful touching of another person. Saying or writing something about someone that damages his reputation is called defamation, Choice (D).

58. **D.** Although elder abuse, drug use, and domestic violence, Choices (A), (B), and (C), respectively, are serious issues, not all states require EMTs to report their suspicions. All 50 states and the District of Columbia mandate the reporting of child abuse and neglect, Choice (D).

59. **A.** Most people are thought to experience various stages of grieving, either for themselves or a loved one who is dying or has died. Those stages include denial, anger, bargaining, depression, and acceptance. Not all people process death in the same way or at the same time.

60. **B.** Hepatitis B is a virus that is transmitted from one person to another through blood, Choice (B). An example of an airborne disease, Choice (A), is the common cold. Hepatitis A can be transmitted through food, Choice (C), such as raw shellfish. Mosquitos are examples of vectors, Choice (D), that can carry diseases such as malaria.

Chapter 9

The Airway, Respiration, and Ventilation

In This Chapter

- Reviewing the structures and functions of the respiratory system
- Assessing patients' breathing and knowing whether to oxygenate or ventilate
- Picking out potential airway and breathing problems

Take a deep breath and hold it for as long as you can, until it's so uncomfortable that it feels like your lungs will burst. When you finally explode and draw in that first panicky breath, let that feeling serve as a reminder of how important your respiratory system is. If it doesn't function well, life literally comes to a standstill.

The national EMT exam makes the importance of this fact abundantly clear in the number and complexity of questions it dedicates to this area. Having the ability to apply your knowledge of the airway, ventilation, and oxygenation to situations quickly, accurately, and confidently is critical. In this chapter, you get the basics on the respiratory system, discover when to oxygenate and ventilate, and figure out how to handle a variety of airway and breathing problems.

Getting an Overview of the Respiratory System

In a sense, the respiratory system serves a very simple purpose: to bring oxygen in and get carbon dioxide out. However, the task is much more complex than that and requires a sophisticated set of structures:

- **The upper airway** (see Figure 9-1a) consists of the *nares* (nostrils), mouth, nasopharynx, pharynx, and larynx. Combined, they work to not only channel air in and out of the body but to warm, humidify, and filter it as well.
- **The lower airway** (see Figure 9-1b) begins at about the level of the vocal cords and includes the trachea, mainstem bronchi, and bronchioles, terminating in the alveoli. The bronchi, bronchioles, and alveoli comprise the lungs. The main function of the lower airway is to produce efficient gas exchange between the alveoli and capillaries surrounding each alveolus (see Figure 9-1c). Blood passing through the capillaries absorbs the oxygen onto red blood cells, and then circulates oxygen to the body's cells. At the same time, carbon dioxide is released into the alveolus, which is then exhaled out of the body.

You need oxygen to produce adenosine triphosphate (ATP), the energy block used by the body, and you need to regulate carbon dioxide so just enough is available to the body and the rest is released to the atmosphere. This process takes place in the alveoli, where the cell walls are thin enough to allow gases to diffuse freely from areas of high concentration to areas of low concentration. So, oxygen diffuses from the alveoli to the capillaries (into the blood), and carbon dioxide diffuses from the capillaries into the alveoli (out of the blood).

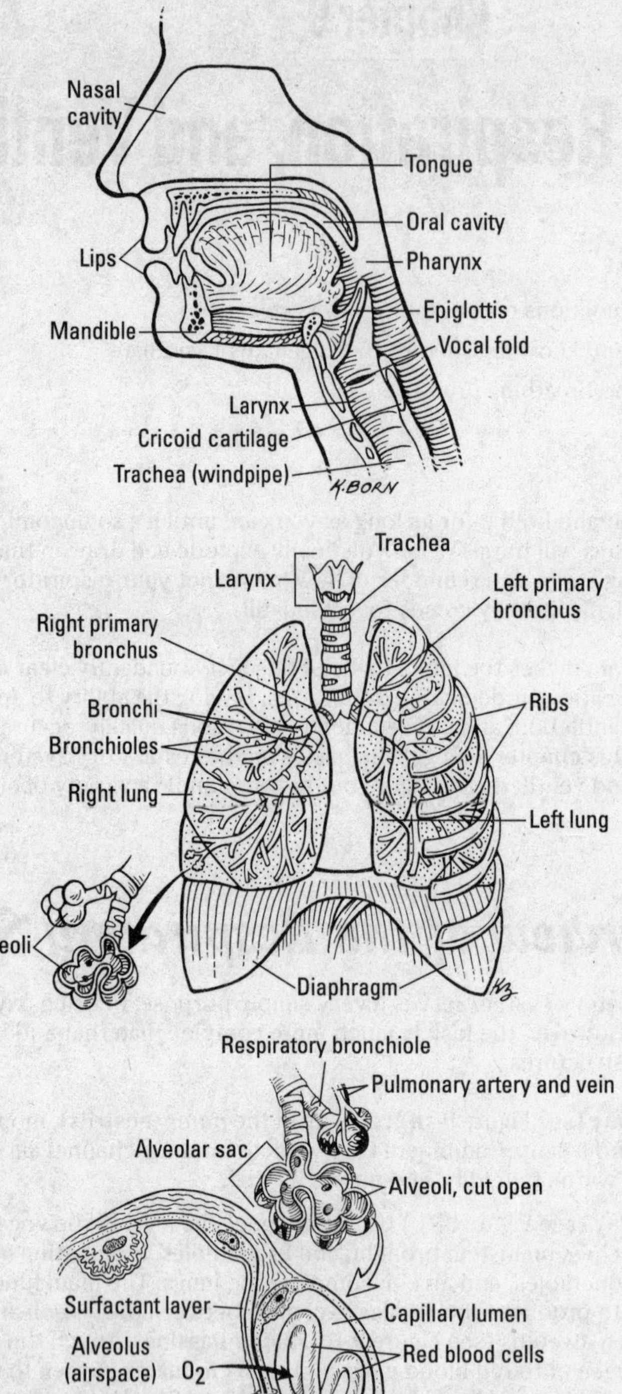

Figure 9-1: The upper and lower airways.

Illustration by Kathryn Born, MA

Of course, the concentration of gases would equalize quickly if the gases just stayed in the alveoli. Breathing, or *ventilation,* is the mechanical effort the body makes to move gases into and out of the lungs. Ventilation occurs with the use of the diaphragm and intercostal muscles (see Figure 9-2):

- **Inspiratory phase:** When these muscles contract, the chest cavity increases in size as the diaphragm moves downward and the ribs are pulled outward by the intercostal muscles. This produces a slight *negative pressure* inside the cavity, causing the lungs to expand and drawing air in. This is the inspiratory phase of ventilation.
- **Expiratory phase:** During the expiratory phase, the reverse occurs. The diaphragm relaxes and moves upward, and the intercostal muscles relax as the chest returns to its resting position. The chest cavity shrinks, creating a *positive pressure* on the lungs. They return to their smaller resting state, pushing air out of the alveoli and back through the lower and upper airways into the atmosphere.

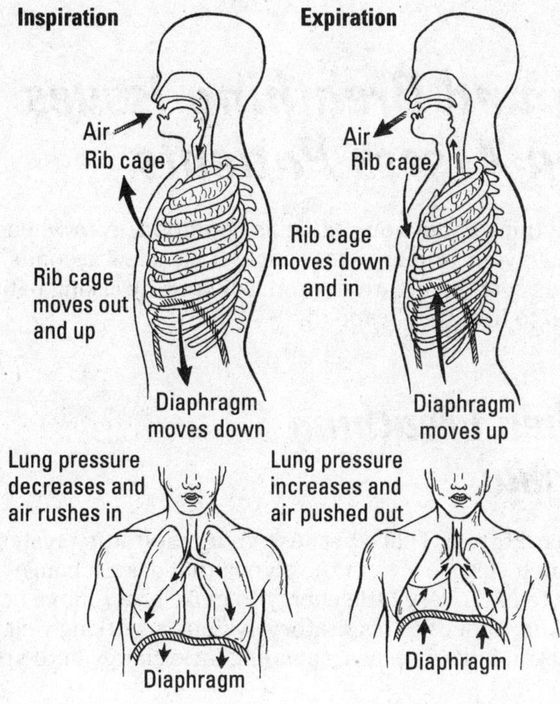

Figure 9-2: The inspiratory and expiratory phases of ventilation.

Illustration by Kathryn Born, MA

Under normal resting conditions, this cycle of inspiration and exhalation occurs about 12 to 20 times a minute, every minute of your life. *Chemoreceptors,* found primarily in the brainstem, detect levels of carbon dioxide and oxygen. They send signals to the brain, which, in turn, trigger an increase or decrease in the work of breathing.

You might think oxygen levels in the body would be the primary driver for respiratory control. But carbon dioxide (CO_2) is the real mover and shaker. That's because CO_2 is used to help create conditions in the body's fluids that are best suited for various life functions. So, in a healthy person, the body depends on detecting a rise in CO_2 more than it depends on a drop in oxygen as a reason to breathe.

Patients who retain CO_2 all the time, such as those with chronic obstructive pulmonary disease (COPD), lose their ability to sense that gas. They end up depending upon *hypoxic drive,* using oxygen levels to regulate their breathing.

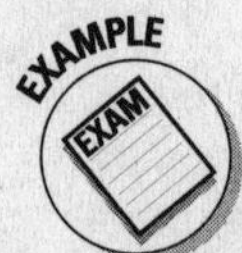

A 30-year-old male is hyperventilating after receiving very emotional news. His breaths are fast and deep. Which of the following statements is most accurate in this situation?

(A) Inhaling too much oxygen will cause breathing to slow, allowing oxygen levels to fall to normal levels.

(B) Inhaling too much oxygen will cause breathing to speed up.

(C) Exhaling too much carbon dioxide will cause breathing to slow, allowing carbon dioxide levels to rise to normal levels.

(D) Exhaling too much carbon dioxide will cause breathing to speed up.

The correct answer is Choice (C). Assuming everything else is normal, as carbon dioxide levels fall within the bloodstream, the brain will signal the respiratory system to slow down, allowing it to retain carbon dioxide and build it back to normal levels. Choice (A) may be true, but only if the patient has COPD and depends upon oxygen levels to control breathing. Neither Choice (B) nor (D) is true.

Knowing the Airway and Breathing Issues to Look for When You Assess Patients

As an EMT, you can't assume anything about your patient's condition, even when he appears "normal" at first glance. In your primary assessment, take a few seconds to consciously evaluate how someone is actually breathing. You can start by asking patients how they are feeling; watch and listen to how they respond.

Understanding when breathing is (and isn't) normal

Ironically, normal breathing is hard to see. That's because your respiratory system is very effective at its job. There's so much surface area in the alveoli that gas exchange is very easy. Therefore, the body needs to exert very little energy to make gases move between the alveoli and capillaries. If everything about the respiratory system is working well, the patient will likely be able to speak in full sentences, spending little energy in the process.

It also takes very little to get the respiratory system to work harder. Suddenly being frightened causes you to breathe a little faster as your body prepares a "flight or fight" response.

Difficulty breathing begins with an increase in rate *(tachypnea).* The patient may breathe deeper *(hyperpnea).* If the condition doesn't improve, *accessory muscles,* such as those in the shoulders and neck, kick in to maximize the chest cavity on inspiration.

If your patient is experiencing a mild level of respiratory distress, you may notice that he has difficulty completing a long sentence, needing to stop midway to take a breath. Or, he may speak more quickly than normal to try to complete a sentence before he needs to take another breath.

In early stages of distress, the patient may want to only sit up; as the condition worsens, the patient may assume a tripod position, holding his upper body up by putting his hands on his knees and straightening his elbows. In really bad situations, the patient may be forced to stand up in order for the diaphragm to contract and push deep into the abdominal cavity.

Deciding when to oxygenate

EMTs used to give oxygen to everyone, regardless of what the complaint was. Chest pain? Give oxygen. Toe pain? Yep, give that gas too! After all, what harm could oxygen do, right? Medical experts have since discovered that inhaling more oxygen than necessary *can* be harmful for certain conditions, and it isn't helpful in situations where it isn't necessary.

Translated, this means that you need to assess the patient for his ability to absorb oxygen and use it. You do this using your powers of observation coupled with a pulse oximeter. If the patient appears to be ventilating adequately (having a good tidal volume and rate, without the use of accessory muscles), check for oxygen saturation levels with your oximeter. Ideally, the saturation level should be between 94 and 99 percent.

What does this mean? If the patient is breathing normally, and his oxygen saturation level is greater than 94 percent, you don't need to administer oxygen. If the saturation level is lower or normal but the patient has mild respiratory difficulty, a nasal canula with oxygen flowing between 2 and 6 liters per minute (LPM) is probably fine. If the patient is working hard to breathe, a nonrebreather mask at 12–15 LPM may be needed. Carefully monitor saturation readings and the patient's level of distress. If things don't improve, you may need to provide manual ventilation (see the next section).

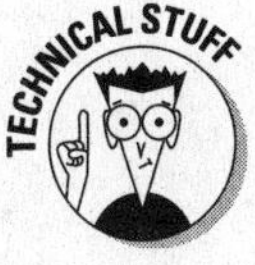

Oxygen is carried on hemoglobin proteins located within the red blood cells (RBCs). Each hemoglobin can carry up to four molecules of oxygen. As hemoglobin picks up oxygen, the color of the RBC changes from a dusky, dark red to a brighter shade. A pulse oximeter can detect these shades of red and calculate the percentage of red blood cells that are carrying oxygen in their hemoglobin. Normal amounts are around 94 percent or higher. Once oxygen saturation drops to about 92 percent, the change in subsequent saturation levels can be quick, dropping to 85 percent or even lower within a few minutes.

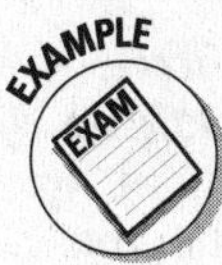

A 42-year-old male is complaining of abdominal pain and cramping after eating a fried chicken dinner. He is alert, with pink, warm, diaphoretic skin. His vital signs include a pulse rate of 92, a blood pressure of 142/90 mm Hg, and a respiratory rate of 18 breaths per minute. His oxygen saturation level is 96 percent. What should you do next?

(A) Administer oxygen at 4 LPM with a nasal cannula.

(B) Administer oxygen at 15 LPM with a nonrebreather mask.

(C) Perform a secondary assessment.

(D) Begin immediate transport.

The correct answer is Choice (C). Based on the patient's chief complaint, relatively normal vital signs, and lack of evidence of respiratory distress, oxygen, Choices (A) and (B), is not indicated. There is also no indication of an emergent condition that requires immediate transport, Choice (D).

Recognizing when to ventilate

To know when to ventilate is to know when the patient crosses the line between respiratory distress and respiratory failure:

- **Respiratory distress:** In respiratory distress, the patient is compensating for a potential hypoxia problem by breathing faster, deeper, and/or harder. By doing so, the patient's mental status remains good, as do his oxygen saturation levels (see the preceding section).

- **Respiratory failure:** If the compensatory mechanisms don't maintain adequate oxygen or carbon dioxide levels, the patient's well-being begins to falter. Mental status changes from alert to confused to unconsciousness as the brain runs out of oxygen or fills with carbon dioxide. Oxygen saturation levels drop below normal. The patient's drive to breathe weakens, causing ventilations to become inadequate. This state, in turn, makes oxygen levels fall even further, creating a vicious cycle. Breathing slows and becomes even more shallow. If left untreated, respiratory failure will deteriorate to respiratory arrest, followed quickly by cardiac arrest.

Recognizing early signs of respiratory failure is key. If the patient looks tired, is having difficulty remaining alert, or his skin becomes very pale or cyanotic, cool, and clammy, it's time to break out your bag-valve mask (BVM) and deliver manual ventilations.

An early sign of hypoxia is anxiety. The brain is so sensitive to oxygen levels that minor changes trigger it to start sending out alerts. If your patient looks or feels anxious, definitely provide reassurance, but also consider whether you're seeing the first signs of a more serious problem.

A 70-year-old female is complaining of shortness of breath that began shortly after a nap. She is alert and appears anxious. She is breathing 30 times per minute and says her fingers and face feel numb. You should

(A) assist with her breathing with a bag-valve mask and oxygen.

(B) provide supplemental oxygen at 4 LPM using a nasal cannula.

(C) have her breathe into a face mask without oxygen attached.

(D) tell her to control her anxiety and that will help with her breathing.

The correct answer is Choice (B). Even though she is breathing quickly, she is alert and communicating with you, which indicates she is getting enough oxygen to her brain. Therefore, she's not in respiratory failure and doesn't require artificial ventilation, Choice (A). However, she may be in true respiratory distress, trying to maintain oxygen levels. The last thing you want to do is to have her rebreathe her own CO_2 and reduce the amount of available oxygen, Choice (C). While she may be experiencing anxiety, she may be hyperventilating for another reason, such as having a pulmonary embolus. Choice (D), although tempting, isn't likely to control her breathing.

Taking Action on Potential Airway and Breathing Problems

Many conditions can affect the airway and breathing, causing someone to become short of breath. And, because the respiratory system reacts to events happening inside the body, many nonrespiratory conditions can cause difficulty breathing as well. I don't cover them all in the following sections, but a good rule of thumb is to always think beyond the breathing tube when a patient is having trouble breathing yet her respiratory system seems okay.

Upper airway conditions

Given that the airway is the only way for air to enter and exit the body, anything that partially or completely blocks it is troublesome, to say the least. Table 9-1 lists common conditions you should be familiar with, their signs and symptoms, and treatment options for each.

Table 9-1 Conditions Affecting the Upper Airway

Problem	*Signs and Symptoms*	*Action Steps*
Anaphylaxis causing major swelling of the upper airway	Exposure to an allergen such as a bee sting or peanuts; drooling; reddened oropharynx; muffled or whispered voice; possible hypotension.	Assist the patient in using an epinephrine injector; administer supplemental oxygen; ventilate as necessary to maintain oxygen saturation.
Croup	Usually occurs in young children; fever; stridor, raspy cough; sometimes relieved with a quick change in air temperature and/or humidity.	Have parent assist with positioning the child comfortably; administer blow-by, humidified oxygen.
Epiglottitis	High fever; drooling; reddened oropharynx; muffled or whispered voice; unable to lie down.	*Don't stick anything into the mouth!* Help the patient into a comfortable position; administer blow-by oxygen.
Foreign body obstruction	Full obstruction: Air is unable to pass by the obstruction. No noise or breathing sounds from airway; skin turns pale to cyanotic; universal choking sign. Partial obstruction: Air is able to move past the obstruction. Patient may be coughing; audible stridor.	Conscious patient: Administer abdominal thrusts (child and adult) or chest thrusts/back blows (infant). If airway is partially obstructed, encourage patient to cough; keep suction available and prepare to act if airway becomes fully obstructed. Unconscious patient: Administer chest compressions (CPR).
Pertussis	Prolonged coughing spells; "whoop" sound when patient takes a deep breath after coughing; more prevalent in children; dark, thick mucous production; 1–2 week history of mild fever and coughing that worsens in duration and discomfort.	Wear personal protective equipment (PPE), including a HEPA mask; administer supplemental, humidified oxygen.
Tongue blocking the airway	Patient has altered mental status or is unresponsive, allowing tongue to relax and block the airway. Snoring sounds may be heard. In severe situations, breathing may become irregular or absent.	Perform head-tilt, chin-lift technique; if neck trauma suspected, utilize a modified jaw-thrust maneuver. Insert oropharyngeal or nasopharyngeal airway to help control the tongue.

A 65-year-old male fell off a stepladder while attempting to replace a light bulb. You find him unresponsive to painful stimulus. He has a large hematoma to his left temple. He has slow, irregular, snoring respirations and his skin is pale, cool, and diaphoretic. After taking manual spine precautions, you should next

(A) apply a head-tilt, chin-lift and insert an oropharyngeal airway.

(B) administer high-flow oxygen with a nonrebreather mask.

(C) apply a modified jaw thrust and insert an oropharyngeal airway.

(D) ventilate with a bag-valve mask with high-flow oxygen.

The right answer is Choice (C). There are indications that a spinal injury may exist (mechanism of injury, a head injury, and a patient who is unable to communicate). A modified jaw thrust will open the patient's airway while minimizing motion to the cervical spine, unlike a head-tilt, chin-lift procedure, Choice (A). The patient's ventilation status is inadequate for simple supplemental oxygen, Choice (B). You'll need to ventilate the patient, Choice (D), but not until after opening the airway.

Lower airway conditions

Table 9-2 lists a variety of common conditions affecting the lower airway structures, causing shortness of breath.

Table 9-2 Conditions Affecting the Lower Airway

Problem	*Signs and Symptoms*	*Action Steps*
Asthma	Episodic respiratory distress; wheezes auscultated during breathing; may have past medical history; may have prescribed inhalers.	Assist with patient's prescribed emergency inhaler if available; administer supplemental oxygen; ventilate if necessary to maintain oxygen saturation.
Bronchiolitis; respiratory syncytial virus (RSV)	Presents mostly in children to 2 years of age; gradual onset of fever, cough, and general weakness.	Wear personal protective equipment (PPE); administer supplemental, humidified oxygen.
Chronic obstructive pulmonary disease (COPD)	Chronic shortness of breath that has abruptly become worse; wheezes, crackles, or rhonchi auscultated during breathing; patient may be thin with an enlarged chest wall (emphysema) or appear bloated and heavy with dusky skin (chronic bronchitis); probable past medical history; may have prescribed inhalers; smoking history.	Assist with patient's prescribed emergency inhaler if available; administer supplemental oxygen; ventilate if necessary to maintain oxygen saturation.
Cystic fibrosis	Genetic condition; chronic illness with acute worsening; heavy mucous production.	Help patient into a comfortable position; suction; administer supplemental oxygen; ventilate as needed to maintain saturation.
Pneumonia	Fever; 1–2 week history of flu or cold symptoms; productive cough with yellow to green sputum production; may auscultate crackles, rhonchi, or wheezes in lung fields; may have chest pain that worsens with cough.	Help patient into a comfortable position; administer supplemental oxygen (consider humidification).

Problem	Signs and Symptoms	Action Steps
Pulmonary edema	Sudden onset; may auscultate crackles or wheezes in lung fields or sounds may be very diminished as condition worsens; if hypertensive, may have jugular venous distension; pedal edema; in worse cases, produces frothy, pink-colored sputum with cough; may have history of congestive heart failure, hypertension, or myocardial infarction.	If blood pressure (BP) is normal or high, assist patient in sitting upright with feet dangling for comfort; administer supplemental oxygen; ventilate as necessary to maintain saturation. Consider continuous positive airway pressure (CPAP).
Pulmonary embolism	Sudden onset; lung sounds remain clear or may have a localized wheeze; may have chest pain; may have tender calf in lower leg; recent history of immobilization such as surgery or a long air flight; oral birth control user or smoker.	Administer supplemental oxygen; ventilate if necessary to maintain oxygen saturation. This condition may mimic psychogenic hyperventilation; do not use paper bag or withhold oxygen.
Spontaneous pneumothorax	Sudden onset; may occur after prolonged coughing or heavy lifting; lung sounds may be normal, or diminished on one side; may experience sharp chest pain; may have history of asthma, COPD, or connective tissue disease.	Help patient into a comfortable position; administer supplemental oxygen.

A 52-year-old female is in respiratory distress. Her heart rate is 104, and her blood pressure is 148/82 mm Hg. She is breathing 24 times per minute and her oxygen saturation level is 95 percent. She tells you that she has been experiencing cold-type symptoms for ten days; during the last two days she has been producing yellow sputum when she coughs. She has a history of asthma, angina, and hypertension, and takes medication for both conditions, including a rescue inhaler and nitroglycerin tablets. You note no accessory muscle use when she breathes. You auscultate her lungs and hear rhonchi. You should

(A) assist with administering her rescue inhaler.

(B) administer oxygen at 4 LPM via nasal cannula.

(C) administer oxygen at 15 LPM via a nonrebreather mask.

(D) assist with administering a nitroglycerin tablet.

The correct answer is Choice (B). The information provided in the question points to pneumonia as the underlying cause of the patient's respiratory distress. There are no signs of an acute asthma attack or angina, so assisting with her medications, Choices (A) and (D), isn't indicated. Her level of respiratory distress is not severe, as indicated by a reasonable oxygen saturation level and lack of accessory muscle use. High-flow oxygen, Choice (C), isn't indicated.

Nonrespiratory conditions

When other, nonrespiratory conditions arise that affect oxygen and/or carbon dioxide levels in the body, the respiratory system attempts to compensate by working harder. Some of the more common ones are listed in Table 9-3.

Table 9-3 Nonrespiratory Conditions that May Affect Breathing

Problem	*Signs and Symptoms*	*Action Steps*
Environmental/industrial exposure to toxic gas or chemicals	Hazardous scene; may involve multiple victims; coughing; nausea, vomiting; may have secretions from eyes, nose, or mouth; lung sounds may be clear or may contain wheezes or crackles; headache, blurred vision (especially with carbon monoxide poisoning).	Operate in cold zone; decontaminate if necessary; remove patient to fresh air; administer supplemental oxygen; ventilate if necessary to maintain saturation.
Metabolic acidosis	Condition resulting from excessive hydrogen ion (H+) buildup in the blood causing high acid levels. The body attempts to shift the acid levels back to normal by buffering H+ with bicarbonate, causing CO_2 to form. The patient breathes faster and deeper (Kussmaul's respirations) to remove the extra CO_2.	None directly. Provide supplemental oxygen if indicated. Don't attempt a procedure that would cause the patient to retain more CO_2, such as breathing into a paper bag or an oxygen mask without oxygen being administered through it.
Myocardial infarction	May have chest discomfort; normal lung sounds; may be elderly, female, or diabetic.	Help patient into a comfortable position; administer supplemental oxygen; ventilate if necessary to maintain saturation.
Opioid (narcotic) overdose	Opioids like heroin and morphine cause altered mental status and suppress the respiratory drive, causing slow, shallow respirations that deteriorate to respiratory arrest.	Insert OPA or NPA to control airway; perform head-tilt, chin-lift maneuver; begin ventilations with bag-valve mask and oxygen.
Psychogenic hyperventilation	Psychological trigger; normal lung sounds; carpopedal spasms; numbness in face, hands, or feet.	Help patient into a comfortable position; coach to control breathing; administer supplemental oxygen. Do not use paper bags or other home remedies.

By no means is this an exhaustive list; just be sure to keep your mind open to the possibility that someone who is having trouble breathing is experiencing a problem not related to the respiratory system.

An alert, 80-year-old male complains of sudden shortness of breath. His skin is pale, cool, and moist. He tells you he began feeling this way about an hour ago, while he was sitting and reading a book. His vital signs include a respiratory rate of 16 breaths per minute, his pulse is 90 and regular, and his blood pressure is 160/96 mm Hg. He has a history of high blood pressure and diabetes, and is allergic to bees. Lung sounds are clear bilaterally. His oxygen saturation level is 97 percent. You should

(A) administer high-flow oxygen via a nonrebreather mask.

(B) place the patient in position of comfort.

(C) encourage him to drink some orange juice with sugar.

(D) assist with an epinephrine autoinjector, if he has one.

The right answer is Choice (B). Although the patient's presentation is vague, his age and a sudden onset of feeling short of breath point to a possible myocardial infarction. Keeping the patient calm and comfortable is key to preserving myocardial tissue. Although the patient feels like he is short of breath, there's little evidence of respiratory distress. High-flow oxygen, Choice (A), is not warranted. He is alert, suggesting hypoglycemia, which Choice (C) alludes to, is not the culprit. There is no evidence of a severe allergic reaction as Choice (D) implies.

Practice Questions about the Airway, Respiration, and Ventilation

The following practice questions are similar to the NREMT EMT exam's questions in this section. Read each question carefully and then select the answer choice that most correctly answers the question. Try to answer each question without looking up the answers, so you can better understand what you do — and don't — know.

1. At a drugstore, an adult patient presents with cool, pale, and diaphoretic skin and difficulty breathing, with wheezing auscultated in both lungs. Bystanders report the patient walked in 5 minutes ago, unable to talk and very short of breath. His heart rate is 126, his blood pressure is 90/60 mm Hg, and his respiratory rate is 24 breaths per minute. He is able to follow simple commands. You should

   (A) administer low-flow oxygen via a nasal cannula.

   (B) perform abdominal thrusts.

   (C) assist the patient with his prescribed epinephrine autoinjector.

   (D) assist ventilations with a bag-valve mask and oxygen.

2. An elderly female presents supine in her bed, alert and in respiratory distress. You can hear audible crackles as she breathes. Her blood pressure is 240/120 mm Hg, her heart rate is 100 and irregular, and her respiratory rate is 22 breaths per minute. You should immediately

   (A) begin bag-valve-mask ventilations with supplemental oxygen.

   (B) place her into a sitting position, with her feet dangling over the edge of the bed.

   (C) administer low-flow oxygen via a nasal cannula.

   (D) turn her left lateral recumbent and administer high-flow oxygen via a nonrebreather mask.

3. A 72-year-old male with a history of chronic obstructive pulmonary disease (COPD) has been increasingly short of breath over the past 24 hours. He reports having a fever, chills, and a cough over the past ten days. His skin is warm, pale, and dry; his breathing rate is 24 times a minute. You should

   (A) administer low-flow oxygen via nasal cannula.

   (B) administer high-flow oxygen via a nonrebreather mask.

   (C) administer medium-flow oxygen via a venturi mask.

   (D) encourage him to cough.

4. A 13-month-old child presents in his parent's arms and is in respiratory distress. The parent reports the child has had a fever, runny nose, and decreasing appetite in the past four days. The child cries when you examine him. He has a nonproductive cough and warm, flush skin. His breathing rate is 30 times per minute, and his heart rate is 120. You should

   (A) assist ventilations with a pediatric bag-valve mask and oxygen.

   (B) suction the nose and mouth with a bulb syringe.

   (C) administer oxygen using the blow-by technique.

   (D) administer pediatric acetaminophen.

5. A 21-year-old male complains of chest tightness and difficulty breathing after a fight with his girlfriend. His respiratory rate is 34, his heart rate is 110, and his blood pressure is 136/90 mm Hg. He feels tingling around his face and in his hands. His skin is pale, warm, and dry. You should

   (A) administer low-flow oxygen via a nonrebreather mask.

   (B) coach the patient to rebreathe his breath with a paper bag.

   (C) help the patient into a supine position.

   (D) administer low-flow oxygen via a nasal cannula.

6. An elderly male presents with sudden stridor, coughing, and wheezing at a restaurant. His skin is pale, warm, and diaphoretic. Patrons report that the patient was enjoying his lunch when this episode began. You detect a strong radial pulse. Your next step is to

   (A) encourage the patient to continue coughing.

   (B) deliver abdominal thrusts.

   (C) administer low-flow oxygen via nasal cannula.

   (D) inspect the patient's mouth.

7. A 72-year-old female presents supine in bed, responsive to painful stimulus by moaning. Her respiratory rate is 12 breaths per minute and shallow. Her heart rate is 126, and her blood pressure is 78/60 mm Hg. You hear diminished lung sounds bilaterally and crackles throughout. Her skin is pale, cold, and clammy. You should

   (A) administer low-flow oxygen via nasal cannula.

   (B) administer high-flow oxygen via a nonrebreather mask.

   (C) ventilate with a bag-valve mask and oxygen.

   (D) have her sit up with her feet dangling off the side of the bed.

8. A 30-month-old child presents sitting on the edge of her bed, appearing short of breath. Parents report she has had a fever and body chills and aches over the past 36 hours. Her skin is hot, pale, and dry. She nods her head when you speak but doesn't say anything herself. You can hear stridor, and you observe that she is drooling. Which of the following procedures should you perform?

   (A) Inspect her mouth, using a tongue depressor.

   (B) Suction her mouth by inserting a rigid-tip catheter.

   (C) Maintain her position of comfort and transport her.

   (D) Administer high-flow oxygen via a nonrebreather mask.

9. A 19-year-old female is having difficulty breathing. You note accessory muscle use. Her respiratory rate is 20 breaths per minute, with a prolonged expiratory phase. Although she appears alert, she can't speak more than one- or two-word sentences. You should

   (A) assist her ventilations with a bag-valve mask and oxygen.

   (B) administer low-flow oxygen via a nasal cannula.

   (C) prepare to suction her airway.

   (D) assist the patient in using her prescribed multidose inhaler.

10. A 24-year-old male is discovered unresponsive on the floor of his bedroom. He does not respond to a painful stimulus. He has a radial pulse rate of 104 and a breathing rate of 5 breaths per minute. His lung sounds are clear. You should immediately

    (A) insert an oral airway and ventilate with a bag-valve mask and oxygen.

    (B) administer high-flow oxygen via a nonrebreather mask.

    (C) determine his blood pressure.

    (D) turn the patient to a left lateral recumbent position.

11. A 35-year-old female is complaining of chest pain and shortness of breath while sitting at her office. You observe that she is breathing 30 times a minute, has a rapid radial pulse, and has pale, cool, dry skin. Her heart rate is 120 and she is alert. This episode began 30 minutes ago while she was preparing for a meeting and has gotten steadily worse since. Which of the following procedures should you perform first?

    (A) Determine the level of stress she had while preparing for her meeting.

    (B) Perform a detailed physical examination.

    (C) Administer high-flow oxygen via a nonrebreather mask.

    (D) Administer low-flow oxygen via a nonrebreather mask.

12. A 56-year-old male is in respiratory distress. He is breathing 18 times a minute, with pursed lips as he exhales. He appears alert. His pulse is 104 and irregular, and his blood pressure is 132/82 mm Hg. You note his skin is pink, warm, and diaphoretic. He is thin, and you can see accessory muscle movement. Wheezes can be auscultated toward the top of his lung fields. You should

    (A) administer low-flow oxygen with a nasal cannula.

    (B) administer high-flow oxygen with a nonrebreather mask.

    (C) ventilate with a bag-valve mask and oxygen.

    (D) assist with his prescribed nitroglycerin tablets.

13. An elderly female presents unconscious on the floor. Her skin is pale, cool, and dry. She is breathing at a rate of 4 times per minute. You can hear snoring sounds when she breathes. She has a faint, slow carotid pulse. You should first

    (A) perform a head-tilt, chin-lift procedure and insert an oropharyngeal airway.

    (B) perform a jaw thrust, and suction with a hard-tip catheter.

    (C) manually stabilize the cervical spine and perform a jaw thrust.

    (D) administer high-flow oxygen with a nonrebreather mask.

14. A 20-year-old male presents prone in bed. Roommates say that he returned from a party earlier that evening complaining of a headache. He is unresponsive to painful stimulus, and vomits when you roll him over to a supine position. You should

    (A) insert an oropharyngeal airway.

    (B) insert a nasopharyngeal airway.

    (C) place the patient in a sitting position.

    (D) suction the airway with a rigid-tip catheter.

15. A patient has overdosed on narcotic painkillers. He is supine in bed and responsive to verbal stimulus by moaning. He curls into a semifetal position when you touch him. Left alone, he has slow, snoring respirations, and he turns pale in color. You should

    (A) insert an oropharyngeal airway.

    (B) insert a nasopharyngeal airway.

    (C) suction the patient's airway.

    (D) manually stabilize the cervical spine.

Answers and Explanations

Use this answer key to score the practice questions in the preceding section. The explanations give you insight into why the correct answer is better than the other choices.

1. **C.** Although the scenario is vague, you have enough information to deduce that the patient is experiencing anaphylaxis. Being at the drugstore, he may have been seeking medications to correct his anaphylactic reaction. His vital signs and poor lung sounds also support a suspicion of anaphylaxis. Although he is critically ill, he's still alert and following your commands, negating the immediate use of a bag-valve mask, Choice (D). He is moving air into his lungs, eliminating an obstructed airway and the need to perform abdominal thrusts, Choice (B). Low-flow oxygen, Choice (A), would be inadequate for his level of distress.

2. **B.** The scenario suggests pulmonary edema as a result of congestive heart failure (CHF). She is alert and doesn't require bag-valve-mask use at this moment as Choice (A) suggests. Low-flow oxygen, Choice (C), is inadequate for her presentation, and turning her left lateral recumbent, Choice (D), isn't as effective as sitting her up to have gravity assist in pooling some of the fluid in the lungs.

3. **A.** The scenario suggests a history of infection, specifically pneumonia. His skin signs suggest that low-flow oxygen will be adequate; any higher concentration, as Choices (B) and (C) suggest, is unnecessary. Coughing, Choice (D), may help the patient to expectorate (produce sputum) but won't necessarily improve the patient's complaint.

4. **C.** Although the child is ill, his vital signs are within the normal range for his age. He is alert and recognizes your presence. Blow-by oxygen may help reduce the respiratory distress, and won't be as claustrophobic to the child as a mask placed over his face. He doesn't need to be ventilated, Choice (A), and bulb suctioning, Choice (B), will likely irritate him. As an EMT you're not permitted to administer acetaminophen, as Choice (D) suggests.

5. **D.** Although his condition appears to be psychogenic hyperventilation, a pulmonary embolus can also have the same signs and symptoms. This possibility makes Choices (A) and (B) potentially harmful. Getting the patient in a supine position, Choice (C), is unlikely to make a difference.

6. **A.** The sudden onset and location of the sound strongly suggest a partially obstructed airway. He's not fully obstructed, so abdominal thrusts, Choice (B), are unnecessary. The priority is to have the patient clear his own airway, rather than inspect his mouth, Choice (D), or provide oxygen, Choice (C). Encouraging the patient to cough and hopefully dislodge the foreign body is the best choice.

7. **C.** Your clinical findings suggest she is in respiratory failure and possible cardiogenic shock. She requires assisted ventilation in order to promote gas exchange. Supplemental oxygen, Choices (A) and (B), won't be enough, and her blood pressure is too low to sit her up as Choice (D) suggests.

8. **C.** The presentation suggests epiglottitis and that soft tissue in the upper airway is swelling. You don't want to take the chance of irritating that airway for any reason, making Choices (A) and (B) inappropriate. She is oxygenating adequately, so even putting a mask over her face, Choice (D), may feel stifling and worsen her stress.

9. **D.** The scenario suggests an asthma attack. She is compensating, making a bag-valve mask, Choice (A), unnecessary at this point. No secretions are reported, making suctioning, Choice (C), unnecessary as well. High-flow oxygen would be better than low-flow, Choice (B), considering her level of distress. However, that choice isn't given for the question, so your best bet is Choice (D).

10. **A.** His breathing rate is inadequate, making bag-valve-mask use necessary. Supplemental oxygen, Choice (B), would be enough only if the patient were moving air in and out of the alveoli. Performing the rest of the exam without intervening in the primary assessment, Choice (C), would be inappropriate. If the patient were breathing adequately, the recovery position, Choice (D), would be an option, but he isn't.

11. **C.** The scenario describes a patient in compensatory respiratory distress. Although there may be some indications of psychogenic hyperventilation, there is also strong suspicion of a pulmonary embolus. Administering the appropriate flow rate of oxygen through the mask is correct, rather than a lower rate as Choice (D) suggests. You may perform Choices (A) and (B) later in the exam, but you need to evaluate her distress early, during the primary assessment.

12. **A.** The scenario suggests a patient with a history of chronic obstructive pulmonary disease (COPD) due to his skin color and body shape. Although he's in distress, he doesn't appear to be in respiratory failure. High-flow oxygen, Choice (B), is unnecessary at this point, as is assisting his ventilations, Choice (C). There's no suggestion of cardiac ischemia, so nitroglycerin tablets, Choice (D), assuming they've been prescribed for the patient, are unnecessary.

13. **C.** You have no clear description about how the patient ended up on the floor, so assume a trauma mechanism until proven otherwise. A jaw thrust will reduce movement of the spine as you open the airway. A head-tilt, chin-lift procedure, Choice (A), is riskier. Snoring respirations are a sign of an airway blocked by the tongue, not secretions as Choice (B) implies. The patient's respiratory rate is too slow for simple supplemental oxygen, as Choice (D) suggests.

14. **D.** The scenario suggests immediate suctioning. You'll likely use an airway adjunct shortly, either Choice (A) or (B), but you need to clear the airway first. Placing the patient in a sitting position, Choice (C), isn't helpful because you'll spend a lot of energy trying to support his body and likely won't be able to do much else.

15. **B.** An overdose on narcotics suppresses the respiratory drive and gag reflex. The patient does respond to verbal stimulus, which implies that he may gag if an oropharyngeal airway, Choice (A), is inserted. Snoring respirations are an indication of the tongue blocking the airway, not secretions, as Choice (C) implies. There are no indications of a trauma mechanism, so you don't need to stabilize the cervical spine, Choice (D).

Chapter 10

Cardiology and Resuscitation Essentials

In This Chapter

- Looking at the basic structure and functions of the cardiovascular system
- Assessing cardiovascular findings and identifying acute coronary syndrome
- Taking care of potential cardiovascular problems

More Americans experience cardiovascular-related medical conditions and emergencies than any other disease. That's the reason why the national EMT examination makes this condition a section unto itself.

It has become clear that emergency medical services (EMS) can make a big difference in the big daddy of cardiovascular disease, the acute myocardial infarction (AMI). Early detection of an AMI, along with safe, rapid transport to a receiving facility of heart attack victims quickly reduces the likelihood of death and promotes a better life long after the event is over.

If AMI is the big daddy, then cardiac arrest is the big momma. Sudden cardiac arrest used to be almost always fatal. However, with early, high-quality CPR and rapid use of automated external defibrillators, EMTs are part of the chain of survival that can reduce the patient's chance of dying.

There are many other causes of chest pain that this chapter explores. Many have signs and symptoms of an AMI. It's not absolutely critical that you can tell the difference all the time; what matters most is making sure that you give each patient the benefit of the doubt as you perform your assessment. In this chapter, you get the basics on the cardiovascular system, discover normal and irregular cardiovascular findings, and figure out how to handle a number of cardiovascular problems.

Checking Out the Cardiovascular System

The cardiovascular system is broken down into three broad areas: the heart, the vasculature, and the blood. They interact closely to be able to create enough pressure in the system to produce *perfusion* (more commonly known as circulation).

Surveying major structures

The *heart* is the sophisticated pump that powers the cardiovascular system (see Figure 10-1). Its four chambers can be divided in two ways:

- Top and bottom, or the atria and ventricles, respectively
- Right and left, or pulmonary and peripheral circulation, respectively

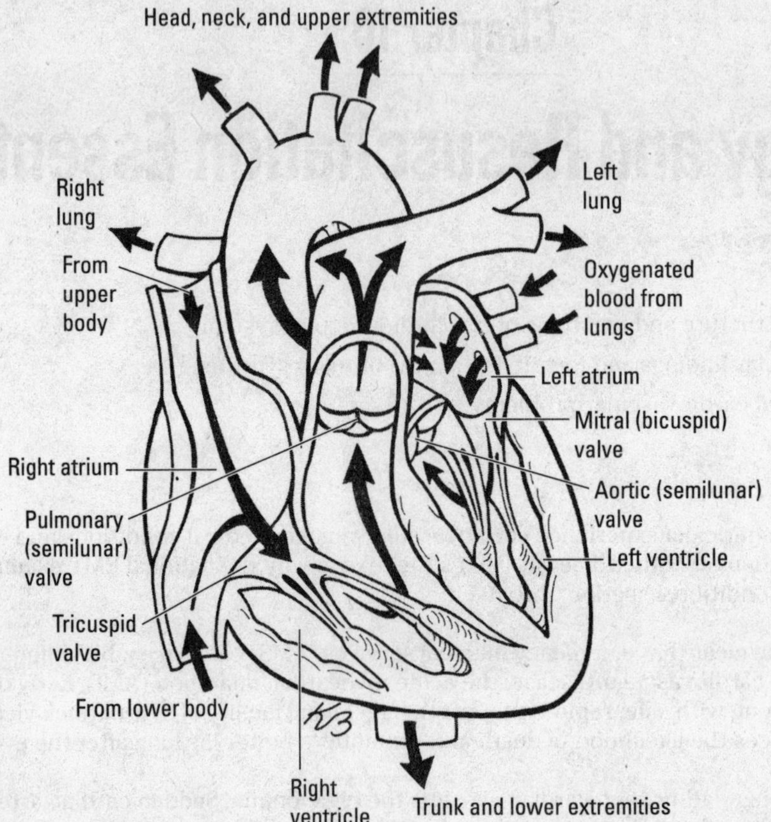

Figure 10-1: The heart's chambers.

One-way valves separate the atria from the ventricles, and pulmonary circulation from peripheral circulation. This structure has the effect of forcing blood to move in one direction only, starting with blood entering the heart from the right atrium and exiting to the body through the left ventricle.

Blood is fluid that's comprised primarily of plasma, which contains mostly water along with various salts, minerals, and proteins. Red blood cells *(erythrocytes)* carry most of the oxygen you need to live. White blood cells *(leukocytes)* fight off infection and are part of your immune system (which I describe in Chapter 11). Platelets begin the *coagulation,* or clotting, process when a tear in the vasculature is detected. Carbon dioxide, nutrients such as glucose, and waste such as urea are carried in the plasma.

You've probably heard the phrase, "Blood is thicker than water." Well, besides having to do with the relatives you're born with, it is indeed true that blood has a consistency, or *viscosity,* that's slightly heavier than water. The cardiovascular system relies on this viscosity to help create pressure within the vasculature.

The *vasculature* is the combination of pipes that the heart pumps blood into, creating pressure. The *arterial* side of the vasculature carries blood away from the heart, either to the lungs via the pulmonary artery to pick up oxygen or to the rest of the body via the aorta to deliver oxygen to the body in the peripheral circulation.

Arteries are made of smooth muscle and have the ability to stretch and snap back to their original shape, which helps tremendously with the flow of blood. They can also constrict and dilate, depending on the demands of the tissue for oxygen and nutrients.

Arteries divide into smaller vessels called *arterioles,* which divide again numerous times and finally terminate in capillary beds within the tissues. Gas exchange occurs at the capillary beds. In Chapter 9, you find out how that happens in the lungs; the process is the same everywhere else. Diffusion of CO_2 and oxygen occurs based on the concentration of each gas between the capillary and the tissue cells.

The heart itself has its own vasculature. Coronary arteries branch off right where the aorta exits the left ventricle, and they supply the heart tissue, or *myocardium.*

Helping to return blood back to the heart is the *venous system.* Blood leaves the venous side of the capillary beds, collecting in *venules.* They, in turn, collect into veins. The veins are much more rigid than the arteries, which helps to maintain blood pressure as blood returns to the heart. Inside the veins are one-way valves that again force blood to travel in one direction.

All together, these vessels create a closed system of pipes that, with the heart acting as a pump, creates a pressure within itself (see Figure 10-2). You measure that pressure with a blood pressure cuff. By measuring the patient's blood pressure early in your assessment, you can get a sense of how well the system is working.

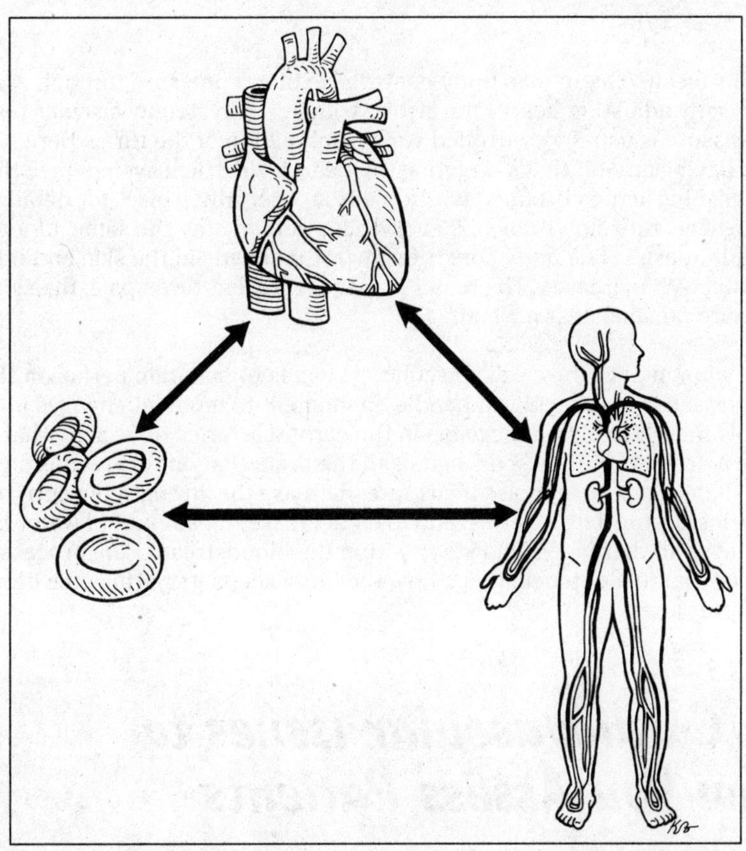

Figure 10-2: The perfusion triangle.

Illustration by Kathryn Born, MA

The heart, blood and vasculature make up a *perfusion triangle,* where all three parts interact with each other to create circulation. In reality, you measure perfusion by assessing the patient's blood pressure.

Understanding blood pressure

One way of talking about blood pressure is with this formula:

Blood pressure (BP) = Cardiac output (CO) × systemic vascular resistance (SVR) (the size of the vasculature)

Before you panic, rest assured — you won't be calculating BP this way! However, the formula quickly illustrates what really counts in maintaining blood pressure.

Cardiac output is the amount of blood that is sent out of the left ventricle in 1 minute. It, too, has a formula:

Cardiac output (CO) = Heart rate (HR) × stroke volume (SV) (the amount of blood squeezed out per contraction)

Again, don't panic — no math is needed here either. But put both formulas together and this is what you get:

BP = (HR × SV) × SVR

What does all this mean? The human body controls its blood pressure through essentially one of three ways: by adjusting heart rate, stroke volume, or systemic vascular resistance. In fact, blood pressure is usually controlled via a combination of the three. Here's an example: A patient is having an AMI that's targeting the heart's electrical system (see the later section "Distinguishing acute coronary syndrome from everything else" for details). The result is that the heart rate slows down. If everything were to stay the same, blood pressure would drop. But it doesn't: The body constricts its arterial beds in the skin and other parts of the body so that SVR increases. The result is that the patient turns pale, the skin cools, and blood pressure remains near normal.

So, if the primary function of the cardiovascular system is to maintain perfusion throughout the body, it makes sense that keeping a handle on moment-to-moment changes in blood pressure controls the system. *Baroreceptors* in the carotid arteries do exactly that. As the receptors sense a drop in BP, they send signals to the brain that, in turn, sends signals to the body to do such things as increase heart rate, increase the strength of ventricular contractions, constrict appropriate arteries, and even decrease the amount of water being filtered by the kidneys so that more fluid stays within the bloodstream. The process is really more complicated, but in a nutshell, that's how the body keeps its perfusion within a very narrow band of pressure.

Knowing the Cardiovascular Issues to Look for When You Assess Patients

So what are the cardiovascular system findings you should look for when assessing the patient? The following sections start with the normal findings, move to irregular findings, and wrap up with acute coronary syndrome.

Recognizing normal cardiovascular findings

You can use yourself as a "normal" picture when it comes to cardiovascular findings. Your normal resting pulse should be strong, regular, and pumping at about 60–100 beats per minute while at rest. You should be able to easily find this pulse by checking your radial artery on the thumb side of your wrist.

While you're feeling the pulse, get a sense of how the skin looks and feels. Unless something is happening to you that I can't see right now, I'd guess that your skin has a normal color; has a normal, warm temperature; and is dry. That's because your skin, an organ of the body, is being adequately perfused. Now, skin can be cooler to the touch when it's cool outside or a little sweaty when you've just finished a workout (or you're panicking about your national exam), but it should return to its normal look and feel within a matter of minutes.

Your blood pressure should be roughly around 120 mm Hg or less systolic and about 80 mm Hg or less diastolic when measured at the distal bicep region of the arm. Many people have blood pressures that are higher than normal *(hypertension)* but live with that pressure. On the other hand, athletes and other fit folks often live with much lower BP. In general, having a lower-than-normal BP is much better than having high BP.

Tightly connected to the cardiovascular system is the respiratory system; what happens in one is often reflected in the other. Under normal conditions, the patient's respiratory rate should be about 12 to 20 breaths per minute without any major effort. When things start to go wrong with the cardiac system, the respiratory system tries to compensate for the issue. Flip to Chapter 9 for more information about the respiratory system.

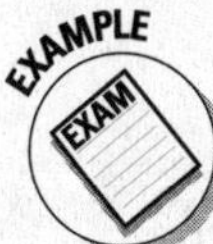

A 73-year-old female complains of chest tightness and difficulty catching her breath. Her blood pressure is 140/90 mm Hg, her pulse rate is 90, and her respiratory rate is 18 breaths per minute. Her skin is pale, warm, and dry; and her oxygen saturation level is 95 percent. Which of the following actions is appropriate?

(A) Lay her supine with her legs slightly elevated.

(B) Place her in a position of comfort.

(C) Administer high-flow oxygen with a nonrebreather mask.

(D) Ventilate her with a bag-valve mask.

The correct answer is Choice (B). While she may be experiencing a medical condition, her vital signs appear to be within normal limits. Keeping her comfortable will help reduce her anxiety and lower body stress. The modified Trendelenberg position, represented by Choice (A), isn't necessary, as her blood pressure isn't low. Her oxygen saturation level is normal, and she appears to be breathing normally; oxygen administration, Choice (C), is not indicated. She is breathing well on her own, so manual ventilations, Choice (D), aren't necessary.

Noting when cardiovascular findings aren't normal

Problems can arise within the cardiovascular system itself, and problems found elsewhere in the body can cause the cardiovascular system to compensate for the issue, sometimes responding so severely that it injures itself. (You find a list of common issues later in this chapter.)

When the body senses that perfusion is or may be compromised, several things happen. Heart rate increases, and the skin turns cool, pale, and clammy. Breathing speeds up too, trying to add more oxygen to the bloodstream and take out excess carbon dioxide. Combine all of these changes and the blood pressure remains as close to normal as possible, even higher than normal sometimes.

If the problem isn't repaired, at some point the cardiovascular system can no longer compensate and begins to fail. Blood pressure falls. The heart slows. The brain, suffering from worsening hypoxia, loses its ability to maintain an alert state; the patient moves from being anxious to being confused and finds it harder to stay awake. As the condition worsens further, the patient becomes unconscious and unresponsive to a painful stimulus.

A 73-year-old female complains of chest tightness and difficulty catching her breath. Her blood pressure is 82/60 mm Hg, her pulse rate is 50, and her respiratory rate is 24 breaths per minute. Her skin is pale, cool, and dry, and her oxygen saturation level is 90 percent. Which of the following actions is appropriate?

(A) Have her sit in a chair.

(B) Administer the patient's prescribed nitroglycerin, if available.

(C) Administer high-flow oxygen with a nonrebreather mask.

(D) Ventilate her with a bag-valve mask.

The correct answer is Choice (C). This patient's vital signs are well outside the ordinary range. She is having difficulty breathing, and her oxygen saturation level is low, making Choice (C) necessary. Her blood pressure isn't high enough to support sitting in a chair, Choice (A), or the administration of nitroglycerin, Choice (B). She is still breathing adequately, so manual ventilation, Choice (D), isn't indicated.

Distinguishing acute coronary syndrome from everything else

The heart is especially sensitive to changes in perfusion. Because of its importance, the heart has a well-developed system of coronary arteries that feed the myocardial muscle. These arteries are fairly small and become easily blocked with a rupture of *plaque* (a layer of fat and minerals that embeds within the inner layers of an artery) or *emboli* (small particles of plaque) that float in from other parts of the body and lodge within the coronary artery itself. If either of these happens, the patient may experience a partial or complete loss of blood flow distal to the blockage. This occurrence marks the beginning of an *acute myocardial infarction* (AMI), or death of cardiac tissue.

As the cardiac tissue becomes *ischemic* (starved of oxygen and becoming more acidic), it sends signals back to the brain. In turn, the brain interprets these signals as the sensation of pressure, burning, tightness, sharpness, or aching. The patient may also feel nauseous, faint, lightheaded, or dizzy. Additionally, because of the close relationship of the lungs and heart, the patient can experience shortness of breath. Because of the way the nerves make their way through the body, the brain may sense related or radiating pain or discomfort to the arms, jaw, or other places in the body.

Sometimes coronary blood flow isn't blocked by plaque or emboli. The patient may have *atherosclerosis,* or narrowing of the arteries that decreases blood flow to the myocardial tissue. Sometimes the arteries themselves can experience a spasm. In these situations the condition known as *angina* may occur. These patients have a lot of the same signs and symptoms as those with myocardial infarction. Usually someone with angina can relieve the symptoms by resting or self-administering nitroglycerin, which dilates the arteries and increases blood flow.

Angina and AMI are part of a spectrum of conditions known as *acute coronary syndrome*, or ACS. Recognizing these signs as early as possible is critical. Because determining the difference between angina and AMI often isn't possible, your safest bet is to assume the worst and treat the patient quickly. Part of that treatment is to transport as quickly and safely as possible to the nearest hospital that's capable of rapidly restoring coronary blood flow, either through angioplasty or fibrinolytic therapy.

A 50-year-old male has a sudden onset of epigastric pressure that comes on without warning. He also has pain in his jaw and feels nauseous. He has a history of ulcers and takes medication for them. He refuses your care, as he believes the discomfort is related to his ulcer history. Which of the following actions is most appropriate?

(A) Assist the patient in taking his ulcer medication.

(B) Advise the patient that he may be having a heart attack.

(C) Stay with the patient until the discomfort resolves.

(D) Begin moving the patient to your ambulance, as time is of the essence.

The answer you're looking for is Choice (B). Although this episode may in fact be a gastrointestinal event, the symptoms also point to possible acute coronary syndrome. As an EMT, you're not authorized to help someone with his ulcer medications, Choice (A). Staying with the patient, Choice (C), isn't feasible, and you can't extricate the patient, Choice (D), without his consent.

Acting on Potential Cardiovascular Problems

Like the respiratory system (covered in Chapter 9), the cardiovascular system can be affected both directly and by conditions outside of it. In the following sections, you discover problems with the heart, vasculature, and blood, and you find out how to handle a cardiac arrest.

Pump problems

In order to work effectively, the heart has to have good blood flow to its muscle via its coronary arteries and an intact electrical system that controls the rate, strength, and timing of the contractions between the atria and ventricles. Table 10-1 outlines the most common heart conditions.

Table 10-1 Conditions Affecting the Heart

Problem	*Signs and Symptoms*	*Action Steps*
Acute coronary syndrome	Described earlier in this chapter; beware of women, diabetics, and older patients having unusual signs such as shortness of breath, sudden weakness, or syncope, or no signs at all other than unexplained diaphoresis.	Find position of comfort; evaluate need for oxygen and administer supplemental O_2 as needed to maintain saturation. If patient has prescribed nitroglycerin and blood pressure is above 100 mm Hg systolic, assist with medication. If authorized, administer aspirin.
Rhythm disturbances: Too fast, too slow, or too irregular	Rates that are too fast or too slow can cause blood pressure to decrease. Radial pulses become difficult to find. Patient may experience chest pain, shortness of breath, or nausea. You may find a pacemaker or an implanted defibrillator under the skin, either in the chest or abdominal area. Irregular heartbeat may also cause blood pressure issues or a lethal rhythm disturbance.	Find position of comfort. Provide oxygen as needed to maintain adequate saturation. Keep an automated external defibrillator (AED) nearby and ready for use if patient loses consciousness and pulse. Note any signs of a pacemaker or implanted defibrillator. If patient becomes pulseless, place AED pads at least 1 inch away from pacemaker or implanted defibrillator.

(continued)

Table 10-1 *(continued)*

Problem	*Signs and Symptoms*	*Action Steps*
Lethal rhythm disturbances	Ventricular fibrillation or ventricular tachycardia that doesn't generate a pulse. Patient is unconscious, apneic, or has gasping respirations; skin is cyanotic, cool, or diaphoretic.	High-quality CPR with at least a 2-inch compression depth and a rate of at least 100 beats per minute. If witnessed, apply AED and follow prompts. Ventilate at a ratio of 2 breaths per 30 compressions.
Cardiogenic shock	Poor cardiac output due to AMI or other condition. Hypotension; cool, pale, and diaphoretic skin; may have chest pain associated with poor perfusion.	Lay patient supine if possible; treat for shock by maintaining body temperature and oxygen saturation.
Congestive heart failure (CHF)	Fluid from capillary beds leaking into the alveoli in the lungs due to too-high or too-low pressure. May auscultate crackles or wheezes in lung fields. May have pedal edema from long-term CHF. If pressure is too high, may have jugular venous distension (JVD). May complain of chest pain or shortness of breath.	If blood pressure is high, place patient in full sitting position with feet dangling if possible. Apply oxygen to maintain adequate saturation levels. Ventilate if patient is breathing inadequately. If patient is in severe respiratory distress and conscious, apply continuous positive airway pressure (CPAP).

It is a warm, humid morning. A 78-year-old woman is attending services at her church when she faints. Church members help her to the floor. She is awake and confused as to the day and time. Her skin is cool, pale, and diaphoretic. She has a blood pressure of 82/50 mm Hg, a heart rate of 100, and a respiratory rate of 20 breaths per minute. She doesn't have any complaints of pain or discomfort and wants to sit up. Which of the following actions is most appropriate?

(A) Assist her to a chair and perform a secondary assessment.

(B) Provide cool compresses to reduce her body temperature.

(C) Provide spinal precautions and transport to an emergency department.

(D) Place her supine on the gurney and transport to an emergency department.

The correct answer is Choice (D). Syncope, or fainting, may be caused by a variety of medical conditions. However, in this case the most serious possibility is an acute myocardial infarction, making Choice (D) the best option. The information doesn't suggest that she is experiencing heat stroke, as Choice (B) implies, nor is there any indication that she may have injured her spine to warrant Choice (C). With her blood pressure low, sitting, Choice (A), may cause her to faint again.

Pipe problems

The body's vasculature can develop leaks that cause fluid to leave the system quickly. On occasion, part of the vasculature can weaken, potentially causing massive failure. Table 10-2 notes common vasculature conditions.

Table 10-2 Conditions Affecting the Vasculature

Problem	*Signs and Symptoms*	*Action Steps*
Aortic aneurysm/ dissection	A weakening in the aorta's wall causing it to bulge out (aneurysm) or tear (dissection) resulting in loss of pressure and bleeding. Patient may complain of sudden tearing or knifelike pain in chest or centered between shoulder blades; may have unequal pulses in arms or legs; may experience a rapid drop in blood pressure, tachycardia, or tachypnea. In rare cases, may have a palpable abdominal mass.	Move patient quickly but carefully; lay supine if possible. Administer oxygen to maintain saturation. Maintain body temperature.
Hypertensive emergency	Sudden rise in blood pressure over minutes to a few hours. Patient may have a rapid onset of headache; a spontaneous nosebleed; sudden ringing in the ears (tinnitus); a strong, bounding pulse; or very high blood pressure.	Place patient in position of comfort; try to keep head elevated. Maintain oxygen saturation levels with supplemental oxygen. Attempt to control any nosebleed by pinching near base of nose and having patient lean forward.
Severe infection (sepsis)	Toxins from bacteria cause vasculature to leak fluids to surrounding tissue (third spacing). Patient may have signs of infection (fever, nausea, vomiting, diarrhea); decreasing oral fluid intake; hypotension, tachycardia, or tachypnea. Skin may be hot, dry, and pale with dark purple-colored areas where microbleeding is occurring (purpura), especially in dependent body areas of the back, buttocks, and legs.	Place patient in supine position and monitor closely for signs of difficulty breathing. If patient is in shock, administer supplemental oxygen to maintain saturation and prevent body temperature loss.
Anaphylaxis	Massive immune response causes vasculature to dilate and leak fluid. Patient may identify source of allergen (a bee sting or peanuts, for example); may aucultate stridor or wheezing; may have hives or swelling of upper airway, hypotension, tachycardia, or tachypnea.	Remove allergen if possible; assist patient with prescribed epinephrine autoinjector; if patient is in shock, administer supplemental oxygen to maintain saturation and prevent body temperature loss.

A 53-year-old male is lifting several boxes at work when he feels sudden, knife-like pain in the middle of his back. He is awake and anxious, with cool, pale, and diaphoretic skin. He has a history of back surgery and hypertension. His radial pulse is weak, fast, and thready; you cannot detect pedal pulses. Of the following suspected conditions, which is most likely?

(A) Aortic abdominal aneurysm

(B) Ruptured vertebral disk

(C) Unsuspected angina

(D) Diaphragmatic hernia

The correct answer is Choice (A). The faint, fast, radial pulse and loss of pedal pulses point to a loss of blood pressure, which isn't likely to result from a vertebral disk rupture, angina, or a diaphragmatic hernia, Choices (B), (C), and (D), respectively.

Fluid problems

If there isn't enough blood inside the vasculature for the heart to pump, perfusion is affected. Table 10-3 notes common conditions related to blood volume.

Table 10-3 Conditions Related to Blood Volume

Problem	*Signs and Symptoms*	*Action Steps*
Dehydration	Loss of water from the blood; causes include excessive physical activity, decrease in oral intake, diarrhea, vomiting, long periods of fever (sweating), and hot environmental temperatures. Patient may complain of weakness or dizziness that may lead to a syncopal episode; cool, pale skin may be dry or wet; tachycardia or tachypnea may be present; may be hypotensive in later stages.	If patient is in shock, administer supplemental oxygen to maintain saturation and prevent body temperature loss. Cool patient if experiencing heat stroke by removing extra clothes and fanning. In most situations, restrict oral intake.
Bleeding	Bleeding in lower GI tract may produce dark, tarry stools (melena). Patients with upper GI bleeding may have bright red or dark, coffee-ground emesis (hematemesis). If significant, patients may appear in shock with cool and clammy skin, tachycardia, tachypnea, or hypotension.	If patient is in shock, administer supplemental oxygen to maintain saturation and prevent body temperature loss. Suction and maintain airway if patient is vomiting.
Third spacing volume loss	Fluids leak into the interstitial tissue surrounding the capillaries, as in sepsis or anaphylaxis. Patient may have signs of infection (fever, nausea, vomiting, diarrhea); decreasing oral fluid intake; hypotension, tachycardia, and tachypnea. Skin may be hot, dry, and pale with dark purple-colored areas where microbleeding is occurring (purpura), especially in dependent body areas of the back, buttocks, and legs. Massive immune response causes vasculature to dilate and leak fluid. Patient may identify source of allergen (a bee sting or peanuts, for example); may have hives, swelling of upper airway, hypotension, tachycardia, or tachypnea.	Place patient in supine position and monitor closely for signs of difficulty breathing. If patient is in shock, administer supplemental oxygen to maintain saturation and prevent body temperature loss. Remove allergen if possible; assist patient with prescribed epinephrine autoinjector.

A 40-year-old female is feeling faint and has difficulty breathing. You auscultate wheezing in both lung fields. Her blood pressure is 85/70 mm Hg, she has a heart rate of 110, and she is breathing 24 times per minute. Her oxygen saturation level is 85 percent. She has a prescribed inhaler for asthma and an epinephrine autoinjector for anaphylaxis. What should you do next?

(A) Assist the patient with her inhaler.

(B) Assist the patient with her epinephrine autoinjector.

(C) Complete a physical examination.

(D) Administer oxygen at 2 LPM with a nasal cannula.

The correct answer is Choice (B). Your findings are consistent with anaphylaxis, and epinephrine is the appropriate intervention for this case. Asthma, which Choice (A) points to, is unlikely to cause low blood pressure. Her oxygen level is very low, so high-flow oxygen would be a better answer than Choice (D). Although you may be able to conduct a full physical examination, Choice (C), that would come after the administration of epinephrine.

Managing a cardiac arrest

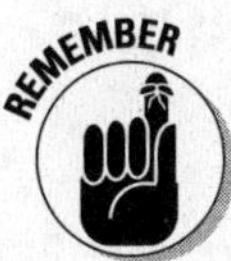

A heart that beats so weakly that it doesn't create a pulse or doesn't contract at all causes the condition known as cardiac arrest. Because there is no blood flow, skin becomes cold and *cyanotic* (blue), and the patient becomes unresponsive to all stimuli. If cardiac arrest continues for more than a few minutes, enough brain cells die to cause permanent death.

Research in the past decade has shown that effective chest compressions are the foundation of successful resuscitation. In other words, during a "working code" everything that is done revolves around the nonstop, high-quality chest compressions. Keep these points in mind:

- After checking to see whether the patient is unconscious, spend no more than 10 seconds to confirm there is no carotid pulse and breathing is absent or inadequate (gasping).
- Begin CPR with compressions, not ventilations. Immediately begin pushing on the chest, while others are assembling other equipment and preparing to ventilate.
- For adults, administer compressions at a rate of *at least* 100 per minute, with *at least* 2 inches of depth, and a *full recoil* of the chest during release. For pediatric patients, compress the chest at least one-third to one-half the depth of the chest.
- For adults, space ventilations so two breaths are provided after every 30 compressions. Deliver just enough to make the chest visibly rise. For two-person CPR on a pediatric patient, space ventilations so two breaths are provided after every 15 compressions.
- Rescuers should switch roles every 2 minutes or 5 cycles of compressions and ventilations, to keep compressions accurate and effective.
- Apply AED pads as soon as possible.
- As soon as the pads are applied, everyone stops and the AED is activated. Follow the prompts and make sure everyone stands clear of the patient. After the AED has analyzed, continue compressions while the AED is charging for defibrillation. When the AED is charged, stop compressions, clear the patient, and deliver the shock. Immediately afterward (or if the AED tells you that no shock is indicated), *immediately begin CPR again.* Do not pause to check for a pulse.

- At the end of the next 2-minute interval, look for signs of effective breathing and check for a pulse. If they are absent, immediately resume CPR. If the AED indicates a shock is needed, continue compressions while the AED charges and then clear the patient and deliver the shock.
- During two-person CPR on a child or infant, the ratio of compressions to ventilations is 15:2. This ratio allows more ventilations to be delivered to the patient.

You and three other trained crew members arrive at a park, where you see a jogger lying on the sidewalk. Two bystanders are performing CPR, with one administering chest compressions while the other is providing mouth-to-mouth ventilations. What should you do next?

(A) Stop compressions and check for a radial pulse.

(B) Stop compressions and apply the AED pads to the patient's chest.

(C) Have other trained crew members take over compressions and ventilations at the end of a cycle.

(D) Apply AED pads during compressions and push the button to analyze when another 5 cycles of compression and ventilations are complete.

The correct choice is (C). You want to minimize interruptions to compressions, and Choice (C) accomplishes this better than Choices (A) and (B). You want to analyze the rhythm as soon as you are able, rather than waiting for 5 cycles of compressions and ventilations to be completed, as Choice (D) indicates.

Practice Questions about Cardiology and Resuscitation

The following practice questions are similar to the EMT exam's questions about cardiology and resuscitation. Read each question carefully, and then select the answer choice that most correctly answers the question.

1. A 68-year-old male has chest pressure and shortness of breath after climbing a flight of stairs. His neighbor is worried and calls 911. The patient is alert and insists that this is an angina episode that will go away on its own. Which of the following questions would be of most benefit in verifying his assertion?

   (A) Are you nauseous?

   (B) Does this pain come on each time you climb these stairs?

   (C) Are you prescribed nitroglycerin?

   (D) Does the pain radiate to your arm or jaw?

2. A man stands up to clear the dishes after dinner. He feels a sharp, tearing sensation in the epigastric region of his abdomen, toward his back. He immediately collapses to the floor. His blood pressure is 100/84 mm Hg, his pulse rate is 108, and he is breathing 24 times per minute. His skin is pale, cool, and diaphoretic. Pedal pulses are absent. You should

   (A) immobilize him to a long backboard.

   (B) assist him to a sitting position.

   (C) move him carefully to a gurney.

   (D) administer the patient's prescribed nitroglycerin.

3. A 72-year-old female presents with "aching" discomfort in her epigastric region that began abruptly 45 minutes ago. She reports a history of hypertension, ulcers, angina, and atherosclerosis. Her pain is a 7 on a 1–10 scale. She self-administered three of her prescribed nitroglycerin tablets, without effect. Her blood pressure is 136/90 mm Hg. You should first

   (A) administer supplemental oxygen.

   (B) administer another dose of the patient's nitroglycerin.

   (C) perform a full secondary assessment.

   (D) determine what other medications are prescribed.

4. A 49-year-old male presents supine in bed, alert, and complaining of lightheadedness, difficulty breathing, and heavy chest pressure that radiates to his arms. His heart rate is 42, his blood pressure is 92/62 mm Hg, and he has a breathing rate of 18 times per minute. You auscultate crackles in both lung fields. You should

   (A) leave the patient supine and administer supplemental oxygen.

   (B) administer the patient's prescribed nitroglycerin.

   (C) sit the patient upright to assist his breathing.

   (D) assist the patient's ventilation with a bag-valve mask and oxygen.

5. A 65-year-old female is supine in bed with difficulty breathing and substernal chest pressure. She is alert and breathing 26 times per minute, with crackles auscultated bilaterally. Accessory muscle use is evident. Her blood pressure is 220/104 mm Hg, her heart rate is 90 and irregular, and she has cool, diaphoretic skin. You should

   (A) assist with her breathing using a bag-valve mask and oxygen.

   (B) sit her upright and administer high-flow oxygen.

   (C) assist the patient with her prescribed hypertension medication.

   (D) keep her supine and administer low-flow oxygen.

6. An 80-year-old male had a syncopal episode while standing during church service. Bystanders assisted him to the ground, where he presents awake, confused, and short of breath. He is pale, warm, and diaphoretic; his blood pressure is 100/70 mm Hg, and his pulse rate is 96. He is breathing 18 times per minute; his lung sounds are clear. Which of the following series of actions would be most appropriate?

   (A) Sit the patient upright and assist him to a gurney, administer oxygen, and perform a full physical examination.

   (B) Move the patient to a cooler spot within the church; loosen his clothing and fan him to promote cooling.

   (C) Keep the patient supine and transfer him to the gurney, administer oxygen, and move toward the ambulance.

   (D) Obtain a complete physical exam and past medical history, administer oxygen, and sit him upright.

7. A 74-year-old male is supine in bed. He opens his eyes when you call his name and is confused as to time and location. His skin is pale, warm, and dry. Family reports the patient has been ill, with vomiting and diarrhea for ten days, and has not been out of bed in the past 36 hours. His blood pressure is 86/64 mm Hg, he has a heart rate of 104, and he's breathing 20 times per minute. His medical history includes diabetes, early stage lung cancer, and a myocardial infarction three years ago. Which of the following conditions is the most likely cause of his presentation?

   (A) Insulin shock

   (B) Septic shock

   (C) Pulmonary shock

   (D) Cardiogenic shock

8. A 34-year-old male presents with difficulty breathing and feeling faint. He came home from a restaurant about an hour ago, felt nauseated, and vomited several times. His pulse rate is 126, his blood pressure is 88/50 mm Hg, and he is breathing 24 times per minute. You auscultate wheezing in both lung fields. His skin is pale, cool, and moist. You should assist with the patient's prescribed

   (A) epinephrine autoinjector.

   (B) multidose inhaler (MDI).

   (C) nitroglycerin.

   (D) insulin injection.

9. A 25-year-old female is confused and slow to respond to verbal commands. Her roommate states that the patient returned from an overseas business trip four days ago and has been experiencing nausea, vomiting, and diarrhea since. You observe yellow-colored, thin emesis in a garbage pail next to the patient's bed. Her skin is warm, pale, and dry. She is tachycardic and tachypneic. Which of the following conditions is the most likely cause of her presentation?

   (A) Gastrointestinal bleeding

   (B) Dehydration

   (C) Food poisoning

   (D) Hypoglycemia

10. A 65-year-old male is sitting at his kitchen table feeling increasingly weak, dizzy when he stands, and nauseated over the past 6 hours. He admits to binge drinking alcohol over the past 72 hours. His skin is pale, warm, and dry. He has neither vomited nor had diarrhea, although his stool has been loose and darker than normal. His medical history includes hypertension, alcoholism, liver disease, and drug abuse. His blood pressure is 98/68 mm Hg, his heart rate is 116, and he is breathing 18 times a minute. His oxygen saturation is 92 percent. You should

    (A) obtain orthostatic vitals, first when sitting and then while standing.

    (B) transport the patient in a sitting position and be prepared to suction as needed.

    (C) transport the patient in a left recumbent position and administer supplemental oxygen.

    (D) administer high-flow oxygen and transport the patient in a sitting position.

11. You are on-scene with a 50-year-old female who is experiencing substernal chest pressure. In mid-sentence she stops talking, rolls her eyes back, and has slow, snoring respirations. Your next step is to

(A) begin deep and fast chest compressions.

(B) apply AED pads.

(C) check for a carotid pulse.

(D) ventilate twice with a bag-valve mask.

12. Bystanders are performing adequate chest compressions on an adult male found down in the middle of a food court at a shopping mall. You are with your partner and are carrying your airway equipment and an AED. You should

(A) take over chest compressions and instruct the bystanders to apply the AED pads.

(B) stop CPR and apply the AED pads yourself.

(C) have bystanders continue chest compressions while you apply the AED pads.

(D) have your partner take over compressions while you prepare the airway equipment.

13. You and your partner arrive at a public pool where lifeguards are performing CPR on a 7-year-old female who was underwater for 10 to 15 minutes. One lifeguard is performing adequate chest compressions, pausing every 30 compressions for the other lifeguard to ventilate the patient with a pocket mask. You should

(A) direct the lifeguards to continue CPR at a ratio of 15 compressions to two breaths.

(B) take over CPR and direct the lifeguards to apply the AED pads.

(C) direct the lifeguards to stop CPR and apply the AED pads.

(D) have your partner take over compressions while you apply the AED pads.

14. You are performing CPR during a cardiac arrest. You stop compressions and push the AED's "analyze" button. After a few seconds the AED announces, "no shock indicated." You should

(A) provide two ventilations with a bag-valve mask.

(B) begin chest compressions.

(C) check for a carotid pulse.

(D) check for breathing.

15. You finish 2 minutes of CPR on an adult patient. You detect a carotid pulse. The patient is not breathing. You should

(A) activate the AED.

(B) ventilate every 5 seconds with a bag-valve mask.

(C) begin chest compressions.

(D) place the patient in the recovery position.

16. Your patient is at her office, complaining of a headache, and "loud ringing in her ears." She is alert, with a pulse rate of 90, blood pressure of 260/110 mm Hg, and a respiratory rate of 16 breaths per minute. She has equal strength and movement in all extremities and speaks without difficulty. She has a medical history of asthma and has an inhaler. Which of the following conditions is most likely to cause her presenting signs and symptoms?

    (A) Trauma to the head

    (B) Hemorrhagic stroke

    (C) Ischemic stroke

    (D) Hypertensive emergency

17. A 1-month-old infant is in cardiac arrest. You and your partner arrive on-scene. Which of the following actions is most appropriate?

    (A) Provide chest compressions using a two-thumb, encircling hands technique, while your partner ventilates every 15 compressions.

    (B) Provide chest compressions using a two-finger technique, while your partner ventilates every 30 compressions.

    (C) Provide 1-inch deep chest compressions at a rate of 100 per minute.

    (D) Provide ventilations with small volume over 3 seconds.

18. A 47-year-old female was asleep when she awoke with an abrupt onset of "tightness" between her shoulder blades approximately 30 minutes ago. Her condition has progressively worsened since it began; it doesn't change with movement or body position. She hasn't had this sensation before. She is anxious and nauseated, but doesn't need to vomit. Her medical history includes hypertension and arteriosclerosis. Her skin is pale, warm, and dry. Her blood pressure is 136/86 mm Hg, her heart rate is 90, and she is breathing 16 times per minute. You should transport her to

    (A) a trauma center with CAT scan capabilities.

    (B) a hospital capable of emergency percutaneous angioplasty.

    (C) her preferred hospital that contains her medical records.

    (D) the closest hospital with rapid lab workup and X-ray capabilities.

Answers and Explanations

Use this answer key to score the practice questions in the preceding section. The explanations give you insight into why the correct answer is better than the other choices.

1. **B.** A hallmark of angina is that it's predictable, meaning the patient can tell when the pain will come on. The other questions can apply to either angina or myocardial infarction, making them less useful in verifying the patient's assertion.

2. **C.** This scenario has the telltale signs of an aortic dissection or rupture. He needs to be rapidly transported to a hospital where he can be evaluated for surgery. There is no indication of a trauma mechanism to indicate Choice (A), and nitroglycerin, Choice (D), may actually worsen the condition. Sitting, Choice (B), may increase the pressure on the already damaged aorta.

3. **A.** If the first three doses of the patient's nitroglycerin weren't effective, it's unlikely that any more doses, Choice (B), will help. The other choices are steps in the assessment process, but first you should apply supplemental oxygen, before moving forward, to ensure that any possible hypoxia is managed.

4. **A.** The patient is experiencing difficulty breathing and has poor lung sounds, making oxygen necessary. The patient's blood pressure is too low to risk having the patient sit up as Choice (C) suggests or to risk administering nitroglycerin, Choice (B). He is alert, meaning he's able to compensate for his respiratory distress, so assisting his ventilations, Choice (D), isn't necessary at this time.
5. **B.** This patient is experiencing pulmonary edema secondary to congestive heart failure (CHF). Sitting her up will assist her ability to breathe. Keeping her supine, Choice (D), won't help. While both Choices (B) and (D) include oxygen administration, the better answer is based upon the body positioning. You're not permitted to administer antihypertensive medications, ruling out Choice (C). Her respiratory rate is adequate, so bag-valve-mask use, Choice (A), is not indicated at this time.
6. **C.** The patient's blood pressure is too low to have him sit up as Choices (A) and (D) suggest. Although the syncopal episode may be simply heat related, which requires cooling, Choice (B), no clear information is provided in the scenario. In addition, a myocardial infarction in elderly patients can often present as a sudden syncopal episode.
7. **B.** The scenario suggests an infection-based condition that has steadily gotten worse. The history of lung cancer implies his immune system is compromised as well. All of this points to sepsis as the root cause of his hypotension. You would expect cool and diaphoretic skin signs for insulin shock, Choice (A), and cardiogenic shock, Choice (D). Pulmonary shock, Choice (C), is a nonsense term.
8. **A.** The scenario suggests that the patient is experiencing anaphylaxis after eating at a restaurant. An asthma attack requiring an MDI, Choice (B), doesn't typically cause such a dramatic change in blood pressure. On the off chance that it's cardiogenic shock, nitroglycerin, Choice (C), is contraindicated. You aren't permitted to inject insulin, Choice (D). Besides, that's for cases of hyperglycemia, not hypoglycemia.
9. **B.** The patient appears to be hypovolemic, secondary to vomiting and diarrhea. The emesis does not appear to contain blood as Choice (A) indicates; food poisoning, Choice (C), usually passes within 8–24 hours. Hypoglycemia, Choice (D), is a possibility, but it's less likely than dehydration in this case because her skin would be cool and diaphoretic, not warm and dry.
10. **C.** Transporting the patient on his side will help him maintain his airway; his oxygen saturation level is low, so administering oxygen will help. The patient is hypotensive; sitting the patient, as in Choices (B) and (D), may worsen his blood pressure. Because the patient is already showing signs of hypotension, orthostatic vital signs, Choice (A), won't provide any additional information and may worsen his blood pressure as well.
11. **C.** You need to confirm the patient is in cardiac arrest by checking the carotid pulse before beginning resuscitation, Choice (A). If she is, you can then begin chest compressions. Applying AED pads, Choice (B), will come next. At the end of 30 compressions, you'll administer two breaths, Choice (D).
12. **C.** If bystanders are performing good chest compressions, allow them to continue so that you can focus on applying the AED pads and activating the device. You don't want to stop chest compressions, Choice (B), and you don't want to tie up yourself and your partner in performing skills that are already being done correctly, Choices (A) and (D).
13. **A.** Pediatric cardiac arrests are thought to be respiratory driven, rather than cardiac driven as in adults. In two-rescuer CPR on a child, more ventilations can be delivered using a ratio of 15 compressions to 2 breaths rather than 30 to 2. You don't want to stop chest compressions, Choice (C), and you don't want to tie up yourself and your partner in performing skills that are already being done, Choices (B) and (D).
14. **B.** Chest compressions that are deep, fast, and continuous improve cardiac arrest outcomes. You want to resume compressions as soon as possible after any intervention. Choices (A), (C), and (D) all delay compressions.

15. **B.** Your patient is in respiratory arrest. Ventilating the patient will provide much-needed oxygen during this stage. Chest compressions, Choice (C), and activating the AED, Choice (A), are not indicated at the moment. You can't ventilate the patient while he's on his side, contraindicating Choice (D).

16. **D.** The scenario describes signs of a hypertensive emergency. Although it's possible she's having a stroke, Choices (B) and (C), her response to a Cincinnati stroke scale test (equal grips, speaks without difficulty) reduces the likelihood. You have no information to suggest a traumatic event, Choice (A), has occurred.

17. **A.** In pediatric, two-rescuer CPR, a ratio of 15 compressions to 2 ventilations is appropriate and improves oxygenation compared to a 30:2 ratio, Choice (B). The compressions should be one-third to one-half the depth of the chest, which is at least 1½ inches deep, not 1 inch as Choice (C) indicates. Ventilation duration is similar to that of an adult, meaning that ventilations are delivered over a period of 1 second each, not 3 seconds as stated in Choice (D).

18. **B.** This patient has all the hallmarks of a myocardial infarction, despite the absence of chest pain. In an MI, time is of the essence. The best place of care for her condition is a facility with emergency angioplasty capabilities to reopen her blocked coronary arteries.

Chapter 11

Medical and Obstetrics/Gynecology Fundamentals

In This Chapter

- Surveying the structures and functions of each body system
- Encountering emergency medical conditions
- Being a medical detective to better understand how to treat your patient

To understand how the body works, you have to look at it as a series of systems that interact to create the state known as *homeostasis* — life, in balance. Every moment of every day, your body tries to keep itself in a constant state of homeostasis. Each system has a very specific series of structures and functions that, under most conditions, are very complementary with each other.

When something goes wrong somewhere in the body, the systems work to compensate and then combat the issue. For example, think about an infection. The body normally does a great job in keeping foreign invaders like viruses and bacteria at bay. But on occasion, one gets through and takes hold somewhere. It multiplies quickly. The body fights back by increasing its metabolism rate and creating a fever to kill the infection. White blood cells in your blood look for and destroy the foreign cells. If the infection is in your gastrointestinal tract, your body speeds up the process of moving food through it, causing you to have diarrhea.

As you can imagine, this battle takes a toll on your body. Other systems also spring into action. Your vasculature dilates, causing blood to pool at the surface of the skin to help dissipate excess heat. Your sweat glands begin to secrete fluid, causing you to perspire as more heat is removed. Your brain triggers your thirst mechanism so that you drink more fluids to replace the loss.

This is a simple example of how the body's organ systems interact with one another. Understanding this interaction helps you better think about what may be causing your patient's signs and symptoms. In fact, you might not look at someone quite the same way as you once did! This chapter describes the body's main systems, lists medical conditions you may encounter, and explains treatments.

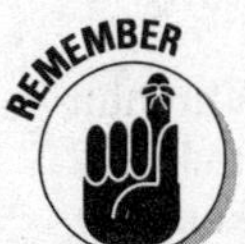

On the EMT exam, don't look for an answer that seems so obviously connected to the patient presentation, especially for medical patients! The chief complaint may be one system compensating for another system's problem. Consider all the information being presented in the question before selecting the best answer.

Introducing the Body's Main Systems

You need to review several organ systems for the EMT exam. Each is comprised of a series of organs and structures, which in turn has a unique series of functions.

As an EMT, you should be knowledgeable about a few structures. Table 11-1 provides an overview of each system. I cover each one in more detail in the rest of this chapter. ***Note:*** The respiratory and cardiovascular systems are so important that they are covered in separate chapters (Chapters 9 and 10, respectively). You may want to take a moment to review them now.

Table 11-1 Overview of Body Systems, Structures, and Functions

System	*Major Organs and Structures*	*Main Functions*
Nervous	Brain, spinal cord, nerves	Fast, short-acting control system Conscious thought
Gastrointestinal	Mouth, teeth, esophagus, stomach, small and large intestines, liver, gallbladder, pancreas, appendix, rectum, anus	Digestion — break down food and absorb nutrients Absorb water Excrete unused food components and unwanted solid waste products
Immune	Thymus, bone marrow	Protection from foreign substances and organisms, such as allergens and infections
Endocrine	Pancreas, ovaries, testes	Slow, long-acting control system
Hematologic	Red blood cells *(erythrocytes),* white blood cells *(leukocytes),* platelets, plasma	Carry oxygen and nutrients to cells and remove carbon dioxide and waste
Urinary	Kidneys, ureters, bladder, urethra	Regulate water balance Excrete unwanted liquid wastes
Reproductive	Male: Testes, urethra, penis Female: Ovaries, uterus, fallopian tubes, vagina, mammary glands	Reproduction (sperm production for males; egg development, ovulation, and pregnancy for females) Secondary sex characteristics (deeper voice, greater muscle growth for males; breast development, higher voice for females)

Feeling Out the Nervous System

Simplistically, the nervous system serves a command and control purpose, primarily by receiving signals from nerves throughout the body, passing them through the spinal cord, processing those signals in the brain, and communicating some type of change in response. Figure 11-1 shows the main structures of the nervous system.

Of course, we're much more than just a bunch of signals moving back and forth. The human brain — which gives us the ability to have conscious thought and engage with our environment in a purposeful, deliberate way — is what makes us stand out from most of the animal kingdom. The human brain is much bigger proportionally to the body compared to most other mammals. It requires a lot of oxygen and nutrients, such as glucose, to function effectively. That's the reason why EMTs evaluate mental status early and often — even simply being sleepy may be an early indication of an oxygenation, ventilation, or circulation issue.

The brain is also sensitive to changes in chemistry, ranging from disease processes like hyperglycemia that causes increased acidity in the blood *(diabetic ketoacidosis)* to recreational drugs such as alcohol, marijuana, and 3-4 methylenedioxymethamphetamine (MDMA, also known as Ecstasy or Molly). Checking for orientation status — awareness of person, place, time, and event — gives you a more precise understanding of how affected the brain is in these situations.

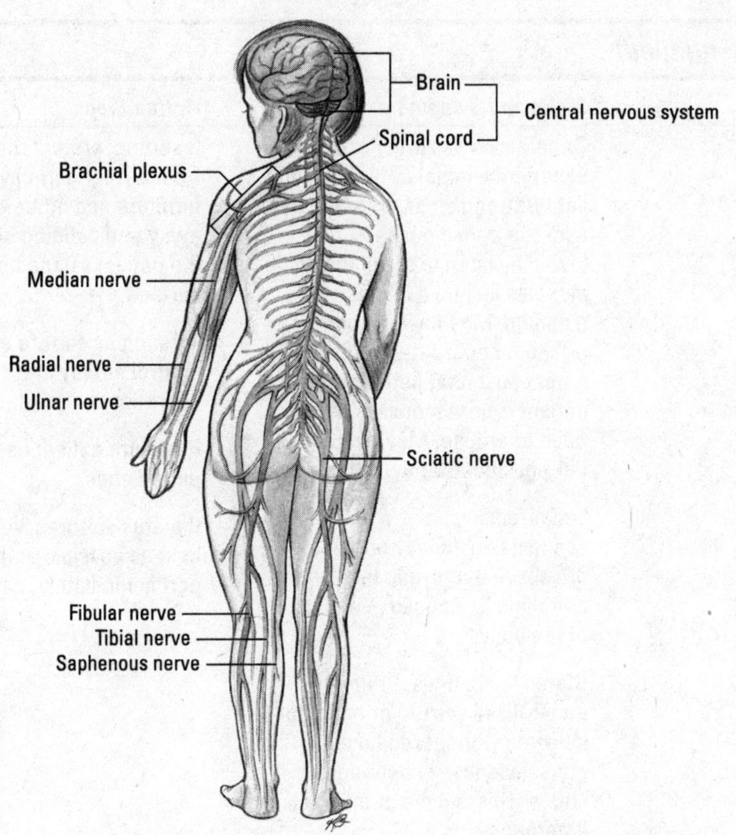

Figure 11-1: The nervous system.

Illustration by Kathryn Born, MA

Because the nervous system can be affected by so many factors, coming up with a full list of conditions that affect it is difficult. However, there are a few illnesses specific to the nervous system that you should recognize quickly and treat. Table 11-2 provides a summary.

Table 11-2 Nervous System Illnesses

Problem	*Signs and Symptoms*	*Action Steps*
Headache	Non–life-threatening conditions such as tension headache or migraine: Generalized discomfort ranging from dull and throbbing to sharp in nature. May be global or focused on one side. May have associated nausea, vomiting. Life-threatening conditions such as hemorrhagic stroke: Rapid onset, severe pain. Projectile vomiting resulting from increased cerebral pressure. Contagious, serious illnesses such as meningitis: May have fever, light sensitivity, vomiting, stiff neck.	Provide quiet, darkened environment. Manage airway: Suction secretions, ventilate with bag-valve mask if needed. Meningitis can be very contagious, spreading through airborne droplets. Wear a HEPA mask and protective eyewear along with gloves if suspected.

continued

Table 11-2 (continued)

Problem	***Signs and Symptoms***	***Action Steps***
Seizure Status epilepticus	Generalized seizure: Patient may experience initial aura (flashing lights, strong smell or taste), then a loss of consciousness, followed by intense twitching of all muscles lasting a few seconds to a minute. May have incontinence or bite tongue. Afterwards, enters post ictal period where patient is unresponsive and difficult to arouse. May not remember episode after awakening. Localized seizure: No loss of consciousness but may not be aware of seizure occurring. Involuntary twitching is focused in one part of the body. Status epilepticus: Prolonged generalized seizure or nonstop seizures without regaining consciousness in between episodes. This is a major medical emergency.	If seizing, protect the patient from further harm by moving furniture and other items away and padding between the patient's head and surface. As soon as seizure ends, control airway and clear oral secretions. Reassure patient as post ictal period ends. If status seizures, ventilate as best as possible and transport immediately.
Stroke: Ischemic stroke: Blockage of an artery in the brain Hemorrhagic stroke: Sudden bleeding in the brain Transient ischemic attack (TIA): A stroke lasting less than 24 hours	Sudden onset of weakness on one side of the body. Facial drooping, difficulty swallowing. Blurred or loss of vision in one eye. Confusion, weakness, dizziness, coma. Sudden, severe headache (more related to hemorrhagic stroke). Speech that's garbled (can't be understood) or nonsensical (clear but makes no sense).	Evaluate using Cincinnati stroke scale. Check blood glucose levels. Maintain airway patency via suctioning, positioning. Administer supplemental oxygen if you see signs of hypoxia. Determine when symptoms began. If patient awoke from sleep, time starts when patient fell asleep. If you can't tell whether you're dealing with TIA or stroke, assume stroke until proven otherwise. If possible, transport to hospital specializing in stroke care.

A mnemonic, AEIOUTIPS, can be used to quickly remember a variety of conditions that can cause altered mental status. Use it when you're asked to determine the underlying cause of a patient's altered mental status. It stands for

- **A:** Alcohol ingestion
- **E:** Epilepsy
- **I:** Infections such as meningitis or sepsis
- **O:** Drug overdoses
- **U:** Uremia of the blood, or kidney failure
- **T:** Trauma to the brain
- **I:** Insulin, or diabetic emergencies
- **P:** Psychiatric emergencies
- **S:** Stroke

A 50-year-old male is unresponsive to a sternal rub. His skin is pale and dry. His blood pressure is 140/86 mm Hg. He is breathing 6 times per minute, with shallow effort, and his lungs sound clear. He has a history of hypertension and diabetes, and recently returned home from the hospital, where doctors repaired a fractured right hip. His medications include an antihypertensive, insulin, and a narcotic painkiller. Which of the following procedures would help you determine the cause of his presentation?

(A) Check for facial symmetry and hand grip strength.

(B) Inspect pupils for size and symmetry.

(C) Inspect the abdomen for injection marks.

(D) Palpate to see whether the surgical site on the hip is painful.

The correct answer is Choice (B). For this patient, AEIOUTIPS provides you with several suspicious possibilities: stroke (hypertension), overdose (narcotic), and insulin or diabetic emergency (patient history). Looking more closely at the information provided, you can see that his slow, shallow breaths may be a result of a narcotic overdose. Choice (B) can help you determine whether his pupils are constricted, which helps to validate that suspicion. You're unable to perform a Cincinnati stroke test, as Choice (A) suggests, because he is unresponsive. Performing the other choices may provide you information, but won't help you determine the underlying cause of the presentation.

Moving through the Gastrointestinal System

The abdomen contains most of the major structures and organs of digestion. In general, they're divided into two categories: hollow organs such as the stomach, gallbladder, and intestines, and solid organs such as the liver, kidneys, and pancreas. If injured or breached, hollow organs tend to spill their contents into the abdominal cavity, possibly causing infection and cell tissue damage. Solid organs contain a lot of blood vessels and tend to bleed if injured.

Food is mechanically broken down by the teeth and chemically taken apart by stomach acid. It eventually becomes a slurry that is moved slowly through the small and large intestines through rhythmical motions known as *peristalsis.* Nutrients and water are absorbed by the walls of the intestines and circulated throughout the body. Eventually all that is left are feces — waste products that the body doesn't need or can't use. They're excreted out the rectum through the anus. Figure 11-2 shows the main structures of the gastrointestinal system.

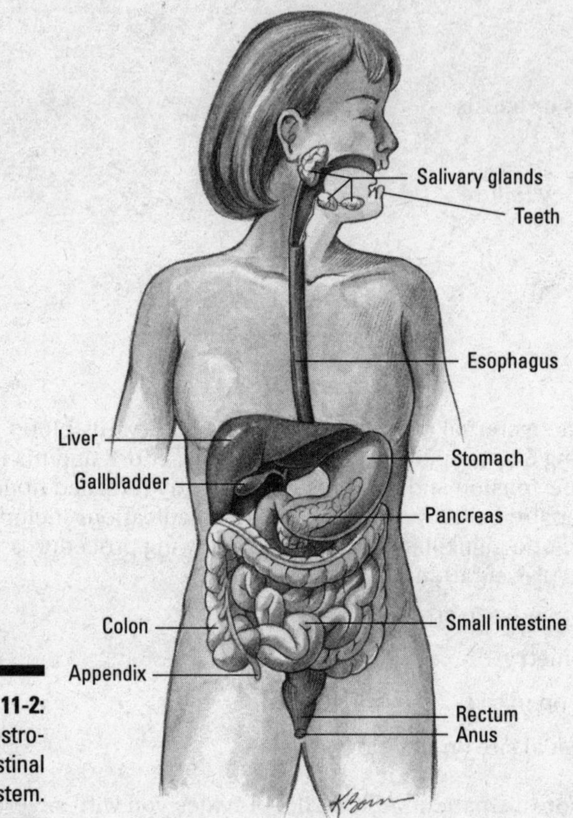

Figure 11-2: The gastrointestinal system.

Illustration by Kathryn Born, MA

Covering the different organs are two layers of tissue: the visceral and parietal membranes. The *visceral membrane* lies on top of the organs; the *parietal* lies against the walls of the abdominal cavity. They slide past each other, allowing the organs to move as we move, yet still maintain their relative positions.

Know the general locations of the abdominal organs. Pain in those areas may be a clue to which organ is involved. For example, right upper quadrant pain may be related to the liver or gallbladder, while right lower quadrant pain may be more specific to the appendix.

Abdominal pain can be hard to diagnose, even for physicians. You're not required to know exactly what is happening when a patient complains of abdominal discomfort. However, having some idea can help you understand whether the patient has a potentially serious medical condition that requires immediate assessment by emergency department staff. Review Table 11-3 for a list of gastrointestinal disorders you should be familiar with.

Table 11-3 Gastrointestinal System Illnesses

Illness or Disease	*Signs and Symptoms*	*Specific Treatment*
Appendicitis	Pain centered in right lower quadrant or beginning around the navel and moving downward over a few hours. Fever, body aches, chills. May feel nauseous, vomit. If appendix ruptures, may cause peritonitis.	Treat for shock if needed by keeping patient supine, administering oxygen, and maintaining body temperature.

Illness or Disease	***Signs and Symptoms***	***Specific Treatment***
Cholecystitis: Inflammation of the gallbladder; often caused by gallstones that block the gallbladder, causing it to swell	Rapid onset of sharp, severe pain in right upper quadrant, radiates to back, right shoulder, or flank 30–60 minutes after a meal rich in fat. May experience nausea, vomiting, indigestion, gas.	Place patient in position of comfort. Avoid anything by mouth.
Esophageal varices/ Mallory-Weiss Syndrome	A weakness in the wall of the esophagus may suddenly burst, causing massive bleeding. Patient vomits large amounts of bright red blood. Shock is likely.	If possible, lay patient in left lateral recumbent position to help keep the airway open. Suction any blood in the airway. Provide supplemental high-flow oxygen using a nonrebreather mask. Maintain body temperature. Rapid transport is needed.
Gastroenteritis: Infection of the GI tract by virus or bacterium	Caused by ingestion of contaminated food or water. Causes nausea, vomiting, and diarrhea. May also cause dehydration, which results in signs of shock.	Treat for shock if needed by keeping patient supine, administering oxygen, and maintaining body temperature.
GI hemorrhage	Depending on where the bleeding site is, patient may vomit blood or, more likely, have blood in stool. If enough blood is lost, signs of early shock may be seen — tachycardia, tachypnea, worsening weakness.	Measure orthostatic vital signs (pulse and blood pressure when laying supine, repeated when sitting, and then standing). Treat for shock if necessary by keeping patient supine, administering oxygen, and maintaining body temperature.
Pancreatitis: Caused by gallstones, alcohol abuse, and other diseases	Deep-set pain in mid-upper abdomen. May experience nausea, vomiting. In severe cases, may cause sepsis or the pancreas to begin bleeding.	Place patient in position of comfort. Avoid anything by mouth.
Peritonitis: Irritation of the membranes lining the abdominal cavity caused by a rupture in the GI tract	Intestinal contents leaking into the abdominal cavity can cause very serious infections. Patient may have fever, nausea, vomiting. Abdomen may become distended, painful to palpitation. In severe cases, may cause septic shock.	Transport patient with knees flexed, may help reduce pain. Treat for shock if needed by keeping patient supine, administering oxygen, and maintaining body temperature.
Ulcers: Small erosions of the stomach lining or duodenum	Burning, pressure, or gnawing discomfort in the upper abdomen or upper back. Comes on shortly after a meal, lasts 2–3 hours. May have nausea, vomiting. May cause bleeding resulting in bloody vomit *(hematemesis)* and/or dark, tarry stool *(melena)*.	If bleeding is significant, there may be signs of shock that you must manage by keeping patient supine, administering oxygen, and maintaining body temperature.

There are also non-GI system causes of abdominal pain. For example:

- An *abdominal aortic aneurysm* (AAA, or triple A) is a sudden weakening of the aorta causing it to bulge out or, in the worst cases, suddenly rupture. An AAA causes severe abdominal pain. The patient's blood pressure may fall quickly, and pedal pulses may be absent. This is a life-threatening emergency that requires rapid but gentle movement of the patient to a hospital.
- Pain from a myocardial infarction (MI; discussed in Chapter 10) may be centered around the epigastric region, midway between the two upper abdominal quadrants. A patient may mistake the discomfort for indigestion. Carefully evaluate the rest of the history of the present illness to see whether an MI may be happening.

A 41-year-old male is complaining of a sudden onset of abdominal pain that began 30 minutes after eating a spicy meal. He describes the pain as feeling sharp, just below his ribcage in the middle of his abdomen. He felt nauseous and vomited, which did not relieve the pain. He is awake and anxious, and his skin is pale, cool, and diaphoretic. He has a faint, fast radial pulse and is tachypneic. You cannot feel his femoral pulse. Which of the following conditions best explains your findings?

(A) Appendicitis

(B) Gastroenteritis

(C) Aortic abdominal aneurysm

(D) Ulcers

The correct answer is Choice (C). Even though this episode came on after a meal, all other signs point to a serious, potentially life-threatening condition. The thready pulse, poor skin signs, and lack of femoral pulses point to a sudden drop in blood pressure. The location of the pain is not associated with appendicitis, Choice (A), which is typically characterized by a slower onset and located in the right lower quadrant or around the umbilicus. Gastroenteritis, Choice (B), and ulcers, Choice (D), don't usually drop blood pressure so dramatically.

Fighting Invaders with the Immune System

The immune system is key to your ability to ward off foreign bodies that can make you sick — bacteria, viruses, and other organisms, as well as proteins that can be irritating to the inside of your body, such as pollen. The following sections describe allergic reactions, anaphylaxis, and infections.

Allergic reactions and anaphylaxis

When it detects an invader, the immune system triggers a series of responses that results in bringing white blood cells to the source, which attack and hopefully kill off the offending body. The immediate area surrounding the source becomes swollen with plasma that's carrying the white blood cells.

This is all well and good, and works very well. However, in some cases the immune system becomes a bit hyperactive, causing the body to shift more fluid than what is needed to do the job. Think of pollen, for example. You and many other people may experience an allergic reaction when exposed to it. Your nose gets stuffy and you may have to blow out mucous. Your eyes get watery and you may end up sneezing and coughing. All of these reactions are ways for the body to try to keep as much of the pollen out of itself as possible.

As annoying as this may be, it's a simple allergic reaction. In more serious allergic reactions, the swelling may be in the skin, causing little red welts called hives or *urticaria* to appear. The skin can become very itchy and the patient may feel very uncomfortable. An antihistamine medication such as diphenhydramine (Benadryl) reduces the intensity of the reaction.

Unfortunately for some people, their immune systems go overboard, causing an anaphylactic reaction. In *anaphylaxis,* the swelling can happen in the upper and lower airways, making it very difficult to breathe. The bronchioles begin to constrict, causing wheezing. A patient may complain of tightening in the throat. The veins may dilate massively, causing blood pressure to fall and plasma to leak into the skin, causing a bloated appearance. Anaphylaxis is a very serious, potentially life-threatening condition. Patients who know they are anaphylactic may be prescribed epinephrine autoinjectors. You may need to assist these patients with their use.

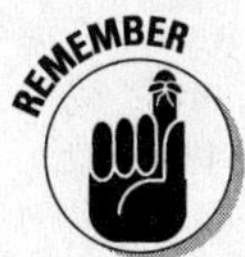

Know the difference between an allergic reaction and anaphylaxis. Assisting a patient with an epinephrine autoinjector can be life-saving in anaphylaxis, but potentially dangerous in a simple allergic reaction because epinephrine puts huge demands on the heart and could cause a heart attack. The benefits outweigh the risk in anaphylaxis, where the blood pressure is very low and you want to improve cardiac outcome. In an allergic reaction, blood pressure is close to normal already, so placing the patient in a position of comfort and monitoring vital signs is appropriate.

A 14-year-old female is anxious and feeling "itchy all over" after eating fried food. She is alert, with pale, warm, dry skin. There are hives on her chest and arms. Her lung sounds are clear and no stridor is evident. Her blood pressure is 110/70 mm Hg, her heart rate is 90, and she is breathing 20 times per minute. She has an allergy to peanuts and has an epinephrine autoinjector and diphenhydramine (Benadryl) tablets with her. You should

(A) continue your secondary assessment.

(B) assist the patient with her epinephrine autoinjector.

(C) administer two diphenhydramine tablets.

(D) lay her supine or left lateral recumbent.

The correct answer is Choice (A). You can come to this conclusion based on excluding the other answers: She's not having an anaphylactic reaction, Choice (B); you are not permitted to assist the patient with nonauthorized medications, Choice (C); and having her lie down, Choice (D), won't have any benefit.

Infectious diseases

The immune system also works to protect you from infectious diseases, which are transmitted from one person to the next. Infectious diseases range from illnesses such as a simple cold to very contagious and serious conditions like tuberculosis and meningitis.

Again, the immune system sends a wide variety of white blood cells to seek and destroy the invading contagion. The body also increases its temperature in the hopes of destroying the foreign cells without damaging too many of its own. If the illness is food or water borne, the GI tract will speed up its process, causing diarrhea.

The immune system works very well to ward off infections. However, sometimes the infection is overwhelming, the immune response is too weak, or toxins are produced when the body is killing the foreign cells. What may have started as a localized infection becomes a generalized one, affecting the entire body. The fever and diarrhea cause dehydration. The vascular system reacts to the toxins by dilating. These two events can combine to cause septic shock. This is a dangerous situation that requires hospital care quickly. As with other forms of shock, treat septic shock quickly by keeping the patient supine, providing oxygen when indicated, and maintaining body temperature.

As an EMT, you want to minimize the chance of receiving exposure to an infection. This means staying healthy yourself so that your immune system functions at its best. Keep your vaccinations up to date. Washing your hands thoroughly after each patient contact, even if you wore gloves, is a highly effective way to break the chain of infection.

Patients experience shock for many reasons. Read all the information that's provided in test questions to determine the underlying cause.

A 47-year-old female is unresponsive in her bed. She has had a cough for a week that produces green-colored sputum, and she's had nausea, vomiting, and diarrhea for 36 hours. She has ovarian cancer and diabetes. Her blood pressure is 84/64 mm Hg, her pulse rate is 110, and she's breathing 24 times per minute. Her skin is hot to the touch, pale, and dry. You should

(A) contact her physician for more information about the ovarian cancer.

(B) sit her up to help her breathe; assist with ventilations.

(C) keep a sheet over her and administer supplemental oxygen.

(D) provide oral glucose and transport in a semi-Fowler's position.

The correct answer is Choice (C). The patient presents in shock, possibly from an infection. Treating for shock is appropriate. She is not awake, so giving her anything orally, as Choice (D) suggests, could compromise her airway. Her blood pressure is too low to have her sit up, and assisting ventilations in that position, as indicated by Choice (B), is challenging. Finding out more about her medical history, as Choice (A) suggests, isn't likely to change the way you treat her condition.

Taking Control with the Endocrine System

As in Aesop's fable, the endocrine system can be compared to the nervous system as the tortoise to the hare. They both perform the same general function — control — but unlike the zippiness of the nervous system, the endocrine system is a much slower but longer-lasting control system. That's good, because the endocrine system controls processes that are longer in duration, such as overall growth, and continuous processes, such as balancing blood sugar levels.

Several organs contain glands that make up the endocrine system (see Figure 11-3). Each secretes a hormone that travels through the bloodstream and causes an effect somewhere else in the body. Hormones cause their effects by connecting with receptors that are found on cell membranes. A specific receptor interacts only with a specific hormone, just as a specific key fits a specific lock.

Of all the different organs in the endocrine system (including the ovaries and the testes), the pancreas is the one you should be most familiar with. That's because it contains the glands that secrete the hormone insulin, which regulates how glucose enters cells. Normally the pancreas functions really well, continuously secreting the right amounts depending on the needs of the body. Patients with diabetes lose this ability; they either secrete much less than what is needed or none at all. As you can imagine, this causes havoc with the body. Without enough insulin, the cells starve for the glucose that is passing right by them, because the key to open the lock that allows glucose to pass into the cell is not available.

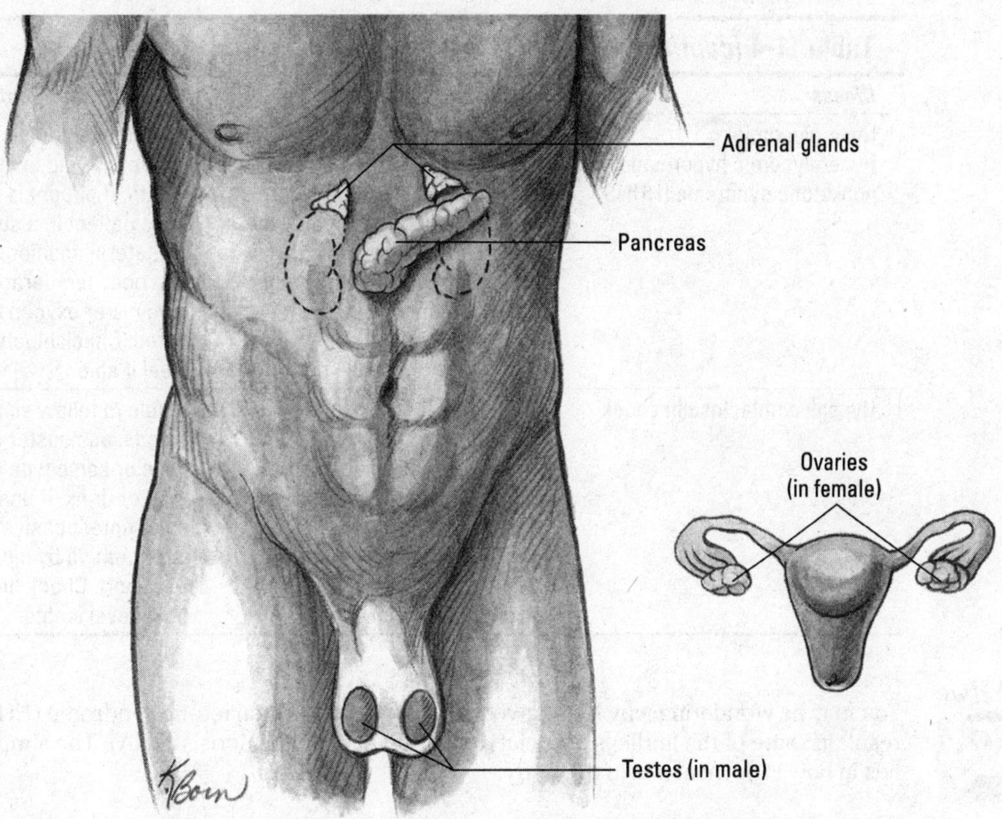

Figure 11-3: The endocrine system.

Table 11-4 lists the different conditions associated with an imbalance between insulin and glucose, their different signs and symptoms, and treatment.

Table 11-4 Diabetic-Related Conditions

Illness	***Signs and Symptoms***	***Specific Treatment***
Hyperglycemia: Diabetic ketoacidosis (DKA)	Warm, flush, dry skin; recent history of excessive eating *(polyphasia),* excessive thirst *(polydipsia),* and excessive urination *(polyuria);* rapid, deep, sighing breathing (Kussmaul's respirations); acetone or sweet smell on the breath; blood sugar level over 300 mg/dL; mental status ranges from confusion to unconsciousness. May show signs of dehydration and shock. Patients are typically insulin dependent.	Place patient in position of comfort. Avoid anything by mouth. If patient is in shock, keep patient in a supine or left lateral position, maintain body temperature, and administer oxygen if indicated. Check blood glucose level if able.

continued

Table 11-4 *(continued)*

Illness	***Signs and Symptoms***	***Specific Treatment***
Hyperglycemia: Hyperglycemic hyperosmolar nonketotic syndrome (HHNS)	Similar to diabetic ketoacidosis, but blood sugar level is higher (600 mg/dL or more) and there is no unusual breathing pattern or smell on the breath. Patients are typically non–insulin dependent.	Place patient in position of comfort. Avoid anything by mouth. If patient is in shock, keep patient in a supine or left lateral position, maintain body temperature, and administer oxygen if indicated. Check blood glucose level if able.
Hypoglycemia: Insulin shock	Cool, pale, and diaphoretic skin; recent history that includes decreased oral intake of food or injecting insulin without eating; blood sugar level below 70 mg/dL; signs may mimic seizures or stroke.	If able to follow simple commands, administer oral glucose or some type of sugary food or drink. If unable to do so or unresponsive, administer nothing by mouth and transport. Check blood glucose level if able.

You may be wondering why hyperglycemic hyperosmolar nonketotic syndrome (HHNS) doesn't result in some of the findings associated with diabetic ketoacidosis (DKA). The simple answer lies in how little insulin is in the body:

- **In DKA,** virtually no insulin is circulating through the body. This condition means that the body cannot use glucose to feed metabolism; it turns to things like fat and protein to create the fuel needed instead. Using these types of molecules isn't very efficient; it creates several byproducts that are toxic if not removed. Some of these toxins are ketone bodies. The body removes these through the respiratory system. The system triggers the exhalation phase of a breath to be longer than normal, like a sigh. These are called *Kussmaul's respirations.* The ketones also have a smell that has been described as "fruity" or "acetone."
- **In HHNS,** enough insulin is circulating to keep the process that DKA causes from happening, but not enough to satisfy all the body's needs. As a result, blood sugar goes much higher than in DKA, and ketones aren't produced in large-enough quantities to trigger Kussmaul's respirations. Unfortunately diabetics with HHNS are much sicker than those with DKA; the death rate is much higher.

Figure 11-4 shows what happens when levels of blood glucose and insulin become unbalanced. When there is more glucose than available insulin, hyperglycemia occurs; when there is not enough glucose, hypoglycemia happens.

A 47-year-old female is responsive only to painful stimulus. Her husband says that she has been feeling ill for several weeks and has been increasingly lethargic in the past 48 hours. She was recently diagnosed with diabetes and takes oral medications to control her blood sugar. Her vital signs include a blood pressure of 104/70 mm Hg, a heart rate of 110, and a breathing rate of 26 times per minute. Her skin is warm and dry. Her pupils are dilated and slow to react, lung sounds are clear, and there is no odor on her breath. Which of the following conditions is most likely the cause of her presentation?

(A) Hypoglycemia

(B) Diabetic ketoacidosis

(C) Hyperglycemic hyperosmolar nonketotic syndrome

(D) Insulin shock

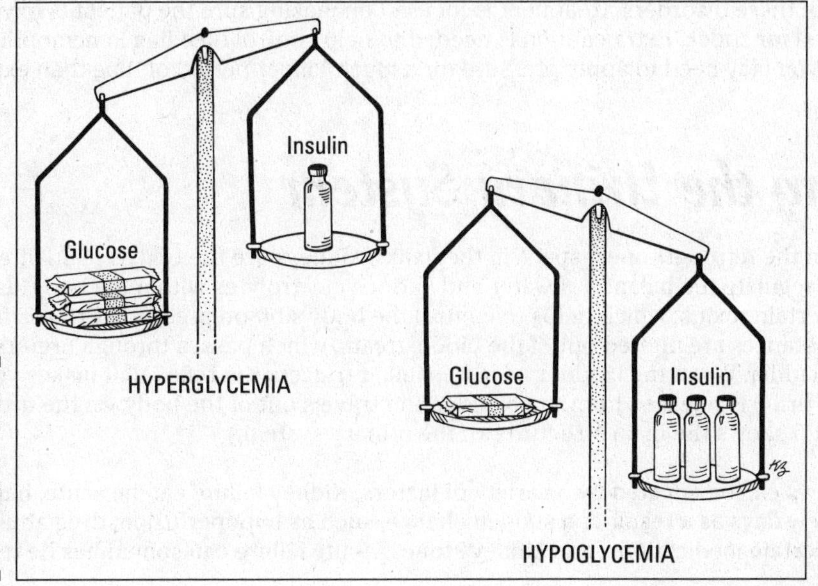

Figure 11-4: Hyperglycemia versus hypoglycemia.

Illustration by Kathryn Born, MA

Choice (C) is the best answer. The long duration of onset is associated with hyperglycemic states, not hypoglycemic as in Choices (A) and (D). You are unable to detect ketone bodies on her breath, and Kussmaul's respirations are not described, ruling out Choice (B).

Getting the Scoop on the Hematologic System (Blood)

Your blood performs several amazing functions. The red blood cells carry most of your oxygen quite efficiently, picking it up only at the alveoli, where it's most abundant, and dropping it off only at the cells, where the concentration is lowest. White blood cells come in different types, but they work in concert to combat infection. Platelets are cells that initiate the clotting process. All of these cells, along with proteins, nutrients, and waste, are carried in plasma, the watery part of blood.

There are several disorders of the blood. However, as an EMT, one condition you should know about is sickle cell disease. Found predominately in African Americans, a genetic mutation causes red blood cells to form abnormally. As a result, these misshapen cells (many look crescent-shaped, or sickle) don't carry oxygen very well. In addition, they can get "stuck" in the capillary beds, causing moderate to severe pain in areas such as bone joints and the abdomen. Treatment is supportive — providing supplemental oxygen, usually low flow with a nasal cannula if oxygen saturation level is low or the patient is in respiratory distress, and keeping the patient as comfortable as possible.

You should also be familiar with clotting disorders:

- **Thrombophilia** is a tendency for blood clots to form, especially in the lower legs. A condition known as deep vein thrombosis (DVT) is often the source of pulmonary emboli, where parts of the clot break off and travel back to the heart, getting lodged in the pulmonary circulation. DVT can cause pain, tenderness, and swelling in the calf area of the lower leg.
- **Hemophilia** is a genetic disease that makes clotting difficult, occurring primarily in men. In other words, patients with hemophilia may spontaneously begin bleeding or, if they become injured, may experience bleeding that is harder to stop.

In either of these disorders, treatment is focused on making sure the patient is oxygenated and treated for shock. Extra caution is needed to help control bleeding in hemophiliac patients; you may need to apply pressure for a much longer period of time than expected.

Considering the Urinary System

Located in the retroperitoneal space in the flanks, kidneys are the body's main filters. They primarily regulate the balance of water and various electrolytes within the body, as well as remove certain toxins, which helps to control the body's blood pressure. Urine is formed as these substances are filtered out of the bloodstream, which passes through ureters into the urinary bladder. When the bladder becomes full, it triggers the reflex that makes you urinate. The urine is released from the bladder and travels out of the body via the urethra. (Figure 11-5 shows the main structures of the urinary system.)

The kidneys can be affected by a variety of factors. Kidney failure can be acute, happening within a few days as a result of a sudden change, such as hypoperfusion, drug abuse, dehydration, certain medications, and kidney stones. Acute failure can sometimes be reversed.

Chronic kidney failure usually results from diseases such as hypertension or diabetes. The condition is usually not reversible. Chronic kidney failure patients require artificial filtering of their blood, called *hemodialysis,* that's done by using a specialized machine. It can also be done at home with special fluids that are pumped into the abdominal cavity. This procedure is called *peritoneal dialysis.*

Signs of kidney failure include swelling around the hands and feet; nausea and vomiting; and in more severe cases, confusion, altered mental status, and seizures.

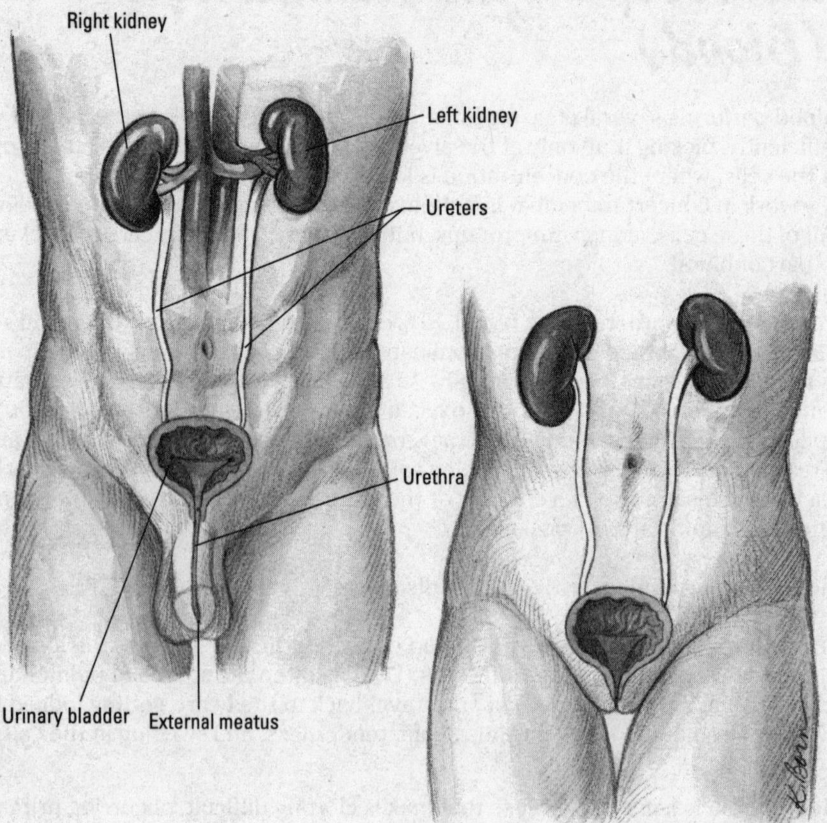

Figure 11-5: The urinary system.

Illustration by Kathryn Born, MA

Dialysis patients are at risk for developing *pulmonary edema* (fluid in the lungs) if they don't perform their treatments according to schedule. If they become short of breath, confirm that their blood pressure is adequate and sit them up to help them breathe. If the blood pressure is too low, lay the patient supine and be prepared to assist ventilations with a bag-valve mask and oxygen.

Patients may not have an ability to urinate normally. In some situations, a urinary catheter, or sterile tube, is passed through the urethra into the bladder, allowing urine to drain passively. Sometimes these catheters can become infected, causing the patient to become sick and weak. Look for signs of fever, chills, and body aches; if there is a Foley bag attached to the catheter, check to see whether the urine is a dark color, very cloudy, or even contains blood. Treatment for this condition is supportive only, keeping the patient comfortable and avoiding anything by mouth.

Sometimes the urine that the kidneys produce is so concentrated that salts clump together, or *precipitate.* As more crystals clump, they form kidney stones that then have to pass through the ureter on the way to the bladder. The stones can get large enough that they become difficult to pass. In addition, they're quite sharp and tear into the sides of the ureter, causing severe pain and bleeding. The pain tends to occur in the flank, the area between the leg and abdomen, and travels downward toward the urethra as the stone passes. In worst-case scenarios, the stone becomes too large to pass, causing urine to back up into the kidney, which can induce kidney failure.

Unfortunately there is little an EMT can do to help with the pain and discomfort of kidney stones. Keep the patient comfortable and transport gently.

An 80-year-old male is lethargic, dizzy, short of breath, and feeling weak. He is bedridden at home after a stroke. According to a caregiver, he has not been well in a week and has had a fever, chills, and body aches. There is a Foley catheter; you note there is a small amount of dark, cloudy urine in the bag. The patient feels very warm to the touch, and has flush, dry skin. His blood pressure is 86/60 mm Hg, his heart rate is 120, and he is breathing 24 times per minute. His oxygen saturation level is 95 percent. Which of the following activities is most appropriate at this point?

(A) Place patient in a semi-Fowler's position and administer high-flow oxygen with a nonrebreather mask.

(B) Place patient in a sitting position and administer low-flow oxygen with a nasal cannula.

(C) Place patient in a supine position and continue with a detailed physical examination.

(D) Place patient in a supine position and prepare to transfer the patient to your gurney.

The best answer is Choice (D). A lot of information is provided in the scenario, but the patient's low blood pressure and fast heart rate indicate shock. The urinary catheter shows signs of infection, which may point to sepsis and septic shock. The patient's blood pressure is too low to have him in a semi-Fowler's or sitting position, as Choices (A) and (B) suggest, and taking more time on-scene, as is the case with Choice (C), delays the time to definitive care. You can further assess the patient in the ambulance during transport.

Cycling through Obstetrics and Gynecology

Obstetrics studies the pregnancy process, from fertilization to delivery. *Gynecology* is the study of diseases that can affect the reproductive system. Together, they represent a variety of conditions specific to the female.

The female reproductive system consists of several organs (see Figure 11-6). A pair of ovaries are the primary organs, generating the hormones that are involved with pregnancy and secondary sex characteristics, and generating eggs. During a menstrual cycle, hormone levels begin to rise, causing an egg to mature and be released roughly halfway through the cycle. The egg is swept into the fallopian tube where, if a viable sperm is present, it may be fertilized and become an embryo. This process is called *conception.*

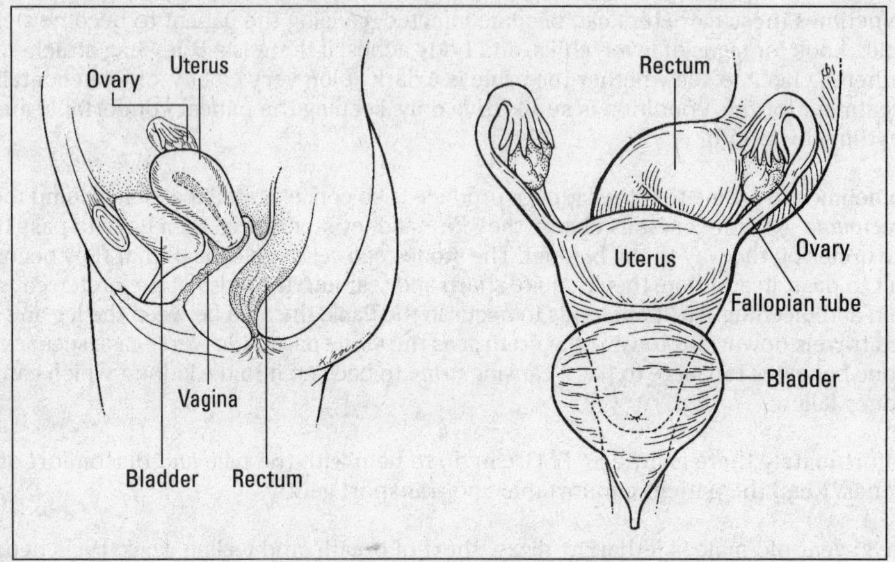

Figure 11-6: The female reproductive system.

Illustration by Kathryn Born, MA

At the same time this process is happening, the uterus thickens in preparation for possible implantation. If no fertilization occurs, the uterus sheds the additional tissue and expels it through the *cervix,* the opening from the uterus to the vagina. This is the bleeding and cramping associated with the menstrual period.

Once the cycle is over, another begins. These cycles are approximately 28 days in length, although the timing varies from one woman to the next.

If fertilization does occur, and the embryo implants within the thickened wall of the uterus, another change in hormone levels signals the body that it is pregnant. Menstrual cycles cease for the next 38 to 40 weeks as the embryo grows and matures. Part of the thickened uterine wall becomes the *placenta,* which transfers oxygen and nutrients from the mother to the developing fetus and carbon dioxide and wastes in the other direction via an umbilical cord. (Figure 11-7 shows the female reproductive system during the menstrual cycle and pregnancy.)

Other changes in the female body also occur, such as enlargement of the mammary glands in the breasts. Many women complain of nausea and vomiting, especially in the first and third phases, or *trimesters,* of pregnancy.

The following sections describe obstetrical and gynecological conditions you need to know about as an EMT.

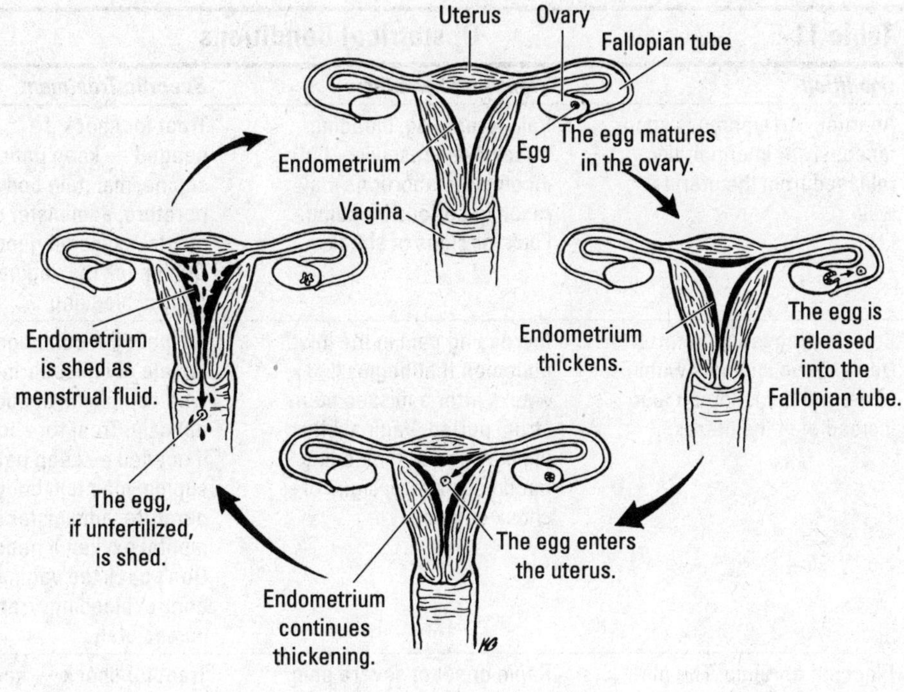

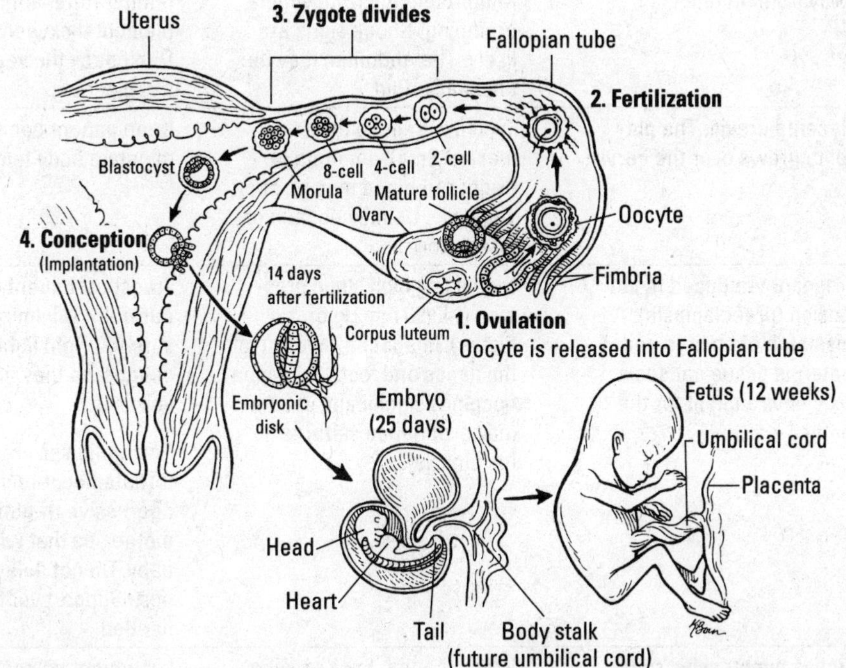

Figure 11-7: The menstrual cycle and pregnancy.

Obstetrics

It's important for a woman to receive regular obstetrical care during pregnancy. Staying healthy and being aware of possible risks that may arise promote a healthy newborn infant. However, several conditions can occur during pregnancy that may require your intervention. Table 11-5 lists these concerns, their signs and symptoms, and possible treatments.

Table 11-5 Obstetrical Conditions

Condition	*Signs and Symptoms*	*Specific Treatment*
Abortion: An embryo is spontaneously or intentionally released from the uterine wall.	Pain, cramping, bleeding. Usually self-resolving, but incomplete abortions may result in serious bleeding. Look for signs of shock.	Treat for shock if needed — keep patient supine, maintain body temperature, administer supplemental oxygen if needed. Don't pack the vagina to control bleeding.
Ectopic pregnancy: A fertilized embryo implants within or around the fallopian tube instead of in the uterus.	Increasing pain in the lower abdomen that begins 6–8 weeks after a missed menstrual period. Vaginal bleeding may occur. If bleeding becomes severe, signs of shock develop.	Suspect the condition in any female of childbearing age who complains of abdominal pain. Treat for shock if needed — keep patient supine, maintain body temperature, administer supplemental oxygen if needed. Don't pack the vagina to control bleeding. Transport immediately.
Placenta abruptio: The placenta abruptly tears partially away from uterine wall.	Rapid onset of severe pain, usually in third trimester. Major bleeding from vagina, cramping. Shock signs are likely. The abdomen may be unusually rigid.	Treat for shock — keep patient supine, maintain body temperature, administer supplemental oxygen if needed. Don't pack the vagina to control bleeding.
Placenta previa: The placenta grows over the cervix.	Typically seen in third trimester. Small amounts of bright red blood may be seen vaginally. Usually no pain or discomfort.	Keep patient comfortable and maintain body temperature.
Pregnancy-induced hypertension (preeclampsia): A mismatch of embryo and maternal tissue causes a toxic environment for the mother.	Increasing high blood pressure (140/90 mm Hg or higher), headache, swelling of the hands and feet. If situation becomes significant, patient may experience seizures (eclampsia).	Transport patient calmly and carefully. Minimize exposure to bright lights or loud sounds, as they may trigger seizures. Eclamptic seizures are life-threatening. Concentrate aggressive treatment on the mother, as that will save the baby. Do not delay transport. Support ventilations if needed.
Supine hypotensive syndrome: Increasing weight of the uterus presses down on the vena cava in the supine position, causing decreased blood flow back to the heart.	When leaning back or lying flat on her back, patient may feel dizzy, faint. Hypotension, tachycardia.	Lie patient on her left side to relieve pressure on vena cava.

Condition	*Signs and Symptoms*	*Specific Treatment*
Trauma during pregnancy: The 20 percent increase of blood volume in the female during pregnancy may mask initial signs of shock. If a mechanism of injury (MOI) exists, assume internal hemorrhage. Later stages of pregnancy also reduce the mother's ability to breathe as the uterus pushes up against the diaphragm. This can cause significant respiratory distress in trauma.	Signs of an MOI to the pregnant abdomen (an improperly worn lap belt in a motor vehicle crash, blunt trauma from a fall or assault, penetrating trauma). Tachycardia, tachypnea. Signs of shock in later stages of bleeding.	Immobilize if needed, place patient onto left side to avoid supine hypotension syndrome. Provide supplemental oxygen if needed. Assist ventilations with bag-valve mask if patient is in respiratory failure. Preserve body temperature by covering patient.

The following sections go into more detail on normal deliveries, abnormal deliveries, and newborn resuscitation.

The normal delivery

Although the majority of newborn deliveries occur within the confines of a labor and delivery suite, there's a chance that you'll be called upon to perform a delivery as an EMT. While that may instill panic in your heart, rest assured that delivery is a normal process and that the vast majority of deliveries are not complicated. Your knowledge, technique, and confidence will go a long way in reassuring the mother-to-be and making the delivery successful.

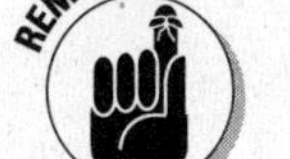
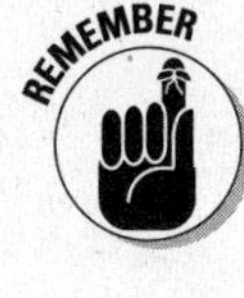

Here are key steps to keep in mind when performing a normal delivery (see Figure 11-8):

1. **There may be a gush of fluid as the amniotic sac breaks and labor begins, as well as a *bloody show* — the mucous plug covering the cervix drops away during a contraction.**
2. **The mother experiences intermittent contractions that become longer and more regular.**

   Contractions are timed from the start of one to the start of the next. These contractions are widening, or *dilating,* the cervix to allow delivery to occur.
3. **Contractions become very strong as delivery begins; the cervix is now fully dilated.**

   If the mother feels the need to move her bowels, delivery is imminent. Prepare your OB kit and find a quiet, private space to perform the delivery.
4. **The baby's head emerges first, face down.**

   Within a few seconds, the head turns sideways as the shoulders twist their way past the pubic bone.

   As soon as the head appears, consider using a bulb syringe to clear the nose and then the mouth of the newborn. Squeeze the bulb first, and then insert the tip into the nares or mouth and release. Repeat until clear.
5. **The head drops down slightly as the next contraction occurs. Very quickly, the shoulders pop past the pubic bone and the newborn is delivered.**

   Use one hand to grasp the legs — the newborn is covered with a slippery substance and is hard to keep a hand on!

6. **Continue to dry and warm the newborn.**

   This action should stimulate spontaneous breathing. The newborn's skin color on the chest should go from a dark red or purple to bright pink within a minute or so of the first breath. The arms and legs may take a few minutes longer to change in coloring.

7. **Note the time of birth and evaluate the newborn's APGAR score at 1 minute and 5 minutes after birth.**

   The highest score is a 10; the lowest is zero. A score of 7 or greater in the first minute is considered normal.

8. **Clamp and cut the newborn's umbilical cord, which is still attached.**

   Clamp the cord with the two clips supplied in the delivery kit. One clamp should be 3 to 4 inches from the newborn's body, the other about 2 to 4 inches away from the first. Cut the cord with a scissor or scalpel.

9. **Wrap the newborn in dry clothing or blankets, and cover the head with the cap in the OB delivery kit.**

10. **If the mother intends to breast-feed her baby, encourage her to do so.**

    Nursing will help the uterus to contract, reducing post-partum (after birth) bleeding.

11. **Prepare for the delivery of the placenta.**

    The placenta delivers 10 to 20 minutes after the newborn. This delivery occurs naturally. Place the placenta into a plastic bag and bring it to the hospital.

12. **Perform fundal massage after delivery to help reduce the amount of bleeding from the uterus.**

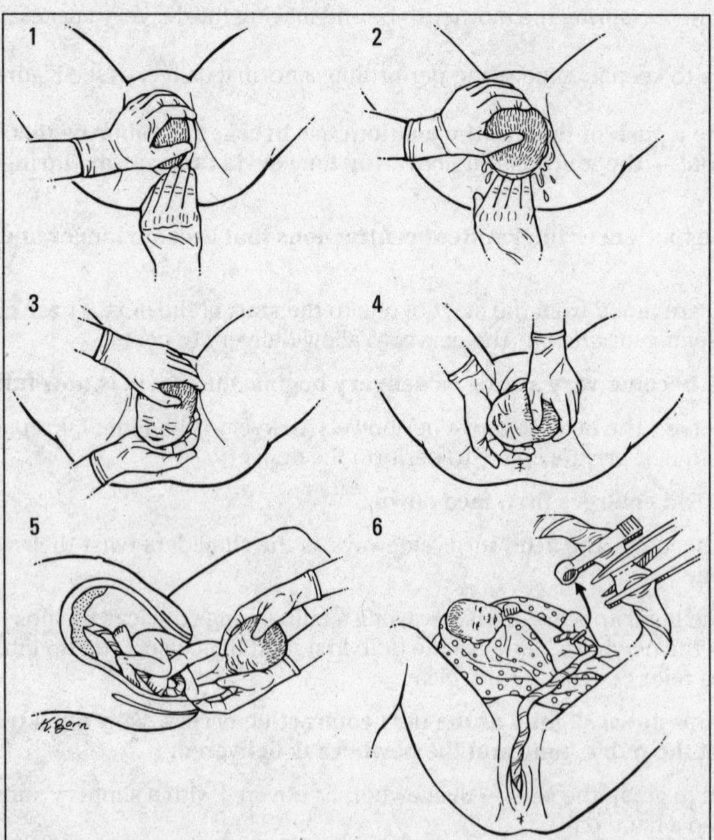

Figure 11-8: A normal delivery.

Illustration by Kathryn Born, MA

An APGAR score is calculated for the newborn at 1 minute, and then 5 minutes after birth, using the following measurements:

	0 points	*1 point*	*2 points*
Activity (muscle tone)	None	Arms and legs weakly moving	Actively moving
Pulse (brachial)	None	Below 100 bpm	Over 100 bpm
Grimace (reflex)	Flaccid	Flexion when stimulated	Active motion
Appearance (skin color)	Blue all over	Body pink, extremities blue	Completely pink
Respirations	None	Slow, irregular	Crying loudly

A score of 7 or better is considered good for a newborn; it's rare for a score of 10 to be assigned right away.

You have just delivered a newborn infant. After suctioning, drying, and warming the newborn, you note that she is crying loudly, is moving all four extremities, and has a brachial pulse of 160. Her arms and legs are blue, while her chest, face, and abdomen are pink. You would rate her APGAR score as a

(A) 3.

(B) 6.

(C) 9.

(D) 12.

The correct answer is Choice (C). She scores a 2 in all categories except for Appearance, in which she scores a 1.

Abnormal deliveries

Unfortunately, on rare occasions a delivery runs into trouble. You can manage a few situations; others require immediate recognition of a serious problem that requires rapid transport to a hospital capable of handling such cases. Table 11-6 details some of the abnormal delivery conditions you may face in the field.

Table 11-6 Abnormal Delivery Conditions

Condition	*Signs and Symptoms*	*Specific Treatment*
Breech presentation	Both legs or buttocks present first.	Cradle the emerging body with one arm while creating a V-shaped space with two fingers to create a small space for the newborn to breathe while the head is still in the birth canal.
Limb presentation	Only one arm or leg appears first.	Nondeliverable scenario. This is a life-threatening event requiring immediate transport.
Multiple births	Strong contractions begin after first birth.	Deliver as normal. There may be more than one placenta to deliver afterwards. Call for additional resources.
Nuchal cord	As head emerges, umbilical cord is wrapped around the neck.	Use palm of one hand to push against the motion of the infant, and use the fingers of the other hand to unloop the cord from around the neck. If you are unable to slip the cord around the head, clamp and cut the cord and remove it from baby's neck.

continued

Table 11-6 *(continued)*

Condition	*Signs and Symptoms*	*Specific Treatment*
Postpartum bleeding	Up to 500 mL is normal. A larger amount is a sign of serious bleeding. Signs of shock may appear.	Treat for shock by keeping patient supine and maintaining body temperature. Administer oxygen if there is respiratory distress or oxygen saturation levels fall below 94 percent. Begin immediate transport.
Prolapsed cord	A loop of the umbilical cord appears first. The newborn's head or shoulder puts pressure on the cord, cutting off circulation.	Nondeliverable scenario. This is a life-threatening event requiring immediate transport. Ensure there is a pulse in the cord. If there is no pulse, place hand in vagina and apply pressure to lift the head off the cord in order to maintain circulation. Placing the mother in a knee-chest position may help take pressure off the cord.

Figure 11-9 shows the different abnormal births described in the preceding table. Regardless which situation presents, remember to remain calm and professional. The mother will be frightened and in pain; your demeanor will help her through a terrifying episode in her life.

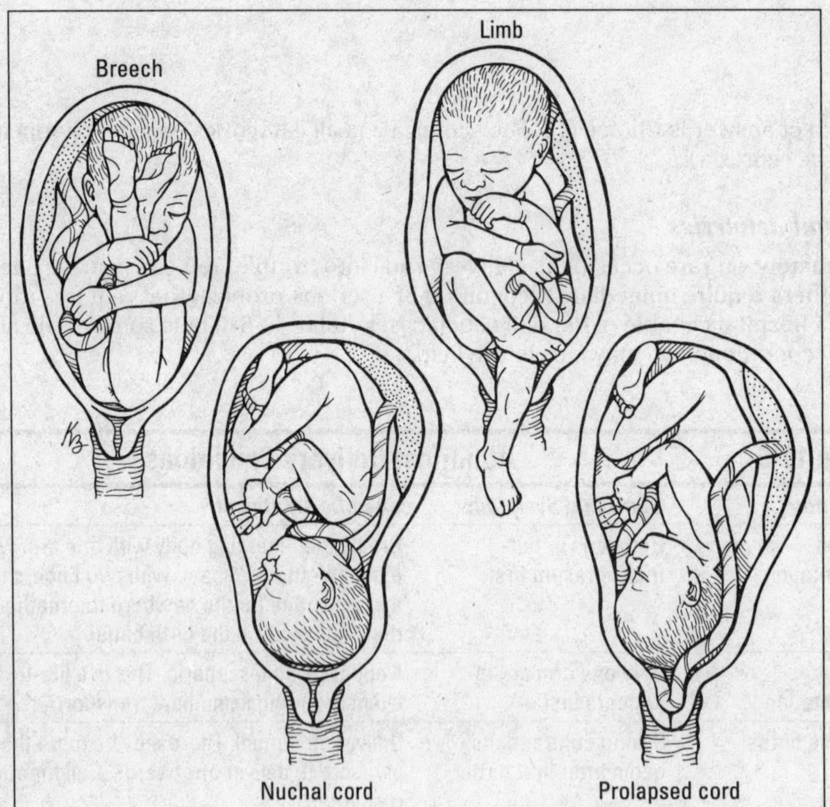

Figure 11-9: Abnormal birth presentations.

A full-term pregnant woman tells you she is in great pain and that she needs to push. When you inspect the vaginal opening, you notice a 5-inch length of umbilical cord protruding from it. You should immediately

(A) open your OB kit and prepare to deliver the newborn.

(B) move the patient to the ambulance and transport rapidly.

(C) check the cord for a pulse.

(D) place the mother in a knee-chest position and deliver the newborn.

The best answer is Choice (C). This is a nondeliverable situation, ruling out Choices (A) and (D). Rapid transport, Choice (B), is indicated, but you want to check for the presence of a pulse in the cord first and, if necessary, relieve the compression of the cord by the newborn's head or shoulders immediately.

Resuscitating a newborn

The vast majority of newborns begin to cry almost immediately after birth. Sometimes there is something abnormal happening, and you need to stimulate the baby to begin breathing or intervene with breathing or circulation. Fortunately, for most newborns, it takes very little effort — you simply have to be aware and prepared to help the infant start breathing. Here are some guidelines (see Figure 11-10):

- An early sign that you may need to resuscitate upon delivery is the presence of meconium. *Meconium* is a dark green/brown bowel movement that is released prematurely in the womb by the fetus in distress. It can cause serious lung illness if inhaled by the newborn. If you see meconium, have bulb syringes ready to suction the nose and mouth well before the newborn takes the first breath.
- The act of drying the skin and suctioning the airway gets most newborns crying and moving. If the newborn is breathing inadequately after 15 to 30 seconds, place an oxygen mask near the face as you continue to suction with a bulb syringe. If breathing doesn't improve or the newborn isn't breathing at all, ventilate with a pediatric bag mask for another 15 to 30 seconds.
- Check for a brachial pulse or for a pulse at the base of the umbilical cord where it enters the newborn's abdomen. A healthy newborn's rate is over 120 beats per minute. A rate between 60 and 100 should trigger the use of a bag-valve mask, because a rate that low is very likely to be respiratory driven. At a rate of less than 60, you need to compress the chest with a two-thumb encircling chest technique. Compress at a rate of at least 100 and ventilate once every three compressions.

  Check the rate every minute or so. It may take only that long to have the heart rate rise to a safe rate and the newborn breathe normally. Regardless, initiate transport as soon as possible.

Gynecology

There are a few female-specific medical conditions you should review. Pelvic inflammatory disease (PID) is an infection that affects the female reproductive system. Bacteria enter the body through the vaginal canal, usually during intercourse, and can infect the uterus, fallopian tubes, and ovaries, causing pain, foul-smelling vaginal discharge, and fever. You may need to move the patient gently and help her achieve a position of comfort during transport.

Sexually transmitted diseases are not life-threatening, but can cause significant discomfort and embarrassment. Chlamydia symptoms may range from nonexistent to low back pain, painful intercourse, and bleeding in between menstrual periods. Gonorrhea may cause painful urination, cramping, and produce a yellow or bloody discharge. Genital herpes may cause painful sores to form within the vagina. Bacterial vaginosis can also cause pain and produce a fishy-smelling odor and discharge. Treatment is supportive only.

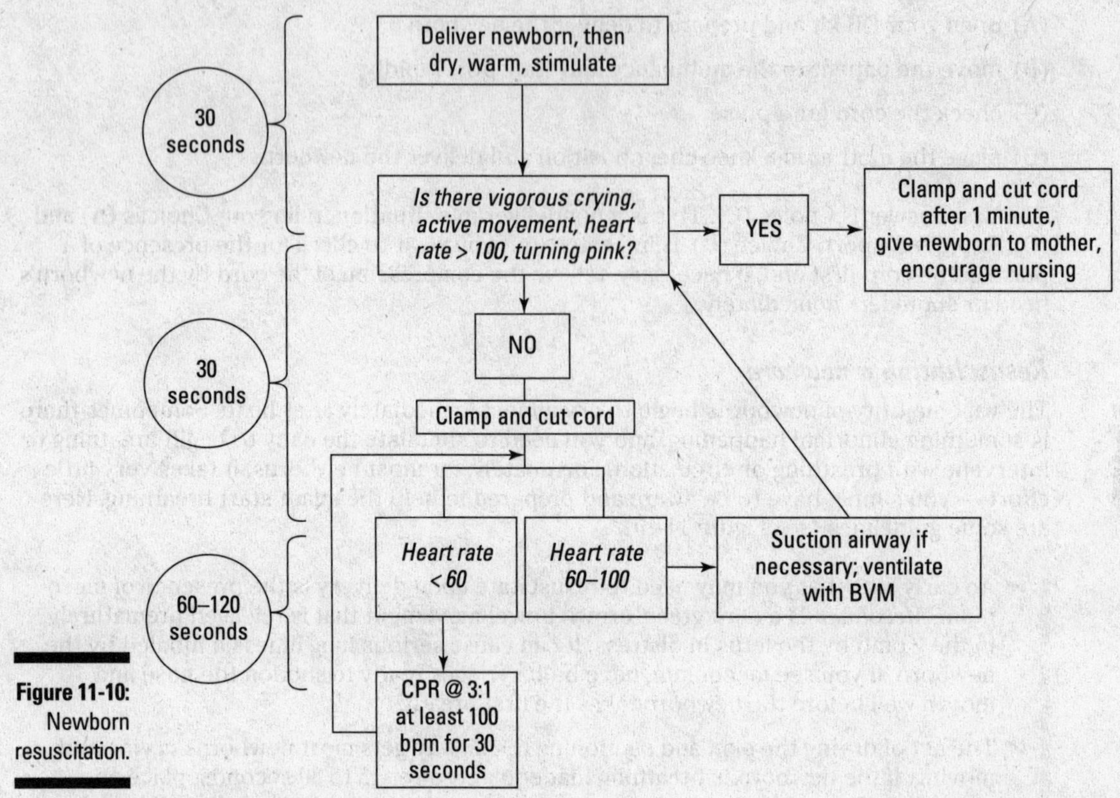

Figure 11-10: Newborn resuscitation.

Vaginal bleeding may be caused by a wide range of conditions, including trauma, spontaneous abortion, ectopic pregnancy, and simply abnormal menstruation. If blood loss is significant, shock may result. It's important to remember that most vaginal bleeding can't be controlled by direct pressure; you should not pack the vaginal canal with dressings or other objects. If necessary, place large absorbent pads at the vaginal opening to help contain the blood. If shock is present, keep the patient supine or left lateral recumbent and maintain body temperature. You may need to administer oxygen if there is respiratory distress or the patient's oxygen saturation level is low.

Boning Up on the Musculoskeletal System

You should be familiar with the basic structure of bone; I review the musculoskeletal system in more depth in Chapter 12.

Bone is a living tissue, made of the protein collagen, which forms a soft framework that looks a little like a sponge. Calcium fills in the gaps, making the outside of bone denser and harder. Bones are spongier toward the center, especially long bones like those found in the arms and legs. Red blood cells are formed within the spongy center and enter the circulatory system.

Most of the bone fractures EMTs see are from trauma mechanisms, such as falls and crashes (covered in Chapter 12). That's because it takes a fair amount of force to cause the bone to fail.

There are some nontraumatic situations where bones become more brittle. Osteoporosis is one disease that causes minerals such as calcium to leach out of the bone structure. It affects women much more than men. In more severe cases, bones can become so brittle that they can break with very little force or even spontaneously fracture. You treat this fracture like any other: Carefully evaluate for distal pulses and sensation, and then splint and immobilize the injury.

Understanding Toxicology

Toxicology is the study of toxic or poisonous substances and their effects on the body. The signs and symptoms associated with toxic exposure and poisoning range very widely, from simple annoyances to life-threatening conditions. As an EMT, your primary goals are to ensure your own safety and identify the possibility of a toxic exposure while preserving the patient's airway, breathing, and circulation.

Toxins and poisons enter the body through the following routes:

- **Ingestion:** Swallowing
- **Inhalation:** Being breathed in
- **Absorption:** Passing through the surface of the skin
- **Injection:** Directly entering the blood stream

As a rule, the fastest route is inhalation; the slowest is ingestion. However, depending upon the substance, any of these routes can cause serious harm.

One number you should always keep handy while working is the one to reach your local poison control center. There are 56 centers across the United States; the universal number is 800-222-1222. Poison control staff have immediate access to a tremendous amount of information about poisonous substances. They can help you identify the substance, determine how dangerous the situation is, and decide whether the patient should seek further attention. They're a great resource for EMS providers in the field.

Table 11-7 lists several toxic and poisonous substances that you should be familiar with, along with their symptoms and treatments.

Table 11-7 Toxic and Poisonous Substances

Substance	*Signs and Symptoms*	*Specific Treatment*
Alcohol ingestion	Recreational sedative that causes initial euphoria followed by sleepiness and an altered level of consciousness; produces slurred speech, loss of balance and coordination, nausea, vomiting. Can dangerously magnify effects of other drugs, especially if they're also sedatives.	Protect airway; prepare to suction if needed. Assist ventilations if needed. Try to determine whether other drugs were involved. Some intoxicated patients can be unpredictably violent; be aware of your own safety.
Carbon monoxide inhalation	Gas that causes headache, nausea, vomiting, sleepiness that worsens into unconsciousness.	If found in a confined space, evacuate patient and yourself to a safe place. Provide high-flow oxygen and assist ventilation if necessary. Consider transport to a bariatric chamber.

continued

Table 11-7 *(continued)*

Substance	***Signs and Symptoms***	***Specific Treatment***
Food poisoning	Onset from within a few minutes to hours of ingestion. Vomiting, diarrhea, abdominal pain, cramping.	Suction as needed. In cases of botulism, patients may suffer respiratory arrest and require assistance with ventilations.
Marijuana, hallucinogens	Mind-altering substances that can be inhaled or ingested. Can cause paranoia, anxiety.	Offer reassurance and remain calm to help reduce anxiety in patient. Try to determine whether there is other drug use.
Narcotic overdose by ingestion, injection, or inhalation	Prescribed painkillers and illegal heroin cause euphoria followed by sleepiness and an altered level of consciousness. In larger doses, patients stop breathing. Constricted pupils; loss of gag reflex; injection sites (track marks) on arms, legs.	If the patient is "nodding," gently stimulate him to keep him breathing spontaneously. If respiratory arrest occurs, insert oropharyngeal airway or nasopharyngeal airway and begin bag-valve-mask ventilations.
Nerve agents	Include pesticides and fertilizers that can be absorbed through skin and chemical weapons that are inhaled. Cause a series of signs that can be remembered as SLUDGE-M (salivation, lacrimation, urination, defecation, GI motility, emesis, and meiosis — constricted pupils).	For a nerve agent attack, EMTs may have specific antidote kits containing atropine autoinjectors to combat the effects on themselves. For pesticides and fertilizers, decontaminate the patient prior to care. Suction as needed and assist ventilations if necessary.
Sedative-hypnotic drug ingestion	Prescription sedative overdoses cause sleepiness that worsens into unconsciousness. Breathing may be compromised. Pupils may become dilated.	Maintain airway patency, ventilate as needed.
Stimulant ingestion	Stimulants such as cocaine, methamphetamines, MDMA, bath salts, and crack can cause paranoia, severe tachycardia, hypertension, and high fevers and can precipitate heart attacks and strokes. Patients may have chest pain, difficulty breathing, and profuse sweating.	Manage airway and breathing; assist ventilations if needed. Be careful of potentially violent behavior.

Handling Psychiatric Disorders and Behavioral Emergencies

At some point in their lives, most people experience some type of behavioral event that makes them act out of the ordinary. In most situations, acute, severe stress is the trigger. Once the trigger is pulled and the stress passes, they return to their normal behavior.

Sometimes the stress is so great that it results in a behavior so out of the ordinary that others become frightened or so concerned that the person is out of control that they contact EMS or law enforcement for assistance.

In many of the cases, you can reassure the patient by speaking with her empathetically and professionally. After the crisis passes, the patient can be more cooperative and coherent, which makes things much easier for you to manage.

However, in some situations you're obligated to take some form of action. A patient may experience acute psychosis — literally being out of touch with reality. Some of your patients may be suicidal, wanting to kill themselves to escape the emotional pain they're experiencing. Others may become so agitated that they try to hurt others, usually unintentionally.

In this state, patients aren't able to determine what's best for them. Law enforcement or authorized social and healthcare providers may need to implement an involuntary hold, which forces the patient to receive acute mental care. As an EMT, you do not have this ability in most states. However, you work alongside others who do, and you help transport the patient to an appropriate care facility.

You may need to physically restrain the potentially violent patient. Doing so is risky and requires training, practice, and a team of people to restrain the patient safely. Don't try to restrain a patient by yourself or with just your partner.

If your patient's behavior is out of the ordinary, take a few minutes first to make sure that there isn't a medical reason. Seizures, low blood sugar, stroke, and brain trauma are just a few reasons why someone may act bizarre or violently. Agitated delirium is an extreme example of irrational behavior with real physical manifestations. These patients may experience hypertension, tachycardia, diaphoresis, dilated pupils, or hallucinations and are generally very hyperactive. If you have to restrain them for their safety and your own, be sure that they end up supine and not prone for transport.

There are many psychiatric disorders. You should consider them just as you do any medical disorder; they require the same level of assessment and compassion. Diseases range from depression and anxiety disorders to bipolar disorder and schizophrenia. You aren't expected to be an expert in understanding these diseases; you primarily want to be able to ensure your safety and the safety of the patient, just as you would with any other patient.

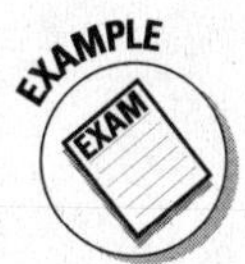

Police have subdued a 33-year-old male who was "acting suspiciously" at a convenience store. They report that as they approached the suspect, he resisted them and a fight ensued. You find the suspect face down on the floor of the store, with his hands cuffed behind his back. He is breathing rapidly and deeply, and his skin is warm, diaphoretic, and pale. He is talking rapidly and is not making any sense; he does not answer your questions. His pulse rate is 130, and his blood pressure is 180/110 mm Hg. Which of the following activities is most appropriate for this situation?

(A) Remove the handcuffs, sit the patient on the gurney, and administer high-flow oxygen with a nonrebreather mask.

(B) Keep him prone on the gurney with the handcuffs, and perform a secondary assessment.

(C) Apply soft restraints, remove the handcuffs, and restrain him supine on the gurney.

(D) Have police transport the patient to the hospital.

The best answer is Choice (C). Medical personnel use a variety of soft restraints to control the movements of an uncooperative patient. Because it's unclear what is happening with the patient, you need to maintain physical restraints, eliminating Choice (A). Keeping the patient prone, Choice (B), may compromise his ability to breathe. This patient has altered mental status and a very high blood pressure; he needs to be medically monitored during transport, making Choice (D) unlikely.

Practice Questions about Medical and Obstetrics/Gynecology Fundamentals

The following practice questions are similar to the EMT exam's questions about medical fundamentals. Read each question carefully, and then select the answer choice that most correctly answers the question.

1. A 50-year-old female is alert but has difficulty speaking clearly and is unable to sit up by herself. She has difficulty raising her right arm when compared to the left. She has a history of diabetes and takes insulin every day. Which of the following is the most likely cause of her presentation?

   (A) Hypoglycemia

   (B) Stroke

   (C) Generalized seizure

   (D) Spinal cord disorder

2. A young adult male presents on the floor of a public bathroom. His skin is warm, diaphoretic, and pale. He responds to painful stimulus by attempting to roll away. There is a scant amount of blood-tinged sputum around his mouth, and he is breathing deeply at 20 times per minute. What should you do next?

   (A) Position him on his side and suction with a rigid catheter.

   (B) Position him supine and assist his ventilations with a bag-valve mask and oxygen.

   (C) Sit him up and provide supplemental oxygen.

   (D) Apply spinal precautions and immobilize to a board.

3. Family members report that an elderly male has garbled speech, difficulty swallowing, and a right-sided facial droop. They also report a similar episode a week earlier that went away on its own. He has a history of diabetes and hypertension. Which of the following treatment plans is most appropriate?

   (A) Encourage the patient to drink orange juice to increase his blood sugar level, reevaluate mental status, and transport if necessary.

   (B) Suggest that the patient is experiencing a transient ischemic attack (TIA) and assist in making arrangements to have patient seen at an urgent care center.

   (C) Suggest immediate transport to an emergency department capable of managing acute stroke.

   (D) Perform a detailed physical examination to determine whether there are any related injuries, immobilize if necessary, and transport to the patient's preferred hospital.

4. You arrive on-scene to find a 25-year-old female unconscious on the floor of her bedroom with generalized tonic-clonic muscle activity. Her roommate reports that when she returned home from school, she heard strange noises from the room and found the patient in the same condition you do. Her skin is hot to the touch, pale, and diaphoretic. She has a rapid pulse at the radial wrist, and you can't see the patient breathe. What is the best approach to managing the patient's condition?

   (A) Expose the patient and apply cold packs to her neck, armpits, and groin.

   (B) Administer supplemental oxygen with a nasal cannula.

   (C) Begin chest compressions and ventilate with a bag-valve mask.

   (D) Extricate the patient and begin transport as soon as possible.

5. A 22-year-old male is at a party when he experiences rapid onset of a severe headache, left ear ringing, and nausea. You find him vomiting in the bathroom and unable to stand. You detect the odor of alcohol on his breath and his pupils are constricted. Which of the following conditions is most likely causing this presentation?

(A) Seizure

(B) Alcohol poisoning

(C) Drug overdose

(D) Stroke

6. After transporting a patient with a fever, vomiting, and a productive cough, what would be the best way for you to reduce the chance of being infected?

(A) Hose down the interior of the ambulance with hot water.

(B) Wash your hands with soap and water.

(C) Spray your hands and face with disinfectant.

(D) Leave the patient compartment fan on for several hours.

7. A 67-year-old male has abdominal pain and is cool, diaphoretic, and pale after vomiting several times over 20 minutes. There is a large amount of emesis that is dark red in color. You suspect that the bleeding is most likely due to

(A) a peptic ulcer.

(B) esophageal varices.

(C) peritonitis.

(D) liver disease.

8. An adult female is curled up on her couch, complaining of severe abdominal pain. The pain is spread throughout her abdomen and hurts worse when she coughs. She has a fever and is nauseous. You suspect her presentation is due to

(A) ectopic pregnancy.

(B) pancreatitis.

(C) dehydration.

(D) peritonitis.

9. A 40-year-old female has a rapid onset of sharp, right upper abdominal pain that radiates to her shoulder blades. She is nauseous but does not need to vomit. Her last meal was about 45 minutes ago. She takes medications for a peptic ulcer. You suspect that she is experiencing

(A) a new ulcer.

(B) acute coronary syndrome.

(C) a gallbladder attack.

(D) a bowel obstruction.

10. An elderly male is complaining of feeling faint and short of breath during a dialysis treatment. His radial pulse is weak and rapid. His skin is cool, dry, and pale. His breathing is rapid and shallow. You should

(A) discontinue dialysis, position the patient supine, and administer supplemental oxygen.

(B) complete dialysis while monitoring the patient's vital signs closely.

(C) place the patient in a sitting position, maintain his body temperature, and finish the dialysis treatment.

(D) have the patient drink fluids and eat a sandwich while the staff discontinues the dialysis treatment.

11. A 22-year-old male has been having increasing, left-sided groin pressure for 8 hours. The discomfort has become so severe that he is unable to sit for any period of time. His urine is dark red in color and contains small clots. You suspect his presentation is most likely due to

(A) a sexually transmitted disease.

(B) a kidney infection.

(C) a kidney stone.

(D) testicular torsion.

12. A teacher reports a 12-year-old child had been "acting out" so she sent him to the school office. The principal called for EMS after the child appeared disoriented and pale. You find the patient to be confused to time and location though he follows commands. His skin feels clammy, and he has a rapid radial pulse. Which of the following treatment plans would be best?

(A) Supplemental oxygen; transport

(B) Heat packs to his armpits and abdomen; supplemental oxygen

(C) Supplemental oxygen; patient's prescribed epinephrine autoinjector; transport

(D) Oral glucose; supplemental oxygen; contact parents

13. A 56-year-old female has had worsening nausea and increasing weakness over the past week. Her husband reports she has been hungry and thirsty, even though her food and fluid intake have been normal. She is responsive to verbal stimulus and is confused to time. Her skin is warm, dry, and flush. Your best treatment approach is to

(A) place the patient in position of comfort and administer supplemental oxygen.

(B) encourage the patient to drink fluids.

(C) expose the patient to promote cooling and administer supplemental oxygen.

(D) administer oral glucose and supplemental oxygen.

14. A 33-year-old female has abdominal and joint pain that has worsened over the past 12 hours. Her pulse rate is 100, and her blood pressure is 116/78 mm Hg. She is breathing 22 times per minute and feels short of breath. Her skin feels warm and dry. Which of the following conditions would most likely explain her presentation?

(A) Hyperglycemia

(B) Sickle cell crisis

(C) Peritonitis

(D) Ovarian cyst

15. An adult male presents with hives on his arms and chest and severe itching after being stung by a wasp. He is alert, his blood pressure is 156/84 mm Hg, and he is breathing at 20 times per minute. You should

(A) administer the patient's prescribed epinephrine autoinjector.

(B) administer supplemental oxygen.

(C) administer diphenhydramine (Benedryl) orally.

(D) transport with lights and siren.

16. A 40-year-old female is short of breath shortly after eating lunch at a new restaurant. She has abdominal cramping and diarrhea. You auscultate wheezing in both lung fields. Her blood pressure is 80 by palpation, and her skin feels cool and clammy. You suspect

(A) food poisoning.

(B) colitis.

(C) gallbladder disease.

(D) anaphylaxis.

17. A welder has a rapid onset of a severe headache, body aches, nausea, and vomiting after finishing a shift on a container ship. She has a rapid radial pulse, pale skin, and is breathing 24 times per minute. You should

(A) complete your exam and transport.

(B) administer oxygen via a nasal cannula.

(C) administer oxygen via a nonrebreather mask.

(D) administer acetaminophen and encourage her to drink fluids.

18. Police have detained an adult male for smashing a storefront window. He is prone with his hands handcuffed behind his back. He is hot to the touch, diaphoretic, and pale. He screams and curses at you. You note his pupils are dilated, his radial pulse is rapid, and he is tachypneic. You should transport the patient

(A) in the same position, on the floor of the ambulance.

(B) on his side, arms handcuffed in front, on the gurney.

(C) prone on the gurney, using soft restraints.

(D) supine on the gurney, using soft restraints.

19. At a party, a young adult female is passed out in a bathroom stall. She is unresponsive to a sternal rub and is breathing at a rate of 6 breaths per minute. Her pupils are 2 mm in size, equal, and nonreactive to light. You find several pill bottles nearby. Her pulse rate is 110 and blood pressure is 122/78 mm Hg. You suspect

(A) narcotic overdose.

(B) barbiturate overdose.

(C) hypoglycemia.

(D) alcohol poisoning.

20. Law enforcement officers report an adult male was staggering and combative outside of a bar. He is sitting in the back of a police car, his arms restrained by handcuffs. You detect the odor of an alcoholic beverage on the man's breath. You see no signs of trauma. He is confused and verbally abusive. You should

(A) have the police transport the person to a hospital.

(B) perform a full assessment.

(C) keep the patient in the handcuffs and transport by ambulance.

(D) allow the police to take the person to jail.

21. Staff at a nursing home report that an 81-year-old resident began to yell and be physically uncooperative about 5 hours earlier. He has a history of Alzheimer's disease, diabetes, hypertension, and alcohol abuse. He is generally cheerful and quiet. You don't find anything unusual during your physical examination. Which of the following explanations for his behavioral change should be your strongest suspicion?

(A) He may be experiencing a stroke that has changed his personality.

(B) There has been a sudden worsening of his Alzheimer's disease.

(C) He is having an episode of hyperglycemia.

(D) He is intoxicated.

22. Family members call 911 for a 75-year-old woman who has overdosed on her blood pressure medications. They report she is typically alert and, other than hypertension, is in good health. The patient appears embarrassed and says she forgot that she had taken her medication earlier and took another dose. You look at the medication bottle and notice that the prescription was filled two days ago and it is empty. Which of the following questions would be important to ask in this situation?

(A) Do you have any other medical history?

(B) Are you allergic to anything?

(C) Are you trying to harm or kill yourself?

(D) Have you been more forgetful recently?

23. A 55-year-old female was sexually assaulted and beaten. She says that she is bleeding from her vagina. You observe that she has lacerations to her head and right forearm that are oozing blood. You should

(A) treat the head and arm injuries only.

(B) apply spinal precautions and immobilize to a long backboard.

(C) bandage the head and arm lacerations, and ask if you can inspect her pelvic area.

(D) inspect the vagina and apply direct pressure to control any bleeding.

24. A 22-year-old female has been complaining of fever and body chills and aches for 24 hours. She has lower abdominal pressure that worsens with palpation. She describes a yellowish vaginal discharge that has an unpleasant odor. Walking makes the discomfort worse. She is sexually active and takes birth control pills. Which condition would best explain her presentation?

(A) Ovarian cyst

(B) Pelvic inflammatory disease

(C) Syphillis

(D) Urinary tract infection

25. A full-term, pregnant woman is in active labor. When she pushes during the next contraction, you notice the top of the head appear, and the umbilical cord appears to be wrapped around the neck. You should

    (A) position the woman on her hands and knees and insert gloved fingers into the birth canal to help the newborn breathe.

    (B) encourage the woman to push harder and cause the cord to slip off.

    (C) stop the forward motion of the delivery with one hand over the newborn's head, while trying to slip the cord off the neck with your other hand.

    (D) use a scalpel to cut the cord, being careful not to injure the newborn.

26. A pregnant woman in her 36th week of pregnancy has severe pain and cramping in her abdominal region. You observe a large number of used tampons and sanitary napkins that are bloody. There is a watery, bloody discharge from her vagina. She is cool, pale, and clammy. Her pulse rate is 130, her blood pressure is 86/50 mm Hg, and she is breathing 25 times per minute. You should

    (A) insert trauma dressings into the vagina and apply direct pressure.

    (B) position her supine, administer high-flow oxygen, and preserve her body temperature.

    (C) open an OB kit and prepare for imminent delivery.

    (D) inspect the tampons and sanitary napkins to estimate the blood loss.

27. A woman is in her 39th week of pregnancy. She is having contractions that are 15 to 20 seconds long, with 2- to 3-minute breaks in between. Which of the following questions will best help you decide whether to transport or prepare for delivery?

    (A) Are you having twins?

    (B) Has your water broken?

    (C) Do you feel the urge to move your bowels?

    (D) Is this your first child?

Answers and Explanations

Use this answer key to score the practice questions in the preceding section. The explanations give you insight into why the correct answer is better than the other choices.

1. **B.** Hypoglycemia, Choice (A), usually presents with altered mental status, along with possible stroke-like symptoms; however, this patient doesn't have an altered mental status. A generalized seizure, Choice (C), also has a change in mental status. A spinal cord injury, Choice (D), doesn't present such an array of signs.

2. **A.** He is breathing with an adequate rate and tidal volume, so use of a bag-valve mask, Choice (B), isn't necessary. He isn't conscious enough to have him sit up and be supported, Choice (C), nor do you know whether his blood pressure is high enough to support that. There is no information to support spinal precautions, Choice (D), at this moment.

3. **C.** Although it's possible that the patient may be experiencing hypoglycemia, Choice (A), the presenting signs also point toward an acute stroke, which requires rapid intervention at a stroke receiving hospital. The same logic goes for the TIA, Choice (B). You want to minimize your time on-scene rather than spend time performing a full assessment and treatment, Choice (D).

4. **D.** Based on the roommate's description and the patient's signs and symptoms, it appears that the patient is in status epilepticus. This life-threatening emergency means early transport is necessary. Delaying transport, as is the case in Choices (A) and (C), delays definitive care. You need to assist her ventilations, not just provide supplemental oxygen, as indicated in Choice (B).

5. **D.** The patient's signs are consistent with a hemorrhagic stroke. Alcohol, Choice (B), doesn't constrict pupils, and a narcotic overdose, Choice (C), causes respiratory depression and altered mental status. The patient's presentation is not consistent with a seizure, Choice (A).

6. **B.** The best way to break the chain of infection is with consistent hand washing, Choice (B). The other choices are either unrealistic, ineffective, or, frankly, dangerous.

7. **B.** A peptic ulcer, Choice (A), bleeds within the stomach, where the blood is digested by the stomach's acid. This causes any hematemesis to appear dark and have a coffee-ground-like texture. Peritonitis, Choice (C), is the irritation of the peritoneum, which doesn't cause bleeding into the gastrointestinal tract. Liver disease, Choice (D), may cause excessive pressure to build within the esophageal varices, but it's the varices that are causing the patient's presentation.

8. **D.** Peritonitis, Choice (D), is the inflammation of the peritoneum, which hurts worse when stretched. Curling into a fetal position helps reduce the stretching and the associated pain. The other conditions, Choices (A), (B), and (C), are not typically relieved by body positioning.

9. **C.** The signs and symptoms are most related to cholecystitis, or inflammation of the gallbladder, Choice (C). The condition worsens shortly after a meal that's high in fat. A bowel obstruction, Choice (D), causes pain to come on slowly, if at all. The signs could point to acute coronary syndrome, Choice (B), but it's less likely. The same goes for an ulcer, Choice (A), where the pain in located more centrally or in the left upper quadrant.

10. **A.** The patient is showing signs of shock, possibly from too much fluid being removed by dialysis. Completing dialysis, as indicated in Choices (B) and (C), may make it worse. Sitting him up, Choice (C), may worsen his blood pressure. It's best not to have the patient eat or drink anything, Choice (D), when he's this ill.

11. **C.** The signs and symptoms point to a kidney stone, Choice (C), which is really more of a crystal with sharp edges. As it passes through the ureter, it tears into its wall, causing bleeding to occur. Testicular torsion, Choice (D), does not cause this, nor does a sexually transmitted disease, Choice (A). A kidney infection, Choice (B), may cause discomfort that's located more posteriorly and higher in the back.

12. **D.** The patient's presentation and history of the present illness is indicative of acute hypoglycemia, or insulin shock. There are no indications of anaphylaxis, Choice (C), or hypothermia, Choice (B). Oral glucose has no negative effect on someone who is able to follow commands and can self-administer the medication, per Choice (D); it's a more effective treatment compared to Choice (A).

13. **A.** The presentation is consistent with hyperglycemia. While oral glucose, Choice (D), isn't likely to hurt the patient, it's not necessary. The patient should receive nothing by mouth, Choice (B), while in your care. The presentation is inconsistent with a heat emergency, Choice (C).

14. **B.** In sickle cell crisis, Choice (B), misshapen red blood cells clump together in the smaller arteries, causing ischemia in local areas of tissue, which is especially felt in the patient's joints and abdomen. Hyperglycemia, Choice (A), takes days to weeks to develop. An ovarian cyst, Choice (D), doesn't cause joint pain, nor does peritonitis, Choice (C).

15. **B.** This patient is experiencing an allergic reaction only. His respiratory rate is slightly elevated, which indicates supplemental oxygen, Choice (B). There are no signs of anaphylaxis, so epinephrine, Choice (A), is contraindicated. You are not authorized by scope of practice to administer Benedryl, Choice (C). An allergic reaction is not life-threatening; emergency transport, Choice (D), is unnecessary.

16. **D.** This patient is exhibiting signs of anaphylaxis, Choice (D). Food poisoning, Choice (A), doesn't cause profound hypotension and bronchoconstriction. Neither does colitis, Choice (B), nor cholecystitis, Choice (C).

17. **C.** The patient is exhibiting signs of carbon monoxide poisoning. High-flow oxygen, Choice (C), is needed to begin displacing carbon monoxide from the red blood cells. Low-flow oxygen, Choice (B), is less effective. Not administering oxygen, Choice (A), isn't helpful. You are not authorized by scope of practice to administer acetaminophen, Choice (D).

18. **D.** To you, the person is a patient, not a prisoner. You must treat him as you do other patients. EMTs don't use hard restraints such as handcuffs, as suggested in Choices (A) and (B), to restrain patients. Keeping the patient prone, Choice (C), may compromise the airway or cause respiratory failure.

19. **A.** The patient's constricted pupils, slow respiratory rate, and altered mental status are consistent with a narcotic overdose, Choice (A). Barbiturates, Choice (B), cause dilated pupils. Neither hypoglycemia, Choice (C), nor alcohol poisoning, Choice (D), causes pupil constriction.

20. **B.** To you, this is a patient, not a prisoner. He is entitled to the same level of care as any other patient. Several medical conditions may explain the patient's presentation, including overdose, severe intoxication, hyperglycemia, and seizures, to name a few. You, not the police, need to transport the patient in your unit to a hospital, eliminating Choices (A) and (D). You should use soft restraints, not handcuffs, Choice (C).

21. **A.** A dementia-related disease doesn't abruptly change, as Choice (B) suggests. Hyperglycemia, Choice (C), takes days to weeks to develop. There are no signs to indicate acute intoxication, Choice (D).

22. **C.** Elements of this scenario description (age, and inconsistency between the patient's story and the empty medication bottle) should make you suspect a possible suicide attempt. You should eventually ask about her medical history and allergies, Choices (A) and (B), but first you need to address the specifics of the situation.

23. **C.** You should evaluate all the patient's traumatic injuries, not just a few, Choice (A), and ensure that no significant bleeding is occurring. Bleeding from the vagina cannot be controlled by direct pressure, Choice (D). There are no indications of a spinal injury, Choice (B).

24. **B.** The fever, abdominal discomfort, and vaginal discharge point to some type of infection, Choice (B). The discharge is not consistent with the other choices.

25. **C.** A nuchal cord can be quickly removed from the infant's neck by slipping a finger under it and pulling it free. Pushing by the mother, Choice (B), may cause the cord to actually tighten around the neck. If the cord doesn't come off easily, you'll need to clamp and cut the cord to free the head, not cut alone, as Choice (D) suggests. Choice (A) is more consistent with the treatment of a prolapsed cord (when a loop of the cord appears first).

26. **B.** This patient may have suffered placenta abruptio or uterine rupture, both of which can result in life-threatening bleeding that can't be controlled externally, ruling out Choice (A). There is no indication of imminent delivery, making Choice (C) inappropriate. Estimating blood loss, Choice (D), doesn't provide any more information about the patient's condition when compared to her poor vital signs.

27. **C.** As the soon-to-be newborn's head nears the vaginal opening, it presses against the mother's anal sphincter, causing her to feel as though she needs to move her bowels, Choice (C). This sensation is therefore indicative of imminent birth. Although the other choices are good questions to ask, they won't help you make a decision regarding transport.

Chapter 12

Trauma Basics

In This Chapter

- Linking injury patterns to the mechanism of injury
- Recognizing injuries that affect the airway, breathing, circulation, and the spinal cord
- Taking care of trauma patients, step by step

Trauma is a disease that harms or kills people during their prime years. In fact, you may know that the modern-day EMT was developed in response to this major cause of death on U.S. highways in the early to mid 1960s.

While you have studied a wide variety of injuries in your EMT training, the ones that I focus on in this chapter are those that happen in the "kill zone" of the head, neck, torso, pelvis, and the upper legs. Although some of these injuries are obvious, others are hidden below the surface and require your detective skills to identify real or potential harm based on the mechanism of injury.

Treating trauma victims is like managing patients with medical conditions (see Chapter 11 for an introduction to medical fundamentals). If the problem has something to do with the airway, breathing, or circulation, it has the potential to cause serious damage. That's why you need to identify the most serious problem early and accurately. Don't be distracted by the minor injuries, even when they may be the most obvious or cause the most pain. In this chapter the focus is on the key elements of good trauma management: determining the mechanism of injury, identifying real or potentially critical injuries, managing them quickly, and beginning transport to the nearest trauma center if necessary.

Relating the Mechanism of Injury to Injury Patterns

In trauma, determining the mechanism of injury (MOI) gives you a jump start in your assessment. Looking for clues as to the nature and amount of force involved in the event can help you predict what injury pattern you may find. The following sections define MOI in relation to force, describe different types of MOI, and show you how to match obvious injuries to hidden injuries caused by MOI.

Connecting MOI and force

A *mechanism of injury* is a description of a force that can cause an injury. Remember Isaac Newton and his three basic laws of physics? They may sound complicated, but in trauma they're pretty easy to understand.

Say that someone is driving a car down a country road. Newton's first law says that an object in motion stays in motion unless acted upon by an outside force. In this example, the car keeps moving down the highway until the driver goes off the road after being distracted by his mobile phone. The car strikes a tree (the outside force) and quickly comes to a stop. However, the driver continues to move forward for another couple of milliseconds, until he, too, is acted upon by an outside force — an airbag and a seat belt, for example.

Hopefully, the driver was smart enough to have this safety equipment, because it was designed to slow him down more gradually than, say, the steering wheel. This slower change in velocity is Newton's second law, which says the faster things move, the more force they have. If the driver was only moving at 25 miles per hour, you might not expect much damage to the car (and the driver.) Change the speed to 50 mph, and now you're talking some serious problems!

Newton's second law actually states that force is a product of the mass of the object and its acceleration. However, what really generates force is the speed of the object and not its mass. Consider the concept of *kinetic energy* (KE), the force a moving object has. The formula for KE is

$$KE = (mass/2) \times velocity^2$$

You don't have to do the math; just recognize that the velocity is squared, meaning that the force increases much more quickly with speed than mass.

Unfortunately for the driver, he was moving at highway speed when he crashed into the tree. He was careless and forgot to put on his seat belt. And did I mention that he was driving a car made in the early 1970s, before there were airbags? All of these factors result in the driver crashing his chest and abdomen into the steering wheel and his forehead into the windshield. The steering wheel bends, and the windshield cracks wildly under the force. More importantly, an opposite force is created by the steering wheel and windshield, causing injuries to the driver's skull, brain, chest cavity, and abdomen. This is Newton's third law: For every action, there is an opposite and equal reaction.

There you have it — Newton's three laws. The MOI is the car crashing into a tree at a high rate of speed. When you size up the scene, you notice that the steering wheel is deformed and the windshield in front of the driver is badly damaged. You also notice he's not wearing a seat belt and there is no airbag. Before you even begin your assessment of the driver, you already have a high index of suspicion that he has serious head, chest, and abdominal injuries based on the apparent MOI.

Don't be distracted by the injuries you can see — it's the ones you don't see that can be lethal. That's why you want to have a clear idea of the MOI. The driver in this example may only have a small laceration to his head, but he may also have a brain injury that doesn't appear until later.

Differentiating blunt from penetrating MOI

Although you may think there are lots of MOIs, they really boil down to two general forms: blunt and penetrating. Each has unique properties. In addition, you have to consider blast MOI, which is a combination of blunt and penetrating MOI.

Blunt MOI

Blunt MOI spreads its force over an area of the body. The skin may or may not be broken open, which can hide injury sites. You need to think beyond the surface and predict what injuries you may find in the following situations:

- **Motor vehicle crashes:** There are a few types of motor vehicle crashes (MVCs):
  - **Frontal:** The front of the vehicle is struck, either directly or offset. The body is flung forward, sometimes in an upward or downward motion. As in the example in the earlier section "Connecting MOI and force," you expect injuries to be focused on the front of the body — the head, neck, chest, and abdomen. There may also be injuries to the arms and legs if they strike the dashboard or steering wheel.
  - **Rear:** The back end of the vehicle is struck, causing the body to lurch backward first, and then whip forward. If the headrest is placed too low, the neck can hyperextend during the first reaction. Injuries to the neck, spine, and pelvis are possible during a rear collision.
  - **Lateral:** The side of the vehicle is struck. The body moves to the side of the impact, causing injuries to the lateral head, neck, shoulder, chest, abdomen, and pelvis.
  - **Rollover:** The vehicle is flipped onto its side or roof after impact. This type of accident can be especially dangerous for unrestrained passengers; they experience multiple impacts with both the inside of the vehicle and any flying objects inside the cabin during the crash, causing a multitude of injuries in a variety of places on the body. Worse yet, they have a good chance of being ejected out of the car during the rollover, and that's likely to produce serious injury or death.
  - **Rotational:** The vehicle spins after impact. Similar to a rollover, the injuries can be highly variable. The initial impact can also cause injuries; for example, say two cars collide in a frontal offset crash, causing one to spin off to one side. It then crashes laterally into a building. If the occupants are not restrained, they will collide with a variety of surfaces within the vehicle, including each other. The injury patterns may vary widely.

Restraints and other safety equipment in motor vehicles are quite good in minimizing injuries in crashes. Victims may not appear to be seriously injured after a horrific crash. However, don't make a snap judgment. Make sure you evaluate the MOI and assess the patient for any potential injuries associated with it.

- **Pedestrians, motorcyclists, and bicyclists, oh my!** Motor vehicles can carry a lot of energy through their mass and speed. People are at a severe disadvantage during a collision when they're on foot, a motorcycle, a bicycle, or another type of wheeled transport.

You need to look for MOI signs of the energy involved in the collision. If the victim was thrown, estimate the distance from where the victim was struck. Damage to the motor vehicle hood, door, or bumper can provide key information. Look for tire skid marks from the motor vehicle — if they occurred before the point of impact, the energy transfer may have been less than expected.

- **Falls:** Falls represent another form of blunt trauma. Acceleration is related to force (as you find out in the earlier section "Connecting MOI and force"), so it's important to determine the approximate height of the fall as a predictor of serious injury. If the distance is three times the height of the patient or more, or at least 15 feet, there is great potential for serious injury.

  Knowing the suddenness of the stop on the other end of a fall is also important. Soft sand, bushes, and other materials that can slow the deceleration improve the victim's chances of escaping serious injury.

  Finally, how the patient lands after falling can help you determine injury patterns. If a person tries to land on her feet after a high fall, not only will she experience possible injuries to her feet, but energy will transmit to her spinal column as well.

- **Falling objects and assaults:** Being struck by bats, falling objects, and asteroids are examples of blunt MOI. Okay, I'm kidding about the asteroids, but the concept is the same: These MOI produce more localized injury patterns to the body. You want to identify the offending object and determine the point of impact on the body and what happened afterward. For example, after the victim was struck over the head with a metal bar, did he fall to the ground? Was he further assaulted? The victim may have numerous injuries in addition to the head (and brain) injury.

Penetrating MOI

Penetrating MOI concentrates its force into a specific area of the body, creating an opening through the skin. Examples of penetrating MOI include

- **Gun shots:** In gun shots, velocity makes all the difference. The faster the bullet, the more damage it can cause. A low-velocity projectile from a small handgun tends to cause damage along its trajectory. A high-velocity projectile from a rifle has a *cavitational,* or pressure, effect, causing tissue to compress and bleed as the bullet passes through.

  A bullet may also be deflected from its path in the body by harder surfaces such as bone. In this case, you may find it harder to predict the injury pattern.
- **Stabbing or cutting:** You can consider a stabbing or cutting to be a very low-velocity penetrating trauma. As such, these injuries tend to be localized to the area.

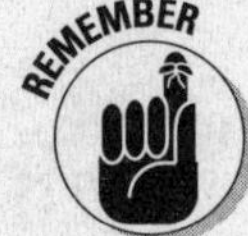

Popular television shows can make penetrating injuries look very dramatic, with blood everywhere. More often than not, bullet and knife wounds bleed very little externally. Most of the bleeding occurs internally, where it can't be seen or stopped.

If you can find out more specifics about the type of weapon used, such as the length of a knife blade or the caliber of a bullet, that's great, but don't waste time trying to track the information down.

Blast MOI

Injuries sustained from an explosion have characteristics of both blunt and penetrating MOIs. Here's the progression:

- **Primary blast wave:** When the explosion first occurs, a wall of air pressure rapidly expands outward in all directions. A victim who is close to the explosion will be struck by this pressure wave, causing blunt injuries to the inside of the body, especially to hollow organs (see the next section).
- **Secondary blast wave:** Immediately behind the primary wave is debris from the explosion itself. It may be the remainder of the original container, shrapnel embedded in a bomb, or glass and other materials from nearby structures. This debris strikes the victim, causing penetrating injuries.
- **Tertiary blast injuries:** If the force of the explosion is great enough, victims can be thrown to the ground or into other solid objects, causing additional blunt and/or penetrating injuries.

Matching obvious injuries to hidden injuries

After you can distinguish different types of MOIs, you can match up different areas of the body to possible injury patterns. Table 12-1 provides an overview of possible injuries; you can review them in more detail in the next few sections. Obvious injuries are those you can see; hidden injuries are ones that require assessment and an understanding of MOI.

Table 12-1 Injuries Organized by Body Area

Body Area	*Obvious Injuries*	*Hidden Injuries*
Head and face	Contusions; abrasions; lacerations; punctures; avulsions; burns; lost or fractured teeth; blow-out eye fractures; foreign bodies; bleeding from eyes, nose, and ears	Epidural hematoma, subdural hematoma, intracranial hematoma, intracranial pressure (ICP), concussion, skull fracture, upper airway swelling
Neck	Contusions, abrasions, lacerations, punctures, avulsions, burns, open neck wounds, cervical spine deformity	Upper airway swelling, soft-tissue bleeding in larynx, subcutaneous emphysema, fractured larynx, cervical spinal cord injury
Anterior chest	Contusions, abrasions, lacerations, punctures, avulsions, burns, open wounds	Pneumothorax (simple and tension); hemothorax; pulmonary contusion; cardiac contusion; commotio cordis; large vessel lacerations; flail chest; rib fractures; traumatic asphyxia; liver, spleen, and upper GI trauma
Anterior abdomen	Contusions, abrasions, lacerations, punctures, avulsions, burns, open wounds, evisceration	Solid organs that bleed (liver, spleen, pancreas, ovaries); hollow organs that rupture (intestines, stomach); mesentery bleeding; pregnancy-related trauma
Pelvis	Contusions, abrasions, lacerations, punctures, avulsions, dislocated hip, proximal femur fractures, genital injuries	Unstable pelvic fracture, bladder and urinary tract injuries, genital injuries (uterus)
Extremities	Contusions, abrasions, lacerations, punctures, avulsions, long bone fractures, dislocations, sprains, strains, amputations	Compartment syndrome, interstitial bleeding, loss of perfusion
Back	Contusions, abrasions, lacerations, punctures, avulsions, spinal deformity, open posterior chest wound	Spinal cord injury, scapula/rib fractures, kidney injury, bleeding into the retroperitoneal space

You probably notice in Table 12-1 that soft-tissue injuries are common to all areas of the body. Don't let these obvious ones blind you to the more serious injuries that are below the skin's surface. Consider the obvious injuries as "road signs" that can point to further problems behind them.

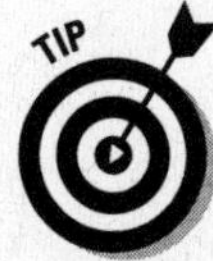

Trauma-related exam questions may ask about which injury you should manage first. Look at all the responses and ask yourself which one is likely to be most *harmful* as opposed to most dramatic. Check out the following example.

A 24-year-old unrestrained driver was involved in a rollover crash of his van. He is lying unconscious outside of the vehicle. He has a deformed left lower leg, swelling in his right thigh, and abrasions across his chest and forehead. His pupils are unequal, he is breathing at 6 times per minute, and his pulse rate is 50. Which of the following actions should you perform first?

(A) Apply a cardboard splint to the lower leg deformity.

(B) Ventilate the patient at 20 breaths per minute with a bag-valve mask and oxygen.

(C) Apply a traction splint to the right thigh.

(D) Administer high-flow oxygen via a nonrebreather mask.

The best choice is (B). Although the lower left leg deformity, Choice (A), and the swelling in the right femur region, Choice (C), may be significant and obvious, the slow respiratory and heart rates, along with the abrasion to the forehead and unequal pupils, indicate the probability of a hidden brain injury that requires your immediate attention. The patient is breathing too slowly for supplemental oxygen only, as Choice (D) suggests.

Investigating Injuries That Affect the Airway and Breathing

The following sections focus on injuries that require rapid identification and, in some cases, immediate action on your part. I am referring to conditions that either block (obstruct) the airway or somehow impair the patient's ability to breathe adequately. Without the ability to move air well, the patient's ability to survive any injury is severely compromised.

Injuries that block the airway

No airway, no life; that's pretty much the message you hear all along in your EMT training. Table 12-2 lists key trauma reasons why an airway becomes blocked and what action you should perform to relieve the blockage.

Table 12-2 Injuries That Block the Airway

Problem	*Signs and Symptoms*	*Action Steps*
Obstructions in the mouth	Blood, other secretions; broken/missing teeth; bleeding from nose	Suction mouth; if possible, position patient lateral recumbent
Tongue obstruction as a result of altered mental status or unconsciousness	Snoring respirations; no breathing sounds; head and neck flexed	Manual spine precautions; modified jaw thrust; oropharyngeal or nasopharyngeal airway; head-tilt, chin-lift if modified jaw thrust is unsuccessful
Soft tissue swelling as a result of heat or chemical burns	Hoarse, muffled, or whisper voice; stridor during breathing; reddened tissues in mouth; excessive saliva/secretions	Maintain an optimal head/neck position that minimizes stridor; sit patient up if no cervical-spine precautions; suction carefully, if at all, to avoid irritating tissue (allow patient to drool)
Impaled object in cheek	Um, something stuck in cheek	Suction as necessary; if airway is blocked, cut object as short as possible and pull it forward through the opening; apply pressure to opening to control bleeding

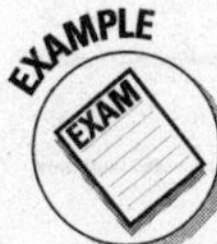

A 35-year-old female strikes a tree while skiing downhill. She is unconscious, with slow, irregular respirations. You can hear snoring. She has a large laceration along the left parietal skull that is oozing blood. You should first

(A) suction her airway for no more than 10 seconds.

(B) apply a head-tilt, chin-lift maneuver.

(C) establish manual spine precautions.

(D) control the bleeding with mild, direct pressure.

The best answer is Choice (C). There is evidence of a significant mechanism of injury, and the patient is unconscious and unable to provide you any information. Therefore, minimizing movement to the spine is important in this scenario. There is no evidence of blood in the airway, making Choice (A) irrelevant. Choice (B) may be required, but only if you are unable to open the airway with a jaw thrust. The bleeding from the laceration is not significant enough to override airway control as the priority, as Choice (D) suggests.

Injuries that make breathing difficult

In order to survive, you have to maintain levels of oxygen and carbon dioxide no matter what. When a patient begins to fail at maintaining ventilation, you need to step in to supplement oxygen or take over ventilation; Table 12-3 details the action steps.

Table 12-3 Injuries That Make Breathing Difficult

Problem	*Signs and Symptoms*	*Action Steps*
Open chest wound, causing air to leak into the chest cavity	Incision or opening on chest wall (don't forget the back!); sounds of air at site (though not always); uneven chest rise and fall; decreased lung sounds on affected side; dyspnea; tachycardia	Seal wound immediately with gloved hand; replace with occlusive chest seal; closely monitor for developing tension under seal and relieve it as patient exhales; if patient is unable to breathe adequately, provide oxygen and ventilate carefully to avoid worsening the problem
Pneumothorax, open or simple, causing a portion of the lung to collapse	Possible diminished lung sounds over affected side; decreased oxygen saturation; dyspnea; tachycardia; possible chest pain	Provide oxygen to maintain saturation; ventilate carefully if patient is unable to maintain
Tension pneumothorax, causing excess air pressure inside chest wall and squeezing the lungs, heart, and great vessels	Diminished lung sounds over affected side; jugular venous distension; unequal chest rise and fall; rapidly falling blood pressure; severe dyspnea and tachycardia	If tension develops after occlusive seal is applied to an open chest wound, lift one side of seal to "burp" the wound and relieve tension. Call advanced life support (ALS) if possible; a paramedic can insert a long needle into the chest to relieve the tension

continued

Table 12-3 (continued)

Problem	*Signs and Symptoms*	*Action Steps*
Hemothorax, causing blood to pool into the chest cavity and squeezing the lung	Diminished lung sounds over affected side; flat neck veins; hypotension (from blood loss); dyspnea and tachycardia	Provide oxygen to maintain saturation; ventilate carefully if patient is unable to maintain
Rib fractures, causing pain	Pain and point tenderness over affected region; pain on inspiration; dyspnea	If possible, place patient in best position of comfort; provide oxygen to maintain saturation
Flail chest, causing loss of chest wall integrity	Pain over affected region; in later stages, paradoxical chest movement, dyspnea	Provide oxygen to maintain saturation; ventilate carefully if patient is unable to maintain adequate tidal volume; some regions suggest splinting with a pillow or bulky dressing to reduce pain

Notice that many of the following trauma conditions have similar signs and symptoms; that's why diagnosis may be difficult. However, also notice that the treatment is very similar for many conditions. As long as you keep that in mind, you'll do okay.

A pedestrian was struck by a motor vehicle that was moving at a high rate of speed. He is anxious and confused, with cool, pale, and diaphoretic skin. You note crepitus on palpation across the right lateral chest wall, from the region of T4 through T10. Breath sounds are diminished over the right side of the chest. His neck veins are flat. His pulse rate is 130, and his blood pressure is 80/60 mm Hg. Which of the following injuries is most likely?

(A) Tension pneumothorax

(B) Hemothorax

(C) Simple pneumothorax

(D) Fractured ribs

The best answer is Choice (B). Bleeding inside the chest cavity can be significant and cause shock. The mechanism of injury, physical findings, and his poor skin and vital signs support this answer. You would expect to see jugular venous distension in Choice (A). Neither Choice (C) nor (D), by itself, would cause such poor vital signs.

Assessing Injuries That Affect Circulation

The circulatory system is responsible for transferring oxygen, carbon dioxide, nutrients, and other wastes to and from every cell in the body. It does so through the interaction of its three major components: the heart, the vasculature (the blood vessels), and blood. The following sections describe the body's circulation (medically known as *perfusion*) and trauma injuries that affect it.

Pump, pipes, and fluid: How circulation works

Think about how water moves through your house or apartment. There has to be a pump that pushes water from your well or your town's water supply into the dwelling. Once there, pipes channel that water to a variety of appliances, from faucets and showers to toilets and sprinklers. There has to be a certain pressure within the system in order to make all the appliances function properly. Lower the water pressure and you have showers that dribble and toilets that clog.

What might cause pressure to fall? It could be the pump at the well or station. Perhaps a break occurred in one of the pipes. Maybe the well ran dry. In any case, unless something changes to compensate for the loss, your water pressure falls and eventually water stops flowing. Not good!

Your body essentially does the same thing with circulation, or perfusion. The heart has to pump at a certain rate and with enough force so that blood is pushed into the vasculature. What's nice about your system is that, unlike a house's plumbing, it automatically tries to compensate for changes in pressure.

Specialized cells called *baroreceptors* are found in the first part of the aorta as it leaves the left ventricle (the *aortic arch;* see the next section for more details). Baroreceptors sense subtle changes in falling pressure and send that information to the brain. The brain interprets these signals and sends commands to the heart to increase both heart rate *(chronotropy)* and contraction of the muscle *(inotropy).* The result is that more pressure is generated out of the heart and into the circulatory system.

Meanwhile, the rest of the body reacts as well. As pressure falls, smooth muscles throughout various parts of the body contract, causing parts of the vasculature to constrict and decrease blood flow from areas of the body that don't need very much circulation during a crisis. Areas such as the skin and gastrointestinal tract are not crucial to the body during low-pressure conditions. The brain, heart, lungs, and kidneys must have blood flow maintained at virtually all costs.

The body also senses, through chemoreceptors in the brainstem, the potential loss of oxygen and worsening ability to remove carbon dioxide. As a result, signals to the diaphragm and intercostal muscles trigger faster breathing.

Put it all together: cool, pale skin; tachycardia; tachypnea. Sound familiar? It should; these are the early signs of shock. When the body can maintain blood pressure and perfusion to the vital organs, it's in compensated shock; when it begins to fail and pressure falls, it's entering decompensating shock. Let it persist long enough, and enough cells will die from lack of perfusion to cause organ failure and probable death.

You may wonder whether the body can compensate for falling pressure by increasing the amount of blood it has. In fact, it does do this by stimulating red blood cell production in the bone marrow. However, it takes days to increase cell production, which is why it's not helpful in the sudden crisis of shock.

Injuries to the heart

The heart's function as a pump can't be overstated; even a small bruise can cause diminished cardiac output. Table 12-4 provides information about potentially serious injuries.

Table 12-4 Injuries Affecting the Heart

Problem	Signs and Symptoms	Action Steps
Myocardial contusion	Possible irregular heartbeat; signs of a myocardial infarction or acute coronary syndrome such as chest pressure or discomfort, radiating pain, shortness of breath	Provide oxygen to maintain saturation; monitor vital signs closely
Commotio cordis	Sudden cardiac arrest caused by a sharp blow to the sternum from an object like a baseball, bat, or fist	Begin CPR immediately and apply an automated external defibrillator (AED) as soon as possible (ventricular fibrillation is the common presenting rhythm disturbance)

Injuries to the vasculature

Rising up from the left ventricle, the aorta is a very large artery that carries blood away from the heart to the rest of the body. It quickly creates the aortic arch, causing it to descend toward the feet. The brachiocephalic, left common carotid, and left subclavian arteries branch off the aortic arch. Collectively they're known as the great vessels. Figure 12-1 illustrates these major arteries.

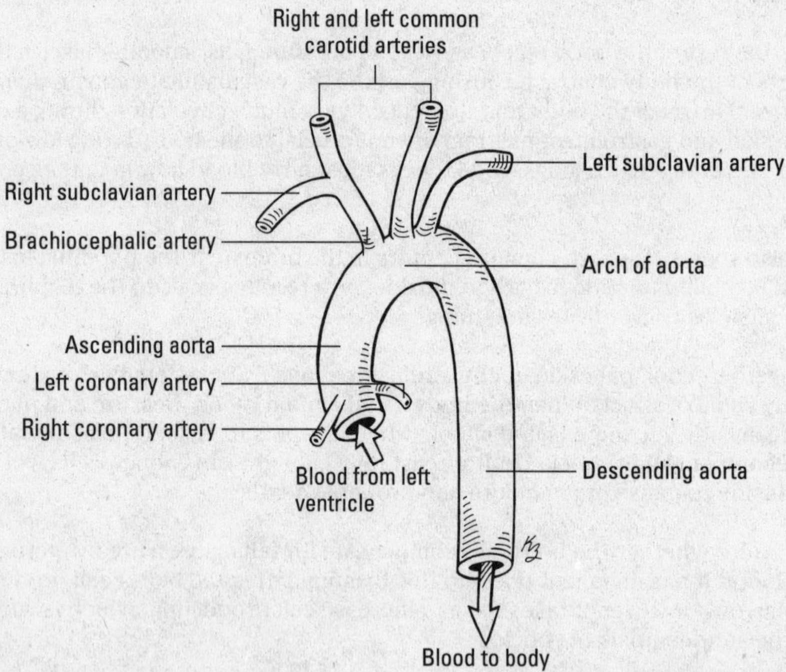

Figure 12-1: The great vessels.

The arch is held up by the ligamentum arteriosum. In major blunt-force trauma, this ligament can act like a knife, causing a tear in the aorta.

Lacerations to the great vessels, or the vena cava, from either blunt or penetrating trauma, cause massive bleeding into the chest cavity. Your patient may appear in severe shock, even though there's little or no external bleeding! Treat for shock and prepare to ventilate the patient if needed.

Lacerations to other major arteries or veins near the femur or in the neck also cause significant bleeding, either externally or internally.

- Specific to the neck region, an open wound can potentially draw air into a vein or artery, causing an air embolism to occur. Just as you would do with an open chest wound, you cover an open neck wound with some type of occlusive dressing.
- Normally, fractures of long bones don't cause major bleeding. However, a broken femur can puncture the femoral artery lying next to it and cause massive bleeding that may require a tourniquet to control. Similarly, bleeding resulting from fractures of two or more long bones, like the tibias of both legs, can become fairly significant when added together.

Controlling any major bleeding you can see is essential. As you discover in the earlier section "Pump, pipes, and fluid: How circulation works," without adequate blood the body can't transport oxygen very well. Fortunately, the steps to control external bleeding are simple:

1. **Apply direct pressure with your gloved hand using gauze or any clean dressing to cause blood to form a clot at the site.**
2. **If direct pressure fails to control the bleeding within a few seconds, apply a tourniquet proximal to the injury site.**

   Note: You may have learned about applying a pressure point or elevating an extremity before applying a tourniquet; these techniques have not been shown to be effective.

You can control external bleeding, but you can't control internal bleeding; the definitive treatment in the field is to rapidly recognize signs of shock, package the patient for safe transport, and move immediately toward a trauma center for surgical intervention.

Some trauma exam questions check whether you know how to properly perform a procedure. See if you can answer this one.

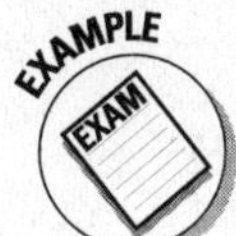

A 17-year-old female was stabbed several times during a fight. She has a 1-inch stab wound to the left side of her neck, which is oozing blood. There is an incision to her left hand, covered with a shirt, which bleeds freely when the shirt is removed. What should you do first?

(A) Use direct pressure to apply a dressing to the hand injury and elevate it above the heart.

(B) Use mild pressure to apply a dressing to the neck injury.

(C) Apply an occlusive dressing to the hand injury.

(D) Apply an occlusive dressing to the neck injury.

The correct answer is Choice (D). Although controlling the bleeding from the hand injury, as noted in Choices (A) and (C), may be tempting, the bleeding appears controlled when the shirt is left on the hand. More importantly, the neck incision has the potential to create an air embolism, so occluding the site as soon as possible is imperative. A gauze dressing can't block the site completely, which makes Choice (B) less effective than Choice (D).

Evaluating Spinal Cord Injuries

Through much of the history of EMS, practitioners have been taught to immediately apply spinal immobilization to patients if the MOI could have caused a possible spinal cord injury. The fact is, the chance of a spinal cord injury is nearly nonexistent when the patient isn't complaining of neck or back pain.

You may think, "Well, I'd rather be safe than sorry. Besides, what harm can a backboard do, right?" Unfortunately, being immobilized to a backboard can indeed cause injuries to the patient! In addition, taking the time to immobilize patients for a low-probability spinal injury while they're experiencing an airway, breathing, or perfusion injury that requires rapid surgical care causes an unnecessary delay on-scene. Finally, if the patient's injuries involve airway or breathing, lying supine on a backboard will only compound the problem.

You get the point: Only immobilize when a blunt force MOI suggests a possible spinal injury *and* you see signs of a possible injury, such as

- Spinal pain or tenderness
- Neurologic complaint (for example, numbness or motor weakness)
- Deformity of the spine

You should also immobilize patients if they exhibit any of the following:

- Altered mental status
- Drug or alcohol intoxication
- Inability to communicate clearly
- Another injury so painful that it can distract the patient's attention from spine pain (distracting injury)

You should not spinal immobilize a patient with penetrating trauma if there is no evidence of spinal injury from the MOI. Spending excessive time on-scene to perform an unnecessary procedure delays transportation to the services of a trauma team, which is what the patient really needs.

This information can be tricky to comprehend. Try the following question to test your understanding.

During a house party, a 29-year-old male falls over the railing of a balcony to the lawn below. He is supine and denies any pain from the fall. You can smell alcohol on his breath, and his speech is slurred. Other than some abrasions to his hands you see no other injuries. You should

(A) immobilize him to a long backboard.

(B) notify the police.

(C) assist him to sit on your gurney.

(D) determine how much he had to drink.

The correct answer is Choice (A). Although the patient denies having any pain or injuries from the fall, there is evidence of an intoxicant that could be masking a trauma condition. Given the MOI, you have to apply spinal immobilization as a precaution.

Compare the preceding question to the following question.

During a house party, a 29-year-old male falls over the railing of a balcony to the lawn below. He is sitting up and denies any pain from the fall. Other than some abrasions to his hands, you see no other injuries. You should

(A) immobilize him to a long backboard.

(B) notify the police.

(C) assist him to sit on your gurney.

(D) determine how much he had to drink.

The correct answer is Choice (C). In this version of the question, there is no evidence of an intoxicant. Even with the MOI, withholding spinal immobilization is appropriate.

Managing Trauma Step by Step

After you review various mechanisms of injury and the critical injuries they can cause (see the sections preceding this one), take a look at the following plan of action that can be used for any trauma patient:

1. **Ensure that the scene is as safe as possible before entry and wear appropriate personal protective equipment.**
2. **Evaluate the scene for signs of the mechanism of injury.**
3. **Look at the patient's appearance and position as you approach.**
4. **If indicated, manually stabilize the cervical spine while you evaluate for airway patency, breathing, and circulation (you guessed it — the ABCs).**
   - Ventilate the patient if needed, right away.
   - If there is major external bleeding, stop it.
   - If there is an open wound to the neck or chest area, block it with your gloved hand or immediately apply an occlusive dressing.
   - If the patient appears in shock, lay the patient supine.

   Note: You may have to do some of these steps almost simultaneously. Other rescuers can help.
5. **Rapidly assess the head, neck, chest, abdomen, and pelvis for injuries described earlier in this chapter.**
6. **If the patient has an actual or potential serious injury, package and begin transport to a trauma center.**

   If you determine that the patient's injuries are not life- or limb-threatening, perform a detailed exam and appropriately manage all injuries prior to transport. This may include splinting extremities, bandaging all wounds, or applying ice packs to sprains or strains.
7. **While enroute, provide supplemental oxygen, obtain a set of vital signs, and note the patient's medical history, medications, and allergies.**
8. **If time permits, perform a detailed, head-to-toe examination looking for minor injuries. If possible, bandage other wounds and splint possible extremity fractures.**

   Fractures can cause a lot of pain and splinting may help.
9. **Constantly reassess the ABCs.**

   They can change quickly if the patient is bleeding internally or is hypoventilating.

Some exam questions check to make sure you have an organized, logical approach to trauma care. Respond to the following example.

A construction worker is caught by the blast of a small, exploding propane tank and thrown 10 feet, landing on his back. He is confused, has difficulty breathing, and has cool, pale, and diaphoretic skin. He has second- and third-degree burns to his arms, anterior chest, and abdomen. He has clear lung sounds. You see multiple lacerations across his face and neck. His pulse rate is 130, and he is breathing 20 times per minute. You should

(A) sit him up, administer supplemental oxygen, begin transport, and dress the burn wounds.

(B) perform spinal immobilization, dress the burn wounds, and begin transport.

(C) perform spinal immobilization, administer supplemental oxygen, begin transport, and dress the burn wounds.

(D) keep the patient supine, administer supplemental oxygen, dress the burn wounds, and begin transport.

The correct answer is Choice (C). This patient is critically injured, with altered mental status and signs of shock (such as poor skins signs and tachycardia). Immediate transport is warranted; perform the minimum level of care on-scene. In this scenario, spinal immobilization and supplemental oxygen should be provided prior to transport, ruling out Choices (A), (B), and (D). Although the burns are serious, their effects on the body won't occur until much later in the process. You can delay treating them until after transport has begun.

Practice Questions about Trauma

The following practice questions are similar to the EMT exam's questions about trauma. Read each question carefully, and then select the answer choice that most correctly answers the question.

1. The patient has sustained a single blow to the head. He is awake, alert, and complaining of a severe headache and neck pain. His blood pressure is 148/84 mm Hg, his pulse rate is 100, and his respiratory rate is 20 breaths per minute. You should

   (A) assist his ventilations with a bag-valve mask and oxygen at a rate of 20 breaths per minute.

   (B) manually stabilize his head and neck and prepare to immobilize the patient to a long backboard.

   (C) immediately transport the patient to a trauma center.

   (D) place the patient supine on a long backboard, with the head slightly lower than the legs.

2. A driver of a vehicle was struck by another vehicle, on her side of the car at the driver's door. There are 8 inches of intrusion into the passenger compartment. She is tachypneic, taking rapid, shallow breaths and complaining of chest pain when she inhales. Lung sounds are diminished over the left side of the chest, which is tender to palpation. Which of the following do you suspect is the most likely injury?

   (A) Left-sided pneumothorax

   (B) Right-sided hemothorax

   (C) Tension pneumothorax

   (D) Diaphragmatic rupture

3. An adult male is complaining of right-sided flank pain after being assaulted 24 hours earlier. There is bruising and swelling to his right lateral abdomen and right lower back. He reports seeing blood when he urinates. You suspect that he may have sustained an injury to his

(A) spleen.

(B) liver.

(C) urinary bladder.

(D) kidney.

4. A young adult woman has been shot. She is alert and sitting on the sidewalk; you notice an open wound to her left anterior chest just inferior to the clavicle. Blood is oozing from the wound. She is coughing up blood and appears to be in respiratory distress. Your first intervention is to

(A) place her in a supine position.

(B) apply gauze to the wound to stop bleeding.

(C) cover the wound with a gloved hand or occlusive dressing.

(D) manually suction her airway.

5. A 19-year-old female was struck by a car as she was walking across the street. She presents approximately 7 feet from the front of the vehicle. You note bruising to her lower abdomen, a hematoma to her left lateral head, and deformity to her right wrist. She is confused and tachycardic with pale and diaphoretic skin. Her blood pressure is 104/78 mm Hg. Which of the following suspected injuries best explains her presentation?

(A) Wrist fracture

(B) Head injury

(C) Pelvic fracture

(D) Punctured stomach

6. An adult male is rescued from a burning apartment by firefighters. He is alert, with his face and body covered with soot. He is coughing, and you hear raspy sounds as he breathes. His respiratory rate is 22 breaths per minute, and he has a pulse rate of 104. You should

(A) administer high-flow oxygen via a nonrebreather mask.

(B) suction his airway.

(C) ventilate with a bag-valve mask and oxygen.

(D) manually stabilize the patient's head and neck.

7. A 32-year-old female fell down a steep hillside while hiking. She responds to verbal stimulus by moaning. Her breath sounds are diminished over the right side of her chest. There is crepitus when you palpate the rib cage. You note her neck veins are flat, and her skin is cool, pale, and moist. Her pulse rate is 130, her blood pressure is 82/60 mm Hg, and she is breathing at a rate of 26 times per minute. Which of the following suspected injuries best explains her presentation?

(A) Flail segment

(B) Fractured rib

(C) Pneumothorax

(D) Hemothorax

8. A 22-year-old male was struck in the face by a heavy object while working. He presents supine on the ground, unresponsive, with blood and broken teeth in the airway. Your next step is to

   (A) measure and apply a cervical collar.

   (B) roll the patient onto his side and suction.

   (C) administer high-flow oxygen using a nonrebreather mask.

   (D) ventilate the patient with a bag-valve mask and high-flow oxygen.

9. A 24-year-old female was stabbed in the third intercostal space of the left lateral chest. She is confused, with cool, pale skin. You note accessory muscle use when she breathes and jugular venous distension (JVD). Her blood pressure is 70/50 mm Hg, and her heart rate is 126. Which of the following possible injuries most likely explains her presentation?

   (A) Hemothorax

   (B) Cardiac tamponade

   (C) Tension pneumothorax

   (D) Simple pneumothorax

10. An adult male has been shot in the neck. He is alert and sitting in a car, tachypneic with a rapid radial pulse. There is a small wound to the right lateral side of his neck, with minor bleeding. He is spitting up blood and can feel and move all extremities. Your sequence of care is to

    (A) cover the wound with an occlusive dressing, have suction ready, and transport in a sitting position.

    (B) cover the wound with an occlusive dressing, apply a cervical collar, immobilize to a long backboard, and transport supine.

    (C) cover the wound with gauze, apply a cervical collar, immobilize to a long backboard, transport supine, and suction as needed.

    (D) cover the wound with gauze, transport in a sitting position, and ask the patient not to cough.

11. A female driver is involved in a head-on collision with another vehicle. There is damage to the steering column, and you note a large contusion to her sternum. She is confused and tachypneic with a weak, rapid, carotid pulse only. Her blood pressure is 112/96 mm Hg, and her respiratory rate is 20 with equal chest rise. There is jugular venous distention (JVD), and her skin is cool and moist. Which of the following possible injuries most like explains her presentation?

    (A) Tension pneumothorax

    (B) Cardiac tamponade

    (C) Myocardial contusion

    (D) Hemothorax

12. A male passenger is sitting in the front seat of a motor vehicle when it's involved in an offset frontal crash. He presents awake and complaining of pressure and tightness in the chest. You note a large bruise over the left lower anterior chest wall that is tender to palpation. His pulse is irregular and rapid; his blood pressure is 156/82 mm Hg, and he is breathing 16 times per minute. You suspect which of the following possible injuries?

    (A) Pneumothorax

    (B) Cardiac tamponade

    (C) Myocardial contusion

    (D) Flail segment

13. A 20-year-old female dove into a pool headfirst and did not resurface. She was removed from the pool by lifeguards who reported she was initially unconscious. She is now awake, confused, and unable to follow your commands. You note a hematoma and abrasions to her left temple. Her heart rate is 68, her respiratory rate is 32 and shallow, and her blood pressure is 90/60 mm Hg. You suspect her presentation is due to

    (A) increased cranial pressure.

    (B) bleeding under the scalp.

    (C) a spinal cord injury.

    (D) a partially obstructed airway.

14. A 72-year-old male driver is involved in an offset, head-on traffic collision. You observe that there is no intrusion into the passenger compartment, the driver's side airbag has deployed, and a seat belt has been used. The patient is awake and complaining of neck pain. His blood pressure is 142/82 mm Hg, his pulse rate is 90, and he is breathing 18 times per minute. His skin is warm and dry. Your physical exam is unremarkable. What would be your best destination decision?

    (A) Transport to the closest receiving facility.

    (B) Transport to the patient's requested destination.

    (C) Transport to a stroke receiving facility.

    (D) Transport to a Level II trauma center.

15. A 68-year-old female is short of breath. Two days ago, she slipped down the two steps in front of her porch, hitting the stair railing with her left side in order to keep herself from falling down. Since this morning she has felt increasingly short of breath, weak, and nauseated. Her skin is pale, cool, and dry. Her blood pressure is 118/68 mm Hg, her heart rate is 100, and she is breathing 20 times per minute. Her lung sounds are clear, and you observe a large bruise lateral to her left upper quadrant. Your treatment would include

    (A) positioning her supine, maintaining body temperature, and administering low-flow oxygen via nasal cannula.

    (B) positioning her in full Fowler's position, administering high-flow oxygen via a nonrebreather mask, and initiating rapid transport.

    (C) positioning her on her right side, administering high-flow oxygen via a nonrebreather mask, and preparing to suction.

    (D) positioning her in a seated position on the ambulance bench seat, being prepared to suction, and administering low-flow oxygen via nasal cannula.

16. A worker is injured in an industrial accident. He is bleeding profusely from a laceration that runs from his right wrist to his elbow. You should first

    (A) apply a tourniquet just above the elbow.

    (B) apply direct pressure to the wound.

    (C) apply pressure to the brachial artery of the right arm.

    (D) elevate the arm above the level of the heart.

17. An adult female was punched in the nose. She is bleeding from both nares. What is the best way to control the bleeding?

(A) Pinch the nostrils and have the patient tilt her head back.

(B) Pinch the base of the nose and have the patient lean forward.

(C) Apply a cold pack to the base of the nose and have the patient lean forward.

(D) Pinch the nostrils and apply a cold pack to the base of the nose.

18. A 25-year-old male was cleaning a glass jar when it broke, causing a laceration to his right palm. He removes a blood-soaked cotton cloth, and you observe a deep, open wound to the palm. There is also a section of avulsed tissue. Blood begins to ooze from the wound. You should

(A) irrigate the site with sterile saline, apply direct pressure with a clean dressing, and bandage the wound after bleeding stops.

(B) apply a tourniquet to the wrist, wait for bleeding to stop, apply a clean dressing, and bandage the wound.

(C) move the avulsed tissue back into place, apply direct pressure with a clean dressing, and bandage the wound after bleeding stops.

(D) put the cotton cloth back, apply a bandage, elevate the arm above the heart, and apply pressure to the radial artery if bleeding continues.

19. An adult male has been shot by an arrow. The arrow entered the right lower abdominal quadrant. There is minor bleeding surrounding the arrow's shaft as it enters the body, and the patient is in severe pain. His blood pressure is 164/92 mm Hg; he has a heart rate of 110 and a respiratory rate of 20 breaths per minute. You should

(A) quickly remove the arrow, apply firm pressure to the wound, and position the patient supine.

(B) carefully remove the arrow, apply firm pressure to the wound, and administer oxygen.

(C) cut off the exposed part of the arrow flush with the skin and cover the site with a moist dressing.

(D) stabilize the arrow in place, place the patient into the position that gives him the most comfort, and administer oxygen.

20. An explosion has injured a worker. He was hit with shrapnel and thrown 5 feet from where he was standing. He is alert and has severe abdominal pain. You observe he has a large open wound across his lower abdomen, and there is a section of bowel protruding from the site. You should

(A) cover the wound with an occlusive dressing and administer oxygen.

(B) cover the wound with a moist dressing and administer oxygen.

(C) push the bowel back into the wound and cover with an occlusive dressing.

(D) immobilize the patient onto a long backboard and immediately transport.

Answers and Explanations

Use this answer key to score the practice questions in the preceding section. The explanations give you insight into why the correct answer is better than the other choices.

1. **B.** Although he may have suffered a head injury, there's no sign of increasing intracranial pressure. Therefore, there's no need to hyperventilate the patient, Choice (A). He does have complaints of neck pain, so while moving him quickly to a hospital, Choice (C), is desirable, you need to immobilize him first. Lowering his head after placing him on a backboard, Choice (D), won't help his situation and, in fact, may make it worse by possibly increasing intracranial pressure.
2. **A.** The MOI and diminished breath sounds lead to a left-sided injury. There are no signs of a tension pneumothorax, Choice (C), nor are there signs of a hemothorax, Choice (B). A diaphragmatic injury, Choice (D), is more likely from a frontal MOI than a lateral one.
3. **D.** The location of the injury points toward the retroperitoneal space, where the kidney is located. This reduces the likelihood of spleen and liver involvement, Choices (A) and (B). Likewise, the urinary bladder, Choice (C), is located more centrally in the lower abdominal region.
4. **C.** An open wound to the chest must be sealed as soon as possible to reduce the chance of additional air leaking into the chest cavity and causing harm. Gauze, Choice (B), won't occlude the wound. You may need to suction her airway, Choice (D), but it appears that she is controlling it with her coughing. Laying her flat, Choice (A), may make her breathing worse. As long as her blood pressure isn't low, she can better tolerate sitting up to breathe.
5. **C.** She is exhibiting signs of decompensating shock with her poor skin, confusion, and a marginal blood pressure. A head injury, Choice (B), wouldn't bleed that much, nor would a stomach injury, Choice (D). Pain from a wrist fracture, Choice (A), wouldn't cause her blood pressure to fall.
6. **A.** Stridor results from some form of obstructed airway. However, because the patient is alert, assisting his ventilations, Choice (C), isn't necessary — yet. There are no indications of secretions to suggest Choice (B), nor any signs of cervical spine trauma that warrant Choice (D).
7. **D.** Her vital signs, along with poor skin signs and altered mental status, indicate a deep state of shock. Massive blood loss, such as a hemothorax, would account for this. A pneumothorax, Choice (C), wouldn't likely cause such profound hypotension, nor would a flail segment, Choice (A), or a fractured rib, Choice (B).
8. **B.** You may need to take all of these measures. However, your *next* step is Choice (B), clearing the airway so that you can further evaluate the patient's breathing ability. Once that is done, you can make a better decision regarding whether to ventilate, Choice (D), or provide supplemental oxygen, Choice (C). Stabilizing the spine, Choice (A), is a lower priority step than managing the airway.
9. **C.** The MOI, along with the JVD and severe hypotension, point to excessive atmospheric pressure inside the chest cavity — a tension pneumothorax. A simple pneumothorax, Choice (D), would not produce JVD. Cardiac tamponade, Choice (B), would produce a narrowing pulse pressure, where diastolic pressure rises and systolic pressure falls. You would expect flat neck veins with a hemothorax, Choice (A).
10. **A.** Open wounds to the neck are like those to the chest — they have to be occluded as soon as possible to reduce the chance of air leaking into the neck tissue or, worse, into a lacerated artery or vein that may then cause a possible air embolus. Despite his injury, the patient's spinal cord does not appear to be affected, eliminating spinal precautions, as noted in Choices (B) and (C). Gauze, as per Choice (D), will not occlude the wound.

11. **B.** The MOI strongly suggests blunt force trauma to the heart. Given the narrow pulse pressure (falling systolic pressure, rising diastolic pressure) and JVD, this scenario points more to a cardiac tamponade than a simple myocardial contusion, Choice (C). A tension pneumothorax, Choice (A), would cause asymmetric rise of the chest during expiration. The presence of JVD eliminates hemothorax, Choice (D).

12. **C.** Bleeding into the cardiac muscle can result in signs and symptoms that mimic a myocardial infarction. There is no sign of a narrow pulse pressure, ruling out cardiac tamponade, Choice (B). Although the injury is tender, there's no indication of crepitus or unusual movement of the chest wall, making a flail segment, Choice (D), less likely. A pneumothorax, Choice (A), isn't known to create acute coronary syndrome–type pain.

13. **C.** The MOI, signs of paralysis, and poor tidal volume, along with a low blood pressure and a near normal heart rate, point to a neurologic shock. Increased cranial pressure would lower the respiratory rate, not increase it, as Choice (A) suggests. Bleeding under the scalp, Choice (B), isn't likely to cause the presenting signs. There's no indication that a partially obstructed airway, Choice (D), exists at the moment.

14. **D.** Although the patient appears to have been minimally injured, his advanced age makes him more susceptible to a worse recovery. Additionally, pain may be masked in an elderly patient, making injuries more challenging to find. These issues make transport to a trauma center a safer decision for the older patient.

15. **A.** The MOI suggests blunt trauma is possible, and her vital signs reflect a possible compensated shock state. Keeping her supine means her heart won't have to work as hard and may improve her pressure. Sitting her up, as in Choices (B) and (D), may worsen her blood pressure. Positioning her on her right side, as noted in Choice (C), makes monitoring the airway difficult in most ambulances because the patient is facing away from you.

16. **A.** This wound is very long, making direct pressure, Choice (B), less likely to work. Pressure points and elevation, as suggested in Choices (C) and (D), have not been shown to be effective.

17. **B.** You want to have the patient avoid tilting her head back, as in Choice (A), because she could end up swallowing blood, which in turn could cause her to vomit — not good! Cold packs, as suggested in Choices (C) and (D), aren't known to control nosebleeds. In addition, putting direct pressure along the base of the nose will control the bleeding; simply pinching the nostrils shut, as in Choice (D), won't.

18. **C.** Bleeding isn't significant at this point, so direct pressure is likely to be adequate; you don't need a tourniquet as Choice (B) suggests. Since the patient removed the cotton cloth, you can replace it with a dressing that is more sterile. Elevating the arm or putting pressure on the radial artery, Choice (D), is neither necessary nor helpful. Finally, irrigating the wound, as in Choice (A), will cause it to bleed again, perhaps profusely, as you wash away the clot.

19. **D.** The impaled object may prevent bleeding in the wound it created; moving it or, worse, removing it, as suggested in Choices (A), (B), and (C), may cause significant bleeding.

20. **B.** The biggest risk to eviscerated organs is that they may dry out, causing significant damage. Keeping the bowel moist and covered can prevent that from happening. There is no need for an occlusive dressing, as suggested in Choices (A) and (C); besides, you don't want to infect the patient with contaminated bowel! Despite the mechanism, there are no signs of spinal trauma, so immobilization, Choice (D), isn't necessary at this time.

Chapter 13

The Scoop on Pediatrics

In This Chapter

- Understanding the differences between children and adults
- Assessing pediatric patients in medical and trauma situations

Kids are not simply pint-sized versions of adults. Any parent can tell you how different it is to interact with their children as they transition from infant and toddler stages to school-age and teenage form.

As an EMT, you need to know what some of these developmental differences are, because they shape your assessment approach for each age group. Anatomical and physiological differences also play a role, not only in the physical findings that you measure but also in the medical and trauma conditions that can be very serious to the child.

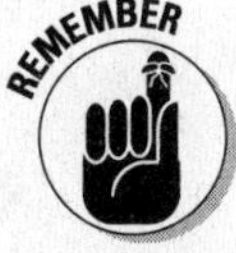

Many EMS providers find that managing pediatric patients makes them most nervous. Part of the reason is that we see them much less frequently than adult or elderly patients. Especially with infants and toddlers, communication can be a major challenge. Finally, you often have more than one individual to take care of; nervous or frightened parents can present problems of their own. Still, the way to overcome these barriers is to be knowledgeable about pediatric conditions, practice the skills and procedures regularly, engage the caregiver in a way that instills trust, and be confident about your ability to assess and manage the situation.

Sorting Out What Makes Children Different from Adults

Besides the obvious differences in size and maturity, there are several key differences between children and adults that affect your assessment approach, scene management, and treatment. These differences are developmental, anatomical, and physiological.

Developmental differences

From the time they are born until they transition to adulthood, children experience rapid physical growth. How they engage with their environment and other humans also changes dramatically. Children can be broadly divided into the following subgroups:

- **Infants:** Birth to 1 year
- **Toddlers:** 1 to 3 years
- **Preschool:** 3 to 5 years
- **School age:** 6 to 12 years
- **Adolescent:** 13 to 18 years

Table 13-1 shows the developmental differences among the groups, as well as their impact upon your assessment and treatment approach.

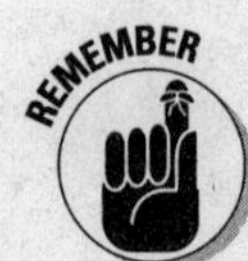

Kids cry when they're hurt or frightened; this is normal. You should be concerned about a child who is unusually quiet or cries weakly during your assessment and care.

Table 13-1 Behavior and Assessment of Children by Age

Age Group	*Developmental Behaviors*	*Assessment and Treatment*
Infants	Easy to separate from caregiver (separation anxiety develops as infant approaches 1 year) Crying a major form of communication, as is touch Well-developed sense of hearing Tracks motion with eyes Being undressed normal, but staying warm is important	If possible, have caregiver hold infant during assessment. Evaluate appearance, work of breathing, and skin color (pediatric assessment triangle, or PAT; see the later section "Assessment tips"). Find pulse at brachial artery. Uncover body as needed but cover back up to preserve temperature.
Toddlers	Begin exploring environment, first by crawling, then walking Do not want to be apart from caregiver (separation anxiety) May need special object to feel safe (toy, blanket) Can speak simply; may understand more than they can communicate Frighten easily; believe they were "bad" and caused situation As they age, less likely to undress	Have caregiver nearby or next to patient during assessment. Perform PAT from a distance; address both child and caregiver. Use simple words and phrases but not "baby talk." Assure toddlers that they did nothing wrong; they were not "bad." Perform physical exam by starting at the feet, to establish trust with toddler. Undress body areas for evaluation but cover up as soon as possible.
Preschoolers	Do not like being separated from caregiver Rapid development of speaking ability Fantastical thinking — pain and injuries may appear overly dramatic to them Do not like being undressed May perceive illness/injury as punishment	Have caregiver nearby or next to patient. Conduct PAT from a distance. Speak to both child and caregiver. Expose areas of the body only when necessary. Use simple words and phrases to question and explain. Reassure preschoolers that the situation is not their fault. Engage more with the patient — ask about what happened.
School-age children	Greater sense of autonomy Can have sustained, sensible discussions Concrete thinking Increasing peer and popularity pressure Modesty is important	Speak to both child and caregiver. Ask patient about medical history and about the events surrounding the current injury or illness. Have school-age children help to make simple decisions. Maintain modesty. Explain as you examine and treat.

Age Group	Developmental Behaviors	Assessment and Treatment
Adolescents	Like to be treated as adults Strong awareness of body image Experiment and take risks	Create private space for questions and examination. Maintain modesty. May need to separate adolescent from caregiver. Have adolescent involved in making more significant decisions. Adolescents may regress when confronted with significant stress. Be prepared to support them as needed.

Anatomical differences

There are several major anatomical differences between children and adults that can affect your assessment and treatment. These differences are more pronounced in younger children (infant through preschool age); they begin to disappear as the children age into school age and adolescence. By the time they are 18, most of the changes are complete. Table 13-2 highlights some of these distinctions.

Table 13-2 Anatomical Findings that Affect Assessment and Treatment

Body System	Anatomical Findings	Assessment and Treatment
Respiratory	Smaller, softer, and shorter upper airway Proportionally larger tongue Flatter nose and face Intercostal and accessory muscles not well developed	Airway is blocked more easily and requires more careful positioning to maintain patency. Pad under shoulders to place head and neck in a more neutral position. May be more difficult to create a mask seal when providing ventilation; continuously check mask seal when ventilating. Children breathe faster as they compensate; slow breathing is an especially bad sign (see the next section for details). Prepare to ventilate earlier in a pediatric situation compared to an adult scenario. May use abdominal muscles to help breathe, causing "seesaw" motion between chest and abdomen.
Cardiovascular	Greater ability to constrict blood vessels Lesser ability of heart to contract Less blood volume	Will maintain adequate blood pressure for longer time than adults, but crash (decompensate) faster; monitor vital signs closely. Does not take much blood loss to cause shock; control bleeding early. Heart rates can be much higher in children.

continued

Table 13-2 (continued)

Body System	Anatomical Findings	Assessment and Treatment
Nervous	More fragile brain tissue Thinner subarachnoid space Brain demands greater amounts of oxygen and glucose	Mental status and level of consciousness key indicators of adequate oxygenation and circulation; pay close attention to how the child interacts. More susceptible to primary and secondary brain injuries.
Gastrointestinal	Liver and spleen less protected by lower ribcage Less well protected by undeveloped abdominal muscles	Greater chance of blunt trauma to internal organs; palpate carefully and thoroughly. Greater chance of shock due to gastrointestinal injuries.
Musculoskeletal	Normal openings in newborn skull (fontanelles) Head proportionally larger to body as compared to adult Proportionally larger occiput Ribcage more pliable, less protective of internal organs Long bones more flexible	May observe normal bulging in infant's head during assessment or may be sign of infection. Younger children tend to fall headfirst, increasing chance of brain injury; check mental status early and often and look through the scalp for signs of an injury. May need to pad more to immobilize spine. Greater chance of blunt trauma to chest and abdomen; palpate thoroughly and carefully. Greater chance of partial (greenstick) fractures of long bones.
Integumentary	Proportionally greater body surface area than adults Proportionally less fat; thinner skin layers	Greater chance of hypothermia when exposed — must keep younger children covered. More serious burn trauma compared to adults.

Physiological differences

Children have incredible demands for oxygen and nutrients as they grow and develop, due to metabolic needs. As a result, children breathe more quickly and their hearts beat faster as compared to adults; blood pressures tend to be lower. Table 13-3 shows the normal ranges in vital signs, based on age.

Table 13-3 Pediatric Vital Signs

Age	Pulse (bpm)	Respiratory rate (bpm)	Systolic BP (mm Hg)
Newborn	120–180	30–50	60–80
6–12 months	120–140	30–40	70–80
1–4 years	100–110	20–30	80–95
5–7 years	90–100	14–20	90–100
8–12 years	80–100	12–20	100–110
Over 12 years	60–90	12–20	100–120

In general, the pediatric patient is usually healthy. Significant problems tend to arise when breathing and/or circulation is compromised. The body attempts to compensate for the problem for as long as possible and then rapidly decompensates when it can no longer do so. You want to be vigilant in observing the child's level of mentation, breathing ability, and circulatory status, as these may change very quickly.

Really fast breathing and heart rates in children are usually compensatory signs, meaning that systems are striving to keep things working as close to normal as possible. A really slow breathing and/or heart rate is alarming — it means that the body is rapidly losing its ability to maintain control. If not corrected, respiratory and cardiac arrest are likely. Consider the following example questions.

A 20-month-old is awake and crying after a motor vehicle crash. She was restrained in her car seat. There is a contusion across her chest in the shape of the harness strap. Lung sounds are clear, her pulse rate is 130, and she is breathing at 30 times per minute. She is pale, warm, and dry. You should

(A) assist her breathing with a bag-valve mask and oxygen.

(B) continue your assessment.

(C) apply a bulky dressing to the chest wall, where the contusion is located.

(D) immobilize the patient to a long backboard.

The correct choice is (B). The child is crying, which is a good sign that she is breathing adequately. Her vital signs, though elevated, are within the normal range of a 20-month-old. She is ventilating adequately, making Choice (A) inappropriate. You have no information to indicate an injury to the chest wall, Choice (C), and using a long board to immobilize a child that young, Choice (D), would require a lot of padding and adjustments to do it correctly. Other devices, specifically, a pediatric immobilization device, would work better.

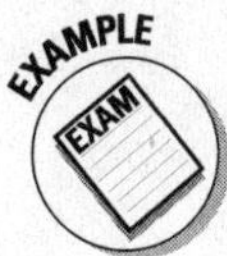

A 2-year-old child is unresponsive. A parent found him unconscious in the bathroom with open pill bottles nearby. His respiratory rate is 10 breaths per minute, and his pulse rate is 60. His skin is cool, dry, and cyanotic. You should next

(A) assist his breathing with a bag-valve mask and oxygen.

(B) provide supplemental oxygen via a blow-by mask.

(C) determine the contents of the medication bottles.

(D) apply AED pads to the patient's chest.

The correct answer is Choice (A). In this case, the patient's breathing rate is too low for this age group. The lack of oxygen may be slowing down his heart rate to a dangerous level. He needs to be ventilated with oxygen quickly. If the heart rate doesn't increase within a few seconds to a minute of artificial ventilation, chest compressions may be needed. Choice (B) won't deliver the oxygen to the cells because he is breathing too slow. You may need to perform Choice (C), but this will not help the child at this point. Choice (D) would be correct if the patient were in cardiac arrest — but he's not.

Managing the Pediatric Patient

The way that you approach pediatric patients is similar to that of any adult patient — you evaluate the scene for any safety issues, perform the primary assessment and treat any life-threatening conditions, decide whether the situation is critical enough to require immediate transport, and then perform a secondary assessment. Given what you know about some of the differences between children and adults (see the preceding section), I point out some key differences in the following sections.

Assessment tips

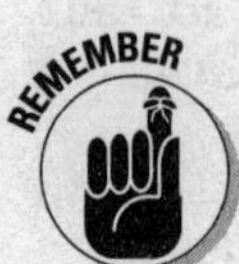

For children ranging from infant to toddlers, performing the pediatric assessment triangle (PAT) can help you to quickly determine how critical the situation is without rushing right up to the child. As you enter the scene, take a moment to look at the following signs (see Figure 13-1):

- **Appearance:** Is the child awake? Crying? Clinging to the caregiver? Those are signs of adequate oxygenation and circulation to the child's brain. You should be concerned about a child who is quiet, crying weakly, not recognizing the caregiver, or sleepy and hard to arouse.
- **Work of breathing:** Keep in mind that fast breathing is fine, so long as the child doesn't appear tired, anxious, or frightened. Be concerned if the child is working hard to breathe, showing signs of accessory muscle use, or seesaw breathing.
- **Circulation to skin:** The skin should have good color. Any mottling, pallor (significant paleness), or cyanosis is a bad sign that requires your immediate attention.

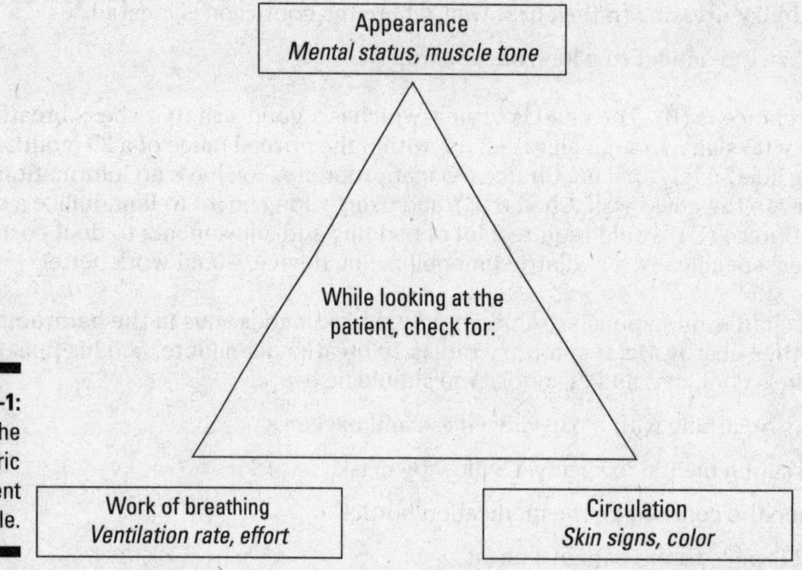

Figure 13-1: The pediatric assessment triangle.

After performing the PAT, you can begin your "close-up" assessment of the child. Here are a few other guidelines for assessing kids of all ages:

- If the toddler or preschool child is not critically ill or injured, performing a toe-to-head physical exam may be less intrusive and frightening to the patient.
- Keep the caregiver close by when evaluating younger patients. Parents can often tell you subtle things they notice about their children. Explain what you are doing when performing an exam or procedure.
- If the child is older, don't ignore what he wants to say or do, and don't keep him out of any discussions with caregivers. Even preschoolers will understand at least some of what you're saying. Absolutely do not hide anything or lie about what you're doing. You'll have a hard time reestablishing any trust with the child once it's broken.
- If the child has a special toy or other object that provides reassurance or comfort, allow him to bring it along. An older child is inquisitive, even if he doesn't feel well. Penlights, a stethoscope, or the back of an ambulance can capture a child's attention and allow you to perform additional exams and procedures.

A parent is holding his 18-month-old infant in his arms. You can see that the infant appears limp, is breathing rapidly, and has pale skin. You should

(A) have the parent hand the infant to you.

(B) perform a toe-to-head assessment.

(C) assess the infant's airway and breathing while in the parent's arms.

(D) ask the parent about the infant's medical history.

The best answer is Choice (A). Your PAT assessment reveals an infant who is very sick. You need to rapidly conduct a primary assessment and provide care as soon as possible. Maintaining the infant in the parent's arms, Choice (C), will inhibit you from assessing the infant fully. Choice (B) is part of the secondary assessment, as is Choice (D).

Medical situations

Several pediatric medical conditions are commonly seen by EMTs. In the majority of cases, your care is supportive — ensure that problems with airway, breathing, and circulation are identified and managed, and help maintain body temperature and oxygenation during transport. In some situations, you may need to intervene quickly. Table 13-4 provides a list of medical conditions, their signs, and specific treatments.

Table 13-4 Pediatric Medical Conditions and Treatment

Problem	*Signs and Symptoms*	*Action Steps*
Foreign body airway obstruction	No air exchange; no crying or other sounds; rapid loss of consciousness, skin turns pale and then cyanotic.	Infant, conscious: Five back blows and chest thrusts. Child, conscious: Abdominal thrusts. Child, unconscious: Perform CPR and attempt to ventilate, check airway to see whether obstruction can be removed.
Croup	Fever; hoarseness; barky cough; difficulty breathing.	Provide supplemental oxygen (humidified if possible). Change in air temperature or humidity may reduce symptoms.
Epiglottitis	High fever; difficult, painful swallowing; drooling; tripod positioning.	Maintain patient's position of comfort. Do not inspect or probe mouth. Provide supplemental oxygen, humidified if possible, using blow-by method (caregiver can help hold the mask).
Asthma	Wheezing lung sounds; difficulty breathing, especially during exhalation; pursed lips, accessory muscle use; coughing.	Maintain patient's position of comfort. Assist with patient's metered dose inhaler if prescribed. Administer oxygen if saturation level is low or patient is having difficulty breathing.

continued

Table 13-4 *(continued)*

Problem	***Signs and Symptoms***	***Action Steps***
Fever	Very warm skin, especially on the chest and abdomen; high temperature using a thermometer; may cause a febrile seizure. Dehydration may be associated with the fever (see "Diarrhea and vomiting" in this table).	Remove most clothing. Be alert for shivering as it may cause the fever to rise. Ice chips may provide comfort.
Meningitis (inflammation of the membranes surrounding the brain and spinal cord)	High fever; neck pain, tenderness, or rigidity; severe headache; hypersensitivity to bright light; nausea, vomiting.	Meningitis can be highly contagious. Wear respiratory protection. Prepare to manage airway and ventilations if respiratory failure occurs (decreasing respiratory rate, decreasing level of consciousness, cyanosis).
Diarrhea and vomiting	If serious, dehydration may set in and cause signs of shock: tachycardia; cool, pale skin; eyes that appear sunken; altered mental status or unconsciousness.	Treat for shock: Maintain body temperature, provide supplemental oxygen, and ventilate if needed. Provide nothing by mouth.
Seizures	Patients with generalized seizures are unconscious during the seizure. Tonic-clonic muscle activity (rhythmic jerking of the limbs, stiffening of the body); patient may be incontinent and/or have bitten the tongue. Will be postictal after seizure ends; may be hard to arouse, confused, and frightened.	Most seizures only last several seconds to a minute. Care is supportive — prevent further harm during the seizure, maintain airway, and provide supplemental oxygen. Status epilepticus are seizures that last more than a couple of minutes or a series of seizures that occur without the patient regaining consciousness. These may be life-threatening. Transport immediately, maintain airway patency, and ventilate with a bag-valve mask and oxygen. Suction may be necessary if secretions become significant.
Altered mental status (AMS)	Younger children: sleepy, lethargic, difficult to arouse from sleep. Unable to maintain interest, easy to separate from caregiver. Irritated, inconsolable. Older children: confusion, lethargy, sleepy. Evaluate for underlying cause: Shock, hypoxia, hypoglycemia, drug ingestion, and head trauma are some possibilities.	Maintain airway patency. Ventilate with a bag-valve mask if in respiratory failure. Use an oropharyngeal airway (OPA) and position the child's airway carefully if unconscious. Keep suction immediately available in case vomiting occurs. Maintain body temperature and transport immediately.

Problem	*Signs and Symptoms*	*Action Steps*
Poisoning	Possible causes of poisoning include medications, household chemicals, intoxicants, and other recreational drugs. Immediate concern is altered mental status (AMS) and loss of airway patency.	Maintain airway, using manual maneuvers and an OPA if necessary. Ventilate if needed. If breathing is adequate, provide supplemental oxygen. Be alert for vomiting. Maintain safety precautions if a hazardous material is the cause of the poisoning.
Respiratory arrest	Not breathing or agonal breaths. Cyanosis. Will cause heart rate to slow.	Insert an OPA and manually position the airway to keep open. Ventilate with bag-valve mask once every 3 to 5 seconds and provide supplemental oxygen. Keep suction immediately available in case patient vomits. Assess for underlying cause. Begin immediate transport.
Cardiac arrest	No pulse, no breathing or agonal breaths.	Single-person CPR, infant: Use two fingers to compress. Two-person CPR, infant: Use thumb-encircling technique. Single-person CPR, child: Use heel of one or both hands. Compress chest to 1/3 to 1/2 depth of chest at a rate of at least 100 beats per minute. Ventilate at a ratio of 30 compressions to 2 ventilations. Two-person CPR, child: Adjust compressions-to-breaths ratio to 15:2. If arrest is unwitnessed, attach an automated external defibrillator (AED) with appropriate size pads after five cycles of compressions and ventilations. Analyze heart rhythm every 2 minutes and administer a shock if indicated. Transport as soon as possible.
Sudden infant death syndrome (SIDS)	No pulse, no breathing. May have signs of death: pooling of blood in lower areas of body (dependent lividity); stiffening of limbs (rigor mortis). Generally no report of any unusual circumstances or events prior to death.	In most situations where death is obvious, treatment is directed toward the family. Try not to disturb the death scene. If there are no obvious signs of death, begin CPR and transport.
Child abuse/neglect	Patient may be quiet, withdrawn, fearful. Most often there are physical signs of trauma (see next section). Other abuse patterns may show signs of neglect such as poor nutrition.	Provide supportive care for any injury. Do not confront caregiver on-scene. Observe the scene and take mental notes. As a mandated reporter, notify child protective services and advise hospital staff of your findings.

A 4-year-old male is sitting in a chair. The parent reports the patient stayed home from school today because of a bad cold. He is looking at you quietly, breathing quickly through his mouth, and drooling. His skin is pale and feels hot. You should

(A) ask him to swallow.

(B) gently insert a flexible suction catheter.

(C) suction with a rigid catheter.

(D) evaluate the patient further.

The best choice is (D). The patient is showing signs of epiglottitis; there is enough swelling of the soft tissues in the back of the throat that he is unable to swallow his saliva without blocking his airway, making Choice (A) inappropriate. Choices (B) and (C) may irritate the swelling, creating a full airway obstruction.

Trauma situations

Trauma is the number-one killer of children in the United States. In general, infants and toddlers are most commonly hurt through falls or abuse. In suspected abuse, there may be multiple bruises in various stages of healing. The caregiver may provide a history of the patient being "accident prone." Injury patterns may be too precise — scald injuries to just the buttocks and legs of an infant, for example.

School-age and adolescent children tend to be hurt through blunt trauma mechanisms involved primarily in automobile crashes or being hit by a motor vehicle while walking or riding a bicycle. Though less frequent, adolescent children are also victims of gunshots and stabbings. Contact sports are another common cause of injuries in children.

Managing pediatric trauma is similar to handling adult trauma (see Chapter 12). Your focus is to

- Preserve the airway and protect the spine.
- Ensure adequate ventilations and oxygenation.
- Minimize the effect of shock by maintaining body temperature and keeping the patient still.

The following sections discuss various trauma situations in more detail.

Head, brain, and spinal injuries

Head and brain injuries are common in children due to the relative larger size and weight of the head. Look for signs of injury to the head and scalp, and control any external bleeding. Signs of increasing cerebral pressure (ICP) include altered mental status, headache, and vomiting. Severe ICP may cause the brain to compress, causing unequal pupils and slowing pulse and respiratory rates. Treatment includes providing spinal precautions, preserving airway and breathing, and performing mild hyperventilation in severe ICP.

While spinal injuries are relatively less common in young children, assessing them in the field can be difficult due to communication issues. Even appropriately sized equipment may be difficult to apply due to sizing and shape issues. Use plenty of padding to help secure the patient to an appropriately sized board. If the child presents in a car seat, consider placing padding around the patient's head and body and immobilize the child within the seat itself, so long as the seat has not been damaged by the crash.

Chest and abdominal injuries

The chest wall is more pliable in children than in adults. This pliability provides less protection to the heart, lungs, and upper abdominal organs such as the liver and spleen. If there is a mechanism of injury (MOI) to the chest, evaluate carefully for signs of internal injury, such as respiratory distress and shock.

The developing abdominal muscles provide little protection for the organs that lie underneath. As a result, abdominal injuries are more common in children with blunt MOI. Children can mask shock symptoms for some time; evaluate the MOI and assess for possible hidden injuries (as I describe in Chapter 12).

Falls and burns

As toddlers master the act of walking, falls are common and can sometimes result in bone fractures. Suspect a fracture if the child guards the injury site, can't put weight on a leg, or is unable to move an extremity without discomfort. Fractures may be incomplete (*greenstick* fractures) because the child's bones are more pliable than those of an adult. Splint any possible fracture the same way you would an adult fracture.

Burns can be especially harmful to children, as their skin is thinner and offers less protection than adults' skin. Treat burns as you would in an adult: Extinguish any burning process first, and then dry and cover with dry, clean dressings to help with pain control. Chemicals may need to be flushed with copious amounts of water. Be careful of your own safety with electrical burns.

The rule of nines in estimating burn surface area (BSA) changes slightly for children to accommodate for different body proportions. Table 13-5 show the differences between infants, children, and adults.

Table 13-5 Burn Surface Area of the Body

Body Part	*Infant*	*Child*	*Adult*
Head	18	12	9
Torso, front	18	18	18
Torso, back	18	18	18
Entire arm	9	9	9
Entire leg	13.5	16.5	18
Genital region	1	1	1

Disaster management for multiple patients

In disaster management, you can use the JumpSTART method to triage children under the age of 8 years and weighing less than 100 pounds (see Figure 13-2).

- Patients who can walk are first categorized as "green" and sent over to the treatment area, where they can be re-triaged.
- Patients with a spontaneous breathing rate between 15 and 45 breaths per minute, a palpable pulse, and an appropriate level of consciousness are categorized as "yellow" and are delayed treatment and transport.
- Patients whose breathing rate is less than 15 or greater than 45, or who begin breathing after airway positioning and five rescue breaths, are categorized as "red" and are treated and transported immediately. This immediate category also includes patients who are breathing, but do not have a palpable pulse, as well as patients who are unconscious or altered.

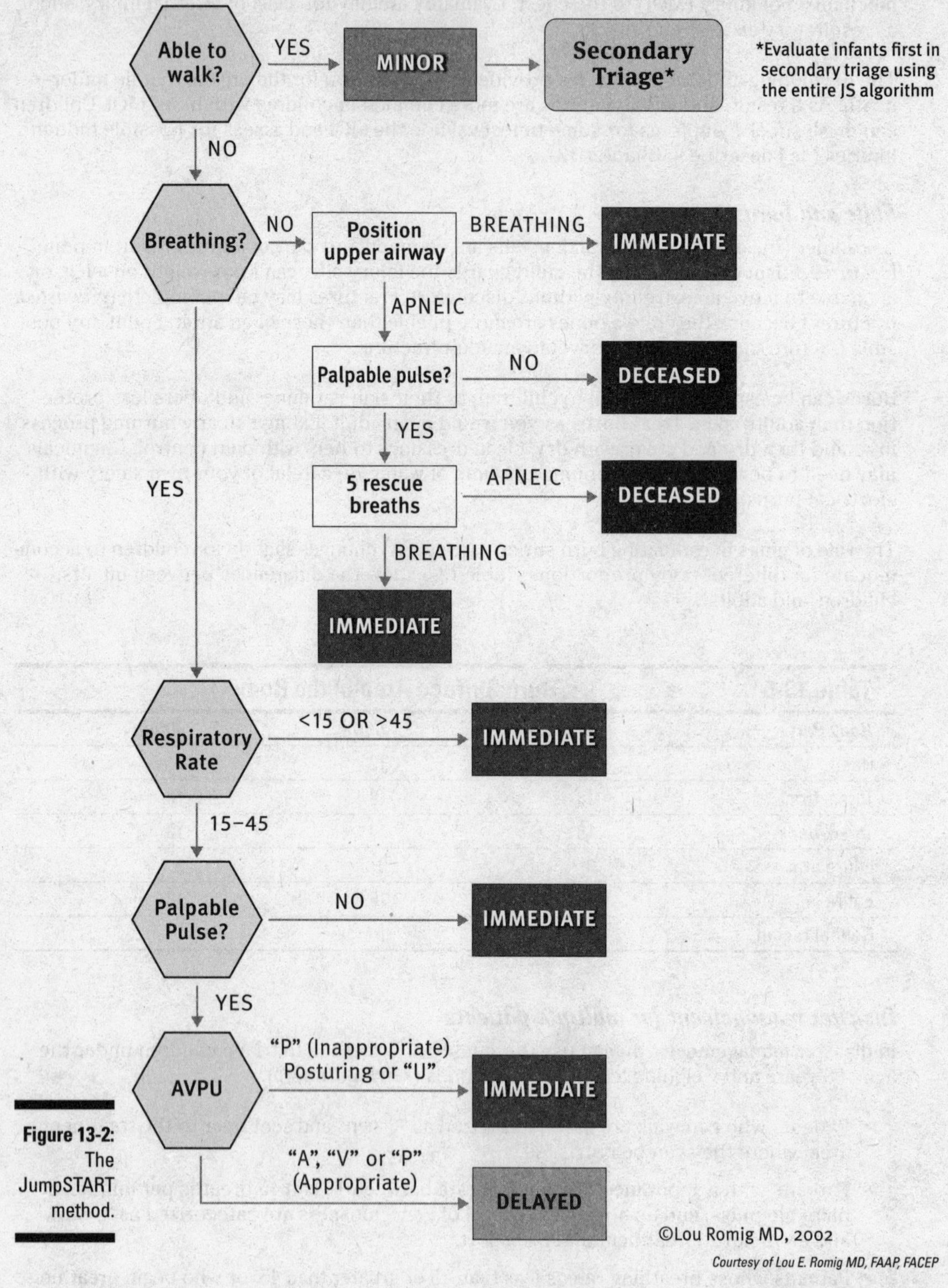

Figure 13-2: The JumpSTART method.

Courtesy of Lou E. Romig MD, FAAP, FACEP

Practice Questions about Pediatrics

The following practice questions are similar to the EMT exam's questions about pediatrics. Read each question carefully, and then select the answer choice that most correctly answers the question.

1. A 6-year-old female presents sitting upright, with difficulty breathing. Her pulse rate is 100, and she is breathing 22 times per minute. Her skin feels hot, she is pale, and there is audible stridor. You should

   (A) position her supine and assist ventilations with a bag-valve mask and oxygen.

   (B) provide supplemental oxygen via the blow-by method.

   (C) assist ventilations with a bag-valve mask.

   (D) inspect her mouth using a tongue depressor.

2. A 7-year-old male is having difficulty breathing after playing in the schoolyard. He is alert, frightened, breathing 24 times per minute, and has a pulse rate of 130. You note wheezing in both lung fields. His skin feels warm and diaphoretic. You should

   (A) help with the administration of the patient's prescribed multidose inhaler.

   (B) help with the patient's prescribed epinephrine autoinjector.

   (C) assist the patient's breathing with a bag-valve mask.

   (D) transport immediately and notify the parents en route.

3. A 14-month-old male is having breathing difficulty. He cries loudly when you examine him. His skin is pale and dry. His heart rate is 128, and he is breathing at a rate of 30 times per minute. You should

   (A) assist ventilations with a bag-valve mask.

   (B) separate the child from his parent.

   (C) have the parent administer supplemental oxygen using the blow-by technique.

   (D) administer high-flow oxygen via a nonrebreather mask.

4. A 20-month-old child does not respond to your presence. She is breathing 12 times per minute, and her pulse rate is 60. She has been having difficulty breathing during the past 12 hours. You should

   (A) assist ventilations with a bag-valve mask.

   (B) have the parent administer supplemental oxygen using the blow-by technique.

   (C) place her in a sitting position and open her airway.

   (D) administer high-flow oxygen via a nonrebreather mask.

5. A 7-month-old female is lethargic and cries when stimulated. She has had a fever, diarrhea, and little to eat or drink in the last 12 hours. Her heart rate is 150, and she is breathing 50 times per minute. You suspect

   (A) respiratory distress.

   (B) respiratory failure.

   (C) compensated shock.

   (D) decompensated shock.

6. A 14-year-old male collapsed after playing soccer for a few minutes. He is unresponsive and breathing 40 times per minute. His pulse rate is 220, and is felt at the carotid artery only. His skin is cool and diaphoretic. You suspect

(A) sudden dehydration.

(B) severe hypoglycemia.

(C) a cardiac rhythm disturbance.

(D) an asthma attack.

7. You evaluate a 5-year-old female at a day-care center. The child has had numerous episodes of "staring into space" over the past 2 hours, lasting a few seconds, followed by confusion and being frightened. Her vital signs are normal. Staff is unable to reach the parent. You should

(A) let the child stay at the center until a parent picks her up.

(B) transport to a hospital while attempting to reach the parent.

(C) administer oral glucose.

(D) wait until the parent is notified.

8. A 4-month-old infant is face up in his crib, pulseless and apneic. There appears to be dark bruising along his back and buttocks. The infant is cold to the touch, cyanotic, and stiff. You should

(A) begin chest compressions and ventilations.

(B) do nothing and transport the infant to the hospital.

(C) provide emotional support for the family.

(D) bring the infant into the ambulance and call police.

9. A 4-year-old female is nauseous, vomiting, and has diarrhea lasting 40 minutes. Her last oral intake was lunch an hour earlier. She has cramping and pain across her abdomen. She is warm and dry to the touch. Which of the following is the most likely cause of her presentation?

(A) Appendicitis

(B) Cholecystitis

(C) Food poisoning

(D) Peritonitis

10. A child falls off his bicycle at a high rate of speed. He has road rash on his hands, knees, and the left side of his body; a contusion on the left parietal portion of his head; and a deformity to his left shoulder. He is unresponsive and breathing 6 times per minute. His pulse rate is 76. What should you do first?

(A) Splint the injured shoulder.

(B) Assist ventilations with a bag-valve mask at a rate of 20 per minute.

(C) Immobilize the patient to a long backboard.

(D) Provide high-flow oxygen via a nonrebreather mask.

11. A 7-year-old falls off an outdoor jungle gym and strikes the right side of his body against a bar when he falls. He is breathing 24 times a minute, and his pulse rate is 120. His lung sounds are clear, and he winces when you palpate his right lateral chest and abdomen. Which of the following injury patterns do you most strongly suspect?

(A) Liver injuries

(B) Rib fractures

(C) Lung injuries

(D) Flail chest

12. A 16-month-old child pulls a pot of boiling water off the stove, burning his entire right arm, the front of his torso, and his entire right leg. The percent of body surface affected by the burn is approximately what percent?

(A) 36

(B) 39

(C) 44

(D) 49

13. A parent reports his 9-year-old child has fallen down a flight of stairs. The child is alert, quiet, and cooperative. His right wrist is deformed, and there are several bruises on both arms and legs. Some are purple and yellow in color, while others are red. You find no other obvious injuries. You should

(A) splint the injured wrist, transport, and further evaluate the bruises.

(B) ask the parent whether the other bruises are a result of the fall.

(C) apply splints to the wrist and legs.

(D) have the parent drive the child to the emergency department.

14. The components of the pediatric assessment triangle (PAT) include

(A) airway, work of breathing, and pulse location.

(B) appearance, work of breathing, and circulation to the skin.

(C) appearance, breathing rate, and pulse rate.

(D) airway, respiratory rate, and pulse rate.

15. You are evaluating a 2-year-old child after a motor vehicle crash. He is crying loudly and reaching for his mother. How would you assess this patient?

(A) Quickly palpate the head, torso, and abdomen for serious injuries.

(B) Take a set of vital signs as soon as possible.

(C) Ask the patient about any medications or allergies.

(D) Perform a toe-to-head assessment.

16. A 3-year-old female ingested liquid drain cleaner. She is alert, frightened, and crying. You note burns around her mouth. You should

(A) position her supine and elevate her legs.

(B) monitor her airway.

(C) determine why the ingestion occurred.

(D) administer activated charcoal.

17. A 9-month-old infant has had a cough, a fever, and diarrhea for 24 hours. Her diaper is dry and her skin feels warm and dry. Her heart rate is 160, and she is breathing 45 times per minute. She cries weakly upon stimulation. Which of the following conditions do you suspect is most likely causing her presentation?

    (A) Respiratory distress secondary to cough

    (B) Respiratory failure secondary to bronchiolitis

    (C) Shock secondary to dehydration

    (D) Shock secondary to cardiac dysthymia

18. During your initial triage of a school bus crash, you have a child who is unconscious and not breathing. You perform a jaw thrust and the patient remains apneic. What should you do next?

    (A) Give five rescuc breaths and reassess.

    (B) Check for a brachial or carotid pulse.

    (C) Declare the patient dead.

    (D) Begin chest compressions.

19. A 10-month-old infant was crawling on the floor when he had a sudden episode of difficulty breathing. His respiratory rate is 30. There is audible stridor. You suspect

    (A) epiglottitis.

    (B) croup.

    (C) foreign body obstruction.

    (D) trauma.

20. A 2-year-old presents with a high fever and repeated vomiting. The parent states the patient has been ill for 24 hours and has become increasingly lethargic. You note red dots spread across the child's face and arms. You should

    (A) remove all the patient's clothing.

    (B) wear an N95 HEPA mask.

    (C) apply cold packs to the patient's groin and armpits.

    (D) put a mask over the patient's mouth and nose.

Answers and Explanations

Use this answer key to score the practice questions in the preceding section. The explanations give you insight into why the correct answer is better than the other choices.

1. **B.** The scenario suggests epiglottitis, which causes swelling of the soft tissues in the upper airway. This patient is not likely to tolerate lying down, as Choice (A) suggests, because the airway may become blocked. Her respiratory and heart rates are normal in her age group, so assisted ventilations, Choice (C), aren't necessary. You don't want to inspect or probe her mouth, Choice (D), if there is epiglottitis, as that may possibly worsen the swelling.

2. **A.** The scenario suggests an asthma attack, which may be resolved with the use of the inhaler. You may need to begin transport after the initial treatment, but don't rush the decision, as in Choice (D). Although it's possible that the child is experiencing anaphylaxis, as Choice (B) suggests, the skin signs and mental status make that suspicion less likely. The respiratory effort is just above the normal range, and the child is alert, making assisted ventilations, Choice (C), unnecessary.

3. **C.** The scenario suggests that the patient is in respiratory distress, not failure. Assisting ventilations with a bag-valve mask, Choice (A), isn't necessary because the child's tidal volume and breathing rate are adequate. You can reduce anxiety in the child by keeping the parent close by rather than separating them, as per Choice (B). High-flow oxygen, Choice (D), isn't indicated for this patient's level of breathing distress, and the mask may worsen anxiety.
4. **A.** The scenario suggests that the patient is in respiratory failure. The slow pulse rate is an ominous sign of impending cardiac arrest. Assisting ventilations, Choice (A), is imperative; supplemental oxygen, Choices (B) and (D), isn't adequate. It will be difficult to keep the patient in a sitting position, Choice (C), because she is unresponsive.
5. **C.** She appears to be dehydrated, although her pulse and breathing rate are just beyond the normal limits. Her breathing rate is a sign of compensating for the reduced circulatory volume, not the primary problem. This eliminates Choices (A) and (B) as answers. If the answer were Choice (D), you would expect the patient to have a very fast pulse and respiratory rate, or the patient to be unconscious with a very slow pulse and respiratory rate, an ominous sign of impending respiratory/cardiac arrest.
6. **C.** The patient's heart rate is much too fast, and the onset too sudden, for dehydration, Choice (A), to be the cause. His loss of consciousness, along with signs of decompensated shock, make Choices (B) and (D) very unlikely.
7. **B.** The scenario suggests a series of generalized absence seizures — no motor activities, but the patient loses consciousness briefly. Although these seizures aren't life-threatening in and of themselves, they can be a sign of something more serious. You should transport the patient under implied consent rather than wait until the parent is contacted, Choice (D). Nothing in the scenario indicates a diabetic situation, as Choice (C) suggests. Leaving the patient, Choice (A), is not an option in this situation.
8. **C.** The infant shows clinical signs of death. You should not attempt resuscitation, Choice (A). Instead, focus on the family's needs during this stressful time. Moving the infant, Choices (B) and (D), would be inappropriate.
9. **C.** Patients with appendicitis, Choice (A), tend to complain about pain around the belly button or in the right lower quadrant. Cholecystitis, Choice (B), is more located in the right upper quadrant. Peritonitis, Choice (D), comes on relatively slowly — over a period of hours to days, not minutes. The timing of the complaints relative to the last oral intake suggests a relationship between the two.
10. **B.** The injury to the patient's head along with the slower heart and breathing rates suggest increased cranial pressure after a blow to the head. Mild hyperventilation is indicated. You will immobilize him, Choice (C), but not until after managing the airway, breathing, and circulation problems. Supplemental oxygen, Choice (D), won't be sufficient without adequate ventilation. You can splint the shoulder, Choice (A), while en route.
11. **A.** Pediatric patients have more pliable rib cages, meaning they tend to bend more when blunt force is applied. This reduces the likelihood of rib fractures, Choice (B). However, the force is transmitted deeper into the body; the liver, Choice (A), is located in the right upper quadrant. The chances of a lung injury, Choice (C), are small, and the respiratory rate is not so fast as to indicate the loss of rib-cage integrity associated with a flail segment, Choice (D).
12. **C.** Using the rule of nines, the front of a child's torso is 18 percent, the right arm is 9 percent, and the right leg is 16.5 percent. Add these percentages together to get 43.5 percent, and then round up to 44 percent.
13. **A.** The varying colors of the bruises are due to time — bruises turn different colors as they age. This suggests that the child has received numerous injuries over a period of time, a possible sign of abuse. Don't accuse the parent on the scene; care for the child and begin transport as soon as you can. You can gently question the child while in the privacy of the ambulance.

14. **B.** The pediatric assessment triangle allows you to quickly size up the child's condition without having to touch or be close — an "across the room" assessment. You can then decide whether the child is critical and needs immediate intervention or whether you have time to perform a full assessment, with the parent nearby to help comfort the child. Choices (A), (C), and (D) all contain some form of pulse check, which must be done up close.

15. **D.** The child appears to be in good condition, based on the pediatric assessment triangle (appearance, work of breathing, and circulation to skin). A rapid trauma assessment, Choice (A), is not indicated at this point. You want to take some time to establish trust with the child so you can evaluate for injuries. A toe-to-head assessment avoids having to inspect the head first, which may frighten the child further. It may be easier to obtain a full set of vital signs, Choice (B), after you establish trust. The patient is too young to respond to specific medical questions as Choice (C) suggests.

16. **B.** The child appears to be stable, despite the ingestion. Keeping her sitting and with a parent will help keep her calm and her airway clear if she vomits; she shouldn't lie down, Choice (A). The use of activated charcoal, Choice (D), in a corrosive ingestion is contraindicated. Knowing the reason why the child ingested the substance, Choice (C), won't change your approach to the patient's care.

17. **C.** The scenario describes a situation where the patient is losing significant fluid due to an infection. The dry diaper hints at little or no urine output. Her breathing rate is in response to hypoperfusion, not the cause of her condition as Choices (A) and (B) indicate. A cardiac dysthymia, Choice (D), generally comes on quickly and is not related to a fever or diarrhea.

18. **B.** In the pediatric triage system known as JumpSTART, you take into account that pediatric patients are very respiratory driven. That is, if you can provide ventilation and oxygenation early, you can slow or reverse a state of arrest. In JumpSTART, if the patient isn't breathing, you open the airway with a jaw thrust or chin lift. If he's still not breathing, you check for a pulse. If the pulse is present, you give five rescue breaths. If the patient begins to breathe, you tag him as immediate.

19. **C.** A foreign body can narrow the upper airway but not block it completely, causing stridor during breathing. Although croup, Choice (B), and epiglottitis, Choice (A), can cause stridor in the upper airway, both take time to develop. No signs of obvious trauma, Choice (D), are described in the scenario.

20. **B.** The patient has signs of Neisseria meningitidis, a particularly dangerous form of meningitis. Meningitis is especially contagious, and you can reduce being exposed by wearing the appropriate mask. Having the patient wear a mask, Choice (D), isn't helpful in reducing cross-contamination. Cooling the patient as Choice (A) suggests is a secondary concern. Applying cold packs, Choice (C), may cool down the body too quickly.

Chapter 14

EMS Operations

In This Chapter

- Practicing EMS within the law
- Keeping yourself safe, healthy, and sane
- Working on a team to resolve an emergency incident
- Operating an emergency vehicle
- Handling large incidents

What makes providers of emergency medical services (EMS) different from other medical personnel is where they practice — in people's homes, places of work, out in the street. Unlike medical professionals who work in hospitals, clinics, or doctors' offices, emergency medical technicians (EMTs) can't control the dangers that accompany unfamiliar environments. However, being aware of the safety issues and responding to them appropriately reduces the potential for harm. This chapter describes important aspects of EMS operations: following medical legal standards, staying healthy and safe, working well with others, handling an emergency vehicle, and being on the scene of a large emergency incident.

Maintaining Medical Legal Standards

No matter where you engage your patient, there is a clear set of medical legal guidelines you should practice religiously, as you find out in the following sections. Ethics and "doing the right thing" apply as well, but it's the law that will either protect you or, if you do the wrong thing, provide patients the ability to be compensated for their losses.

Grasping the basic legal tenets of medical practice

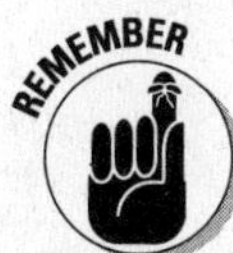

The basics of understanding your legal role as an EMT are grounded in the following three legal terms:

- **Scope of practice:** Your state laws dictate what medical procedures you can perform, as well as what you cannot do. For example, you can ventilate a patient with a bag-valve mask and oxygen, but you can't ventilate a patient with an endotracheal tube.
- **Standard of care:** The way that you perform a particular procedure or technique is the way most other EMTs would do so under similar circumstances. The standards of care that apply range from being very regional (for example, system protocols that provide guidance while you are at work) to nationwide (CPR standards, for example).

- **Duty to act:** You are required to perform your scope of practice to the level of the standard of care. This includes nonclinical aspects of the job, such as keeping a vehicle stocked, responding to an emergency call, transferring the patient to receiving staff at a hospital, or allowing a patient to refuse medical care.

Avoiding negligence

If you breach your duty to act (see the preceding section), the patient may be able to file a lawsuit against you for negligence. To prove negligence, the patient has to be able to prove four things happened:

1. You had a duty to act.
2. There was a breach of that duty.
3. There was an injury.
4. The injury (physical, emotional, or both) was a result of the breach, or causation.

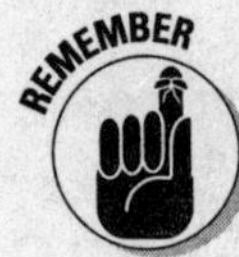

All four elements must be proven in order for a suit to be successful. For example, when you were transferring your patient to the gurney, you lost your footing and dropped her to the floor. Fortunately, she wasn't injured by the fall. No negligence occurred in this case because the patient wasn't injured and you didn't perform above or below your level of training; you didn't breach your duty to act.

A 35-year-old male has been shot in the chest. He is unconscious; has cold, diaphoretic, and pale skin; has a rapid carotid pulse; and is tachypneic. You apply occlusive dressings to the single open chest wound, but overlook a bleeding, open wound to the patient's back during your assessment. The patient survives his wounds and takes a long time to recover. The patient sues you for negligence. Overlooking the back wound would be an example of

(A) duty to act.

(B) breach of duty.

(C) injury.

(D) causation.

The best answer is Choice (B). Part of your training requires you to inspect the back for an injury, which you failed to do in this scenario. You had an obligation to respond when called, Choice (A), which is unrelated to overlooking the back wound. The gunshot wounds are examples of an injury, Choice (C). With regard to Choice (D), if you had controlled the bleeding sooner by identifying the back wound early, you may have reduced the extent of his shock condition (as indicated by his vital signs), possibly reducing his recovery time.

Getting the proper consent

You must establish the right to render care to the patient. This can be expressed consent, where the patient is able to indicate he wants your help. Or, it can be implied consent, when the patient is unconscious or otherwise incapacitated and it would be reasonable to ask for help. Only adults are capable of providing consent; children must be judged by the legal system to be emancipated minors in order to give consent.

Adults who are unable to determine their own medical care may have a court authorize another adult to act on their behalf. The person making such decisions has *durable power of attorney.*

If you don't obtain consent and proceed to treat and/or transport, you may end up being accused of battery (touching the patient without consent) or false imprisonment (kidnapping or holding someone against his will). If you threaten a patient or otherwise make the patient fearful of possible bodily harm, you are committing assault.

Understanding slander and libel

Speaking poorly about someone's character is known as *slander.* Writing poorly about someone's character is *libel.* For example, stating that a patient is "just drunk" to a receiving nurse could be seen as a slanderous statement; documenting that the patient was "drunk" or "intoxicated" can be seen as a libelous statement.

Dealing with refusals of care and/or transport

An adult, under most circumstances, has the right to refuse your treatment and transport. You have to determine whether the person is capable of making such a decision. This includes determining whether the patient is alert, oriented, and understands the consequences of not accepting your care. You also have to assess whether any existing circumstances are impairing the patient's judgment, such as intoxication or a language barrier.

Documentation is crucial in patient refusals. It includes having the patient sign a form that affirms her right to refuse further treatment and, in many circumstances, the signature of a witness that verifies the patient did sign the form.

Maintaining confidentiality

You are required to protect the patient's right to privacy in matters related to treatment and personal information. Federal law known as the Health Insurance Portability and Accountability Act (HIPAA) sets strict guidelines (and financial penalties!) regarding who you can share information with, which is usually limited to other medical professionals directly involved with the patient's care. This means no talking about private patient information to other crew members or your family or friends, as well as doctors and nurses in the hospital who will not be providing care to the patient. The patient has to authorize the sharing of information with a signed release form.

Respecting advanced directives

Patients with terminal illnesses may legally request that no "heroic" or aggressive interventions be done if they die, or are dying from, that illness. The request is in written form and is generically known as a "do not resuscitate" (DNR) directive.

DNR doesn't mean you shouldn't treat the patient at all. You may still be required to provide supportive care and comfort. You may also need to start resuscitation during a cardiac arrest when the DNR paperwork is not available. Check with local and state policies and procedures to find out what you should do.

Steering clear of abandonment

Once you have established contact with your patient, you are obligated to stay with the patient until you release the care to an equal or higher medical authority. This person may be a paramedic who intercepts your unit or the nurse at an emergency department. Releasing a patient includes making a verbal report with the person who is receiving your patient and following up with a written report. If you fail to do so, you may be liable for abandoning your patient.

Complying with mandatory reporting

In most states, there are laws that protect the health and welfare of children and so-called dependent adults, usually older patients and adults who are unable to make independent decisions. As an EMT, you're required to report suspected cases of abuse or neglect to specific departments, such as child or adult protective services. Immunity from prosecution is provided to protect you in case your suspicions turn out to be inaccurate.

You may be obligated to make a report in other situations as well, such as criminal circumstances like rape or domestic violence, or special clinical scenarios such as at-home births. These vary from one state to the next. Your instructor should provide you information that is relevant in the area where you will be practicing; check state regulations regarding your role as a mandated reporter.

Coping with crime scenes

EMTs often respond to situations where a violent crime has been committed, such as physical assaults, shootings, or stabbings. Your priority is to treat the patient to the best of your abilities; while doing so, try to avoid contaminating scene evidence as much as you can. For example, try not to cut through bullet or knife holes in clothing as you take it off the patient. Do not pick up anything in the area that you don't absolutely need to, including any items you may discard such as plastic wrappers on cervical collars. Do your best to avoid disturbing the scene. Your local police will be very appreciative.

Documenting your cases

You are required to document what you observed about the patient and the environment, the findings that you assessed, the care you provided, and any changes in the patient's condition while in your care. Documentation may be done either on paper forms or electronically with a computer, laptop, or tablet. The following are key things to keep in mind when documenting:

- **Document completely.** Use the CHART or SOAP method to capture all the details. Don't leave anything blank. Cross out, and initial if possible, any sections that are not relevant.
- **Document consistently.** Each patient care report (PCR) should begin and end very similarly. A standardized method of documentation will have you describe the patient, your findings, your treatment, and any changes to the patient's condition in a methodical way. The more consistent you are in documenting your assessment and treatment, the more accurate and faster it becomes.

- **Document just the facts.** Don't give your opinion or interpretation of what you saw or heard. For example, your patient is not "drunk." He has "slurred speech, is unable to maintain his balance, and has an odor similar to alcohol on his breath." This will help you avoid being charged with libel — you're simply recording what you saw, heard, smelled, and felt.
- **Spell correctly and use good grammar.** You are transmitting information to not only other healthcare professionals, but also quality improvement personnel, police investigators, and, most importantly, attorneys who want to make you look less than professional in a lawsuit. Messy documentation is often interpreted as messy patient care, no matter how well you treated the patient.

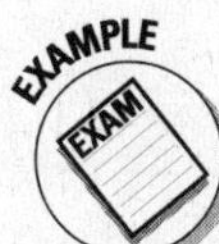

The emergency department is extremely busy when you and your partner arrive with a noncritical patient. As you wait in an exam room for a nurse to take your report, your dispatcher pages you for a "cardiac arrest, CPR in progress" at an address two blocks away from your location. You should

(A) move your patient to the hospital bed and let the staff know you are responding to a cardiac arrest nearby.

(B) notify the dispatcher that you are unable to respond to the call.

(C) have your partner respond to the call.

(D) have your partner stay with the patient while you respond to the call.

The best answer is Choice (B). Choice (A) can be construed as abandonment because you did not provide a report to a specific person who took over care of the patient. Having either of you respond without the other partner, as Choices (C) and (D) suggest, can be construed as a breach of duty because it is customary and within the standard of care to send an ambulance with two crew members.

Staying Healthy, Sane, and Safe

EMS is a physically demanding profession and has more than its share of dangerous work environments. It requires you to stay in good physical shape, keep a positive attitude, and be aware of the dangers that surround you while you're working.

Being fit for the job

Lifting and moving patients can be difficult. Unconscious patients are literally dead weight that is difficult to control. Injured patients may need to be immobilized to a long backboard and carried down several flights of stairs. Many EMS patients are obese. Even the equipment bags can be heavy. You need to be physically fit and strong enough to avoid seriously injuring yourself or your partner. You also need to be smart enough to call for additional resources when you're unable to perform a lift without assistance.

If you drive around in an ambulance all day, finding ways to exercise, stretch your muscles, and maintain your back strength is challenging. It's even more difficult to eat right and avoid the fats and salts so common in fast food.

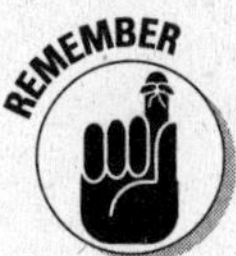

You need to develop discipline to exercise and maintain a healthy diet and lifestyle. Smoking is a no-no, as is excessive alcohol consumption. Exercises that help you to strengthen the back, abdominal, and leg muscles are easy to do and don't require expensive training equipment. Chances are there will be someone at your future EMS workplace who can provide tips and guidance on a realistic workout and diet routine. You can also search the Internet for articles and videos on these topics; combine and enter terms like "EMT," "workout," and "video" in your browser.

Handling the stress of the profession

EMS is a rewarding career. You have the honor of being present at the beginning of a new life as well as the end of a life. In between, you experience situations that most people never will. These conditions can bring on emotional stress that can be difficult to acknowledge and deal with.

It's important to recognize signs of stress that can be harmful to you. These include

- Being short tempered to coworkers, family, and friends
- Being unable to concentrate
- Sleeplessness or excessive sleeping
- Loss of appetite, interest at work, or interest in relationships
- Increased use of alcohol or recreational drugs
- Feelings of hopelessness, constant anxiety, sadness, or guilt

Dealing with stress is different for everyone. Some find comfort in discussing their feelings with people they trust. Others exercise. Adjusting your work schedule or taking time off work can help reset your outlook on life. Whatever you do, make sure it's a positive and healthy way to cope with stress.

Many EMS organizations provide assistance to their employees who may be under a great deal of stress after a serious event like a pediatric cardiac arrest or multiple-casualty event involving many deaths. This assistance may include *critical incident stress management,* or CISM. CISM may include a situational *defusing,* which occurs immediately after the event is over. It gives supervisors an opportunity to check in with employees to see how they're managing any stress or emotions. If the event is significant, there may be a *critical incident stress debriefing* (CISD), which usually occurs 24 hours after the event. There may be follow-up with mental health professionals in case the employee experiences post traumatic stress disorder (PTSD).

Stress while working can be especially dangerous. You may create a situation where your feelings provoke or worsen a confrontation. Don't overreact to what the patient says or does! Take a deep breath and be sure not to take things personally. The patient doesn't know you, and you won't be going home with him, so why get angry over what is said?

Knowing that safety is job one

As an EMT, you enter people's homes or workplaces, work in the middle of a roadway, or handle patients affected by a hazardous materials incident or major catastrophic event. You must maintain a constant state of alertness to safety hazards that exist in the environment.

Some safety concerns are common, such as trip hazards, slippery surfaces, and obstructions like low ceilings and overhead wires. Others are more serious, such as cars moving past you or downed electrical wires. Some are violent in nature — aggressive patient behavior, items that can be used as weapons, or large crowds who aren't pleased with your work.

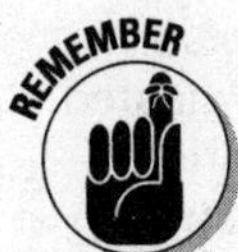

It's critical that you remain observant and be prepared to act or react to maintain scene safety for yourself, your crew, and your patient, in that order. If you can't establish or maintain scene safety, you're not obligated to begin or maintain patient care until it's safe to do so.

Your safety extends to communicable diseases. Maintain your immunizations and make sure you undergo periodic testing for exposure to diseases such as tuberculosis.

Hand washing is still considered to be the best way of reducing your exposure to communicable diseases. Using soap and water or an alcohol-based gel or foam is an effective hand-washing method. Spend at least 15 seconds scrubbing your hands continuously before rinsing. Wash even if you wore gloves.

You should be wearing gloves when physically touching patients. If the patient is coughing, consider wearing a HEPA mask to reduce your chance of catching an airborne illness. You may also wear protective eyewear if blood or other bodily fluids are present. Gowns can help keep these fluids off you.

Communicating Well with Others During an Emergency

With all the discussion about safety, stress, and physical activity on an emergency scene, things may seem to be a bit out of control — which they can be! EMS providers are trained to bring control to chaos. Staying calm, functioning within a team, and being able to communicate quickly, clearly, and empathetically with patients, family, friends, and bystanders will get you through even the craziest of calls.

Working on a team

Working completely alone as an EMT is extremely rare. Even in those circumstances, you'll likely be interacting with other healthcare and public safety providers at some point during a call. More likely, you'll be functioning as a member of a team. It may be a single partner, a fire engine crew, or even an emergency department staff — regardless of the size, everyone has a role to play.

Every team has a leader and one or more followers. Both roles are vital to the success of the team.

- **When you're the leader:** As team leader, you are responsible for the overall health and safety of the team. In small teams, you may need to perform some of the scene functions, such as performing the patient assessment or collecting information from bystanders. In larger teams, you may have more team members who can perform most of the scene functions, which allows you to monitor the overall progression of the incident. The role of team leader is decided by the crew prior to arriving at the scene, to avoid any possible confusion in front of the patient or bystanders.

Now, I'm not suggesting that you make every decision on the scene. Part of being a successful team leader is to solicit input from other team members. For example, say you're developing a treatment plan for the patient. You may consider turning to your partner and saying something like, "I think we need to immobilize the patient to a backboard and provide some oxygen, maybe 4 liters per minute, with a nasal cannula. What do you think?" This way, you may gain some additional input or other information that you may have missed during your exam.

- **When you're the follower:** Team leaders can't lead if there's no one to follow them. Followers, or team members, need to perform their functions well and in a coordinated fashion. A lot of tasks need to be performed during an emergency incident — patient assessment, treatment, extrication, moving equipment, talking with bystanders, just to name a few. To accomplish these tasks with the least amount of effort and time takes practice and a commitment to excellence. As you gain experience, you'll end up not only listening carefully for direction from your team leader, but also anticipating what task will need to be done next.

Interacting with others on the scene

EMS providers deal with human beings. You need to be able to listen attentively and communicate clearly. These skills come naturally to some, while others need to work at them. If you're part of the second group, take a deep breath and relax. You can learn how to do this part of the job through diligence and lots of practice.

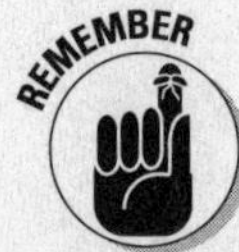

The most important people you need to communicate with are your patients. Keep in mind why you're there with them in the first place — no one calls for EMS because she's having a great day! No matter how minor an injury or illness may seem to you, it was a big enough deal for her to ask you to come. Be empathetic with your patients. Put yourself in their shoes and be supportive and respectful. Remember the golden rule: Treat others the way you want to be treated.

Often, there are family members, friends, coworkers, and bystanders who are witnesses to the emergency incident. Some can be deeply affected by what they observe. This is especially true when someone is critically ill or injured, or dead on-scene. You need to pay some attention to others on the scene to explain to them what's happening. You have to work delicately — privacy issues do apply, even in these situations — but tending to others helps to relieve some of the fear and anxiety that they feel during such a crisis.

Just as no EMT ever really works alone, no EMS agency works alone. By definition, EMS is a community-based endeavor. Without people in the community getting sick or injured, there would be no need for EMS.

Think about this: When people call for EMS, they don't get a choice of who comes to take care of them. Regardless of who it is, they expect to be treated with respect, compassion, and good-quality care. Living up to that expectation can be a challenge!

To foster great relations with your community, engage them outside of emergency calls. From open houses to low-cost or free CPR or first-aid training, find different ways to show your "customers" how much you care for them. When the time comes, they'll be supportive of you!

Understanding Emergency Vehicle Operations

You may respond to emergency medical incidents in a variety of vehicles, such as ambulances, fire engines, or even your private vehicle if you volunteer as an EMT. Regardless of what it is, the vehicle must be ready to go at all times. Keeping your vehicle in tip-top condition requires preparation and ongoing maintenance.

Maintaining equipment levels and vehicle readiness

Professional emergency vehicles must be stocked with the appropriate type and levels of equipment. For ambulances, your agency or your regulatory body may have specific requirements for what needs to be available. Medical supplies, such as medications, often have expiration dates that require you to replace them when necessary.

The ambulance should be cleaned continuously. You transport sick patients, and the patient compartment is an ideal place to grow contaminants. Use approved cleaning solutions and techniques to wipe down the sides and floor of the patient compartment. A solution made of one part sodium hypochlorite (bleach) mixed in ten parts water can be used to disinfect carrying equipment such as gurneys and long backboards. Pay attention to so-called "grab" surfaces — door handles, side bars, and, in the front of the ambulance, control buttons and switches.

The vehicle itself should be checked daily for its ability to be driven. You don't need to be a mechanic to do this; a daily operational checklist may include activities such as

- Inspecting common fluid levels, such as oil, radiator, brake, and power steering fluids.
- Inspecting the tires for wear and tear.
- Starting the engine and checking the fuel level.
- Turning on the emergency lights and noting if any have failed.
- Testing the siren, air horn, and regular vehicle horn.
- Checking the running lights, signal lights, and headlights.
- Putting the vehicle in drive and testing the parking brake and vehicle brakes.

Driving an ambulance

Perhaps the most dangerous part of an emergency incident is responding in the emergency mode. Statistics show that your chances of being injured or killed while driving with lights and siren on is far greater than in your private vehicle or driving routinely. Part of the reason is that emergency vehicles such as ambulances are heavier and have higher centers of gravity than regular vehicles, making them difficult to handle at high speeds.

Additionally, modern vehicles are well insulated, which makes hearing a siren very difficult. Drivers can also be distracted given the level of technology being used in motor vehicles, such as cellphones. Drivers in other vehicles may react unpredictably when surprised by an emergency vehicle that "suddenly" appears in their rearview mirror.

These and other factors require you to drive with due regard for other drivers while operating your emergency vehicle. Driving with lights and siren on doesn't give you authority over other drivers. In most states, the use of emergency lighting simply requires others to yield the right of way. Many states still require you to adhere to the normal driving regulations, even in an emergency response. It simply makes sense to avoid acting crazily while responding to an emergency call. Your partner, your crew, and others driving around you will all appreciate it.

Here are a few guidelines for driving and parking an ambulance:

- Before heading to the call, determine the best route to get there. Sometimes the shortest route isn't the best one! Factor traffic and road conditions into your route planning.
- Use your seat belt, both in the front and back of the ambulance. If you're the driver, don't be distracted by the radios, GPS, or computer terminals that are part of most ambulances today. Have your partner guide you to the call and operate the communications equipment so that you can focus on operating the vehicle.
- If you're the first to arrive at a vehicle crash, you may need to use your vehicle as a protective barrier to oncoming traffic. Turn the steering wheel so that if the ambulance is struck from behind, it will veer away from the incident scene, not into it.
- If another emergency vehicle is on the scene by the time you arrive, park your ambulance so that you have more direct access to the patient compartment. Put on your reflective vest and very carefully depart the vehicle.
- Some scene calls require you to size up homes, apartments, office buildings, and other commercial buildings to locate the best route of entry and exit. Sometimes the front door is not the best way! For example, hotels often have larger service elevators toward the rear of the building that make moving a gurney and equipment much easier.
- If multiple vehicles are on-scene, park in such a way as to avoid being blocked by them. This may mean parking farther away than normal and walking into the scene with your gear. Hopefully, other responders on the scene will assist you when you're ready to leave.
- Driving patients to a hospital requires a smooth ride. Most ambulances are built on heavy-duty van or truck chassis, which are inherently stiff and uncomfortable for riders. Drive as if you have something delicate balanced on the gurney. Accelerate, turn, and brake slowly. Time traffic lights so that you don't have to stop at every one. Choose routes that minimize stops, hazards, or rough road surfaces.

Very rarely do you need to drive patients to the hospital in emergency mode. The time you save is minimal, and whether it saves lives is unclear.

Using air medical services

Many, if not most, EMS systems have access to an air medical service to transport critically ill or injured patients over distances that would take significantly longer to travel by ground ambulance. Most air medical transports are done by specially configured helicopters staffed by a wide range of medical personnel, including paramedics, nurses, and physicians.

The decision to use a medical helicopter is not an insignificant one. It's costly to the patient and incurs a greater risk of injury and death due to an aircraft crash. For these reasons, helicopters are usually dispatched under specific criteria, usually when the chance of a critical illness or injury is high, and the time it will take to transport in a helicopter is far less than the time ground ambulance transportation will take.

The time interval is important to understand. It takes many minutes to ready a helicopter for takeoff. Once the air crew arrives overhead, it takes time to circle the scene to look for hazards, land the aircraft, and reduce the speed of the rotors in order to load the patient. The helicopter crew will need to reassess the patient and possibly perform additional treatments before moving the patient to the aircraft. It takes a few more minutes to load the patient into the helicopter, and then more time again to power up the unit and take off. Once it arrives at the hospital landing pad, it has to repeat the same procedure as it did before in order to land safely.

This time interval can be reduced by dispatching the helicopter at the same time as ground crews to an emergency scene where the chance of needing a helicopter is higher. In very rural areas, this may allow the air unit to arrive at about the same time as ground crews, saving time.

Performing light rescue

Depending on where you work, you may be required to know how to perform simple rescue operations. These may include breaking a car window safely with a window punch, prying open a stuck car door with a pry bar, or stabilizing a vehicle that is on its side with cribbing. At the very least, when at the scene of a motor vehicle crash, you must make sure that the ignition is turned off and that the vehicle is in park before you begin your assessment and treatment.

You are responding to an emergency call using your lights and siren. As you approach a busy intersection, you observe that the traffic light facing you is red. The traffic crossing through the intersection is not stopping. You should

(A) proceed into the intersection at the same rate you are traveling.

(B) stop at the light and wait for traffic to stop.

(C) use your air horn while continuing into the intersection.

(D) slow down and proceed through the intersection.

The best answer is Choice (B). Using your lights and siren does not allow you to drive without due regard for other drivers. Choices (A) and (D) will place you at great risk for a crash; an air horn, Choice (C), may not be heard by drivers who are moving across the intersection until they are directly in front of you.

Managing Large Incidents

Incidents that overwhelm local, immediately available resources are commonly called *mass casualty incidents* (MCI). These can take the form of a major vehicle crash with multiple patients, a fire or hazardous materials incident that sickens many people, or a weather-related event such as a tornado or flash flood. In such events, the normal rules of engagement are suspended and attention is focused on taking care of the greatest number of patients with the limited amount of resources.

An incident management system (IMS) is used to coordinate the resources. An IMS is able to scale up or down, depending on the size of the incident and pool of available resources. An incident commander (IC) (or one from each agency on-scene, working together in a unified command structure) interacts with other section leaders to coordinate scene activities and resources.

The EMS section focuses on providing medical care, with a medical group supervisor reporting to the operations leader, who in turn reports to the incident commander. Under the medical group supervisor are several key positions:

- **Triage officer:** Determines which patients need to be taken care of first
- **Treatment officer:** Oversees the care provided on-scene
- **Transport officer:** Coordinates with hospital resources and communications to send the right patients to the right facilities
- **Staging officer:** Coordinates arriving ambulances, which may be staged some distance away from the actual scene

As a rule, the crew from the first ambulance to arrive at an MCI will assume the roles of medical group supervisor and triage officer. The second ambulance crew will fill the roles of treatment and transport officers. If multiple ambulances are needed to transport patients, one member of the third ambulance crew will be the staging officer, while the other member assists with the treatment area.

You may have realized that this scenario means the first few ambulances may not be transporting patients right away, which seems counterproductive. It's not — as major incidents unfold, sorting out who is most injured and needs to be transported immediately may take some time. This strategy also allows more effective use of the available medical resources.

The following sections cover triage and hazardous incidents.

Triage

Triage is a French word that means "to sort." In mass casualty incidents, triage is used to decide which patient receives the most immediate care, who can wait to be treated, and, sadly, who is beyond help. Many EMS systems use a triage system called START, which stands for Simple Triage and Rapid Treatment (see Figure 14-1).

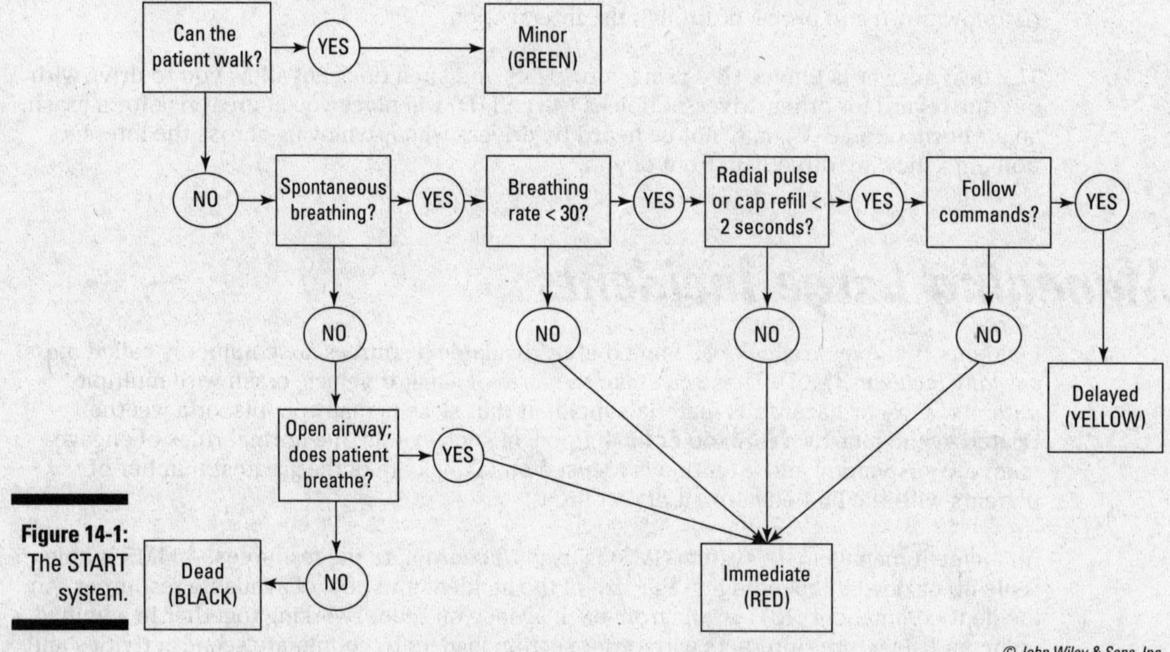

Figure 14-1: The START system.

START depends upon several basic parameters. The patients are categorized by severity as immediate, delayed, minor, and deceased; these correspond to colors on triage tags to enable rapid visual assessment of triaged patients.

Triage begins with directing patients who can walk under their own power to an area where they can be reevaluated for their actual injuries. These patients are categorized as "green" or minor. With the remaining, nonambulatory adult patients, you apply the following rules:

1. **Is the patient spontaneously breathing?**

   If YES, go to Step 2. If NO, open the airway and reassess. If still not breathing, the patient is dead and categorized as BLACK. If the patient begins to breathe, then the patient is RED, or immediate.

2. **Is the breathing rate less than 30 breaths per minute?**

   If YES, go to Step 3. If NO, then the patient is RED.

3. **Is there a radial pulse, or is capillary refill less than 2 seconds?**

   If YES, go to Step 4. If NO, then the patient is RED.

4. **Does the patient follow commands?**

   If YES, the patient is YELLOW, or delayed for treatment. If NO, then the patient is RED.

This process takes only a few seconds to apply, allowing you to triage a large number of patients in a short period of time. Triage tags or tape is used to label the patients as you process them.

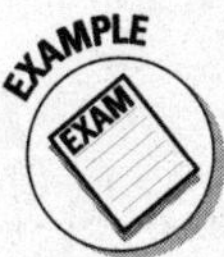

An explosion has occurred at a local manufacturing plant. You are the triage officer. A patient walks up to you with an amputation of the right arm at the elbow. There is a pant belt looped around the remaining arm. It is oozing blood. The patient's skin is pale and cool to the touch; he is breathing 30 times per minute, and his radial pulse rate is 100. Using START triage, you would categorize this patient as

(A) black.

(B) green.

(C) yellow.

(D) red.

The best answer is Choice (B); as distressing as this patient's injury is, he is walking and therefore triaged into the minor, or green, category. In the initial triage phase, he wouldn't fit into any of the other categories. However, it's likely that upon reaching the treatment area, he'll be retriaged and probably moved into a more urgent category.

Hazardous incidents

The modern world is filled with a near-infinite number of chemicals that are used to make our lives better, safer, and more convenient. An unfortunate side effect is that many of them are also hazardous to health; companies worldwide spend billions of dollars to minimize spills and accidents.

EMS responds to hazardous events regularly. Unless you are specifically trained, equipped, and responsible for mitigating the hazard, your job is to notify others of a possible hazardous incident and keep unauthorized personnel from entering.

Operate only within the *cold zone,* where there is no contact with the hazardous material. Patients are decontaminated in the *warm zone* by specialists who are trained to perform this task. Hazmat technicians mitigate the actual problem within the *hot zone.* (Check out all these zones in Figure 14-2.)

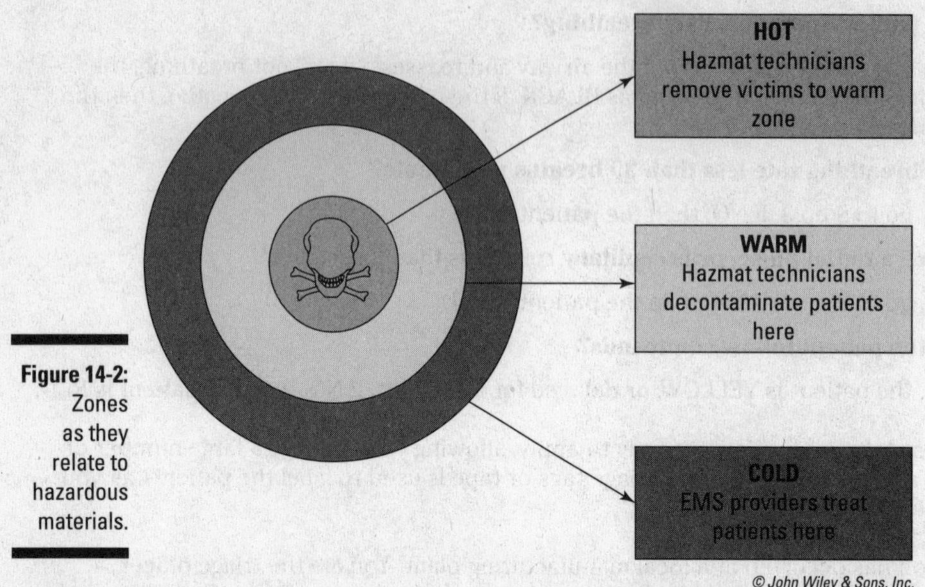

Figure 14-2: Zones as they relate to hazardous materials.

Make sure patients are decontaminated before transporting them to hospitals. It does no good to bring the disaster to the emergency department!

Practice Questions about EMS Operations

The following practice questions are similar to the EMT exam's questions about EMS operations. Read each question carefully, and then select the answer choice that best responds to the question.

1. You and your partner have just finished a shift and are off duty. The station pager goes off, signaling another call. No one is available to respond. Your partner does not want to go back in service. Which of the following statements is most correct?

   (A) There is a duty to act, and you must respond.

   (B) This may be an ethical issue, but not a legal issue.

   (C) Good Samaritan laws will protect you in not responding.

   (D) Your partner could be held liable for negligence.

2. A 55-year-old patient has sudden syncope. He is evaluated by EMTs at his home. He is alert, with pale, dry skin. He refuses their care and offer of transport. He subsequently experiences a cardiac arrest and dies. His family sues the EMTs for negligence. Which of the following statements is most correct?

   (A) Because the EMTs failed to consider the potential seriousness of the condition and an injury occurred, they are liable.

   (B) There was a breach of duty when the EMTs did not take the patient to the hospital.

   (C) The patient has a right to self-determination and to make decisions about his care.

   (D) There was no duty to encourage the patient to receive further medical care.

3. A 40-year-old female is at her office. She is confused, but cooperative. She is refusing your care and offer of transport. Her vital signs are normal and there are no obvious signs of illness or injury. You should

(A) advise her of possible negative outcomes of her decision.

(B) request police to respond.

(C) treat and transport.

(D) have coworkers transport her.

4. You are treating a 47-year-old female who is unresponsive, hypotensive, and breathing at a rate of four breaths per minute. One family member, who has power of attorney, wishes only supportive care for the patient. Several other family members are upset and begging you to begin resuscitation. You should

(A) move the patient to the gurney and begin transport.

(B) assist ventilations with a bag-valve mask and oxygen.

(C) contact police to question the family.

(D) administer supplemental oxygen.

5. You're evaluating a patient with altered mental status when he becomes agitated and attempts to strike you. You should immediately

(A) step back and prepare to retreat if he becomes more violent.

(B) grab his arm and restrain him.

(C) have you and your partner grab his arms and torso.

(D) call for police assistance.

6. A patient has a fever and a productive cough. Your best way to avoid being infected is to

(A) have the patient be tested for serious airborne diseases.

(B) wash your hands after transporting the patient.

(C) place a mask over the patient's face.

(D) wear eye protection.

7. After a call you note blood on the metal rails of the gurney, as well as the mattress. You should

(A) use hot water and soap to clean the affected areas.

(B) sterilize the gurney.

(C) use hand sanitizer to clean the rail and mattress.

(D) use a bleach-water solution to wipe down the gurney and mattress.

8. Your partner is tired, short-tempered, and treating his patients with disrespect. You are aware that he is having issues with his marriage and he has been working a lot of overtime. Which of the following ways of handling the situation would be most appropriate?

(A) Ignore the behavior, as the situation is none of your business.

(B) Report his behavior to the supervisor.

(C) Ask him how he is doing and offer to help.

(D) Talk with his wife to mediate a discussion with your partner.

9. You and your partner are preparing to remove a 300-pound patient from the third floor of a house. Which of the following approaches would be safest?

   (A) Use a stair chair to carry the patient.

   (B) Request that additional resources respond to the scene.

   (C) Have family members assist you in moving the patient.

   (D) Use the gurney to help move the patient.

10. While responding to an emergency call using lights and siren, you approach an intersection. The traffic light begins to change from green to yellow as you approach. You should

    (A) slow down and prepare to stop if needed.

    (B) speed up and proceed through the intersection before the light turns red.

    (C) maintain your speed and prepare for an emergency maneuver if necessary.

    (D) use your airhorn to clear the intersection.

11. You are 8 minutes away from a report of a major rollover auto crash. The incident is 45 minutes travel time by ground ambulance to the trauma center and 10 minutes to the community hospital. A medical helicopter can be over the incident location within 10 minutes of dispatch. You should

    (A) request the helicopter to respond to the community hospital while you transport the patient to that location.

    (B) request that the helicopter respond to the scene.

    (C) arrive at the scene, evaluate the situation, and request the helicopter if necessary.

    (D) transport the patient to the trauma center.

12. As you arrive at the scene of an industrial building, you note a person lying on the ground near several metal containers. Other persons are nearby, coughing and holding their hands over their mouths. You should

    (A) begin assessing the person lying on the ground.

    (B) ask the coughing individuals to move away from the scene.

    (C) stop your vehicle.

    (D) administer supplemental oxygen to those who are coughing.

13. A driver is trapped in her passenger car after a crash. As firefighters are preparing to extricate, you determine that the patient's breathing is slow and shallow. The radial pulse is absent. You should

    (A) maintain spinal stabilization during extrication.

    (B) use a short backboard or vest device to extricate.

    (C) administer high-flow oxygen via a nonrebreather mask.

    (D) apply AED pads and prepare to defibrillate.

14. You arrive at a parking lot where an infant has been left alone in a passenger car. The air is quite warm and humid. Through the windshield you observe that the infant's eyes are closed. You're not sure whether the infant is breathing. You should

    (A) attempt to find the owner of the car to unlock the doors.

    (B) call for a rescue squad for extrication.

    (C) break the window farthest away from the child with a hand tool.

    (D) cover the car with a tarp to shield it from the sun.

15. According to START, which of the following presentations should be treated first?

(A) An adult female with an amputated arm, bleeding, crying, breathing 20 times per minute.

(B) An adult male with no obvious injuries, apneic after a jaw thrust.

(C) A young child with a fractured femur and a radial pulse rate of 90.

(D) A teenage male, altered, with cool, pale, and diaphoretic skin and a carotid pulse only.

16. You are the second unit to arrive at a multicasualty incident. You should

(A) assume the role of transport officer.

(B) assume incident command.

(C) respond to the staging area.

(D) begin triaging victims.

17. At the scene of a hazardous materials incident, patients should be decontaminated in the

(A) hot zone.

(B) warm zone.

(C) cold zone.

(D) washdown zone.

18. You are evaluating a terminally ill patient who is having difficulty breathing. Family members report having a "do not resuscitate" (DNR) form for the patient, but they are unable to find it. You should

(A) do nothing until the form is located.

(B) do nothing and document the circumstances.

(C) provide appropriate care until the form is located.

(D) have family members sign a new DNR form.

19. Under what circumstances can you legally release confidential patient information?

(A) When a detective needs information about a suspect

(B) At the family's request

(C) When the media is recording in a public space

(D) When the patient is competent and signs a release form

20. An apartment building landlord lets you into an apartment, where you find an elderly female who has fallen but is uninjured. She lives alone; you note her apartment is filthy and there is little food in the refrigerator. She is confused and unable to recall her medical history or medications. Your best course of action is to

(A) assist her to a chair and clean up her apartment.

(B) file a report with adult protective services.

(C) notify the police of possible criminal activity.

(D) transport her to a specialized nursing facility.

Answers and Explanations

Use this answer key to score the practice questions in the preceding section. The explanations give you insight into why the correct answer is better than the other choices.

1. **B.** Since you are off duty, and there is no expectation of your response, there is no legal duty to act in this situation as Choice (A) suggests. Good Samaritan laws, noted in Choice (C), only protect your actions on the scene of a medical incident. Because no duty to act exists, negligence, Choice (D), does not apply.
2. **C.** There was a duty to act in this event — the EMTs were on duty and responded, contrary to Choice (D). Based on the scenario, the patient had the ability to legally refuse medical care and/or transport. The crew could have been liable if they had forced him to go to the hospital, Choice (B). There is no indication that the crew failed to perform an adequate assessment, as Choice (A) suggests.
3. **C.** The patient does not have the capacity to make the decision Choice (A) suggests. This allows you to treat and transport under implied consent. She shouldn't be transported by coworkers, Choice (D), because they're not able to monitor her medically and can't help her if her condition suddenly worsens. Having the police respond, Choice (B), wouldn't alter the situation, as they have no jurisdiction in medical matters.
4. **A.** The family member with power of attorney has the legal right to make decisions for the patient. Providing any intervention that may prolong the life of the patient, as in Choices (B) and (D), would be inappropriate. Medical direction, Choice (C), would have little to say in this situation.
5. **A.** Your immediate maneuver is to avoid being injured. Calling police, Choice (D), can be your next step after you retreat. Trying to restrain the patient yourself or with a partner, as in Choices (B) and (C), is risky.
6. **B.** The single best way to reduce cross contamination is to wash your hands, even if you wear gloves. Choice (A) doesn't keep you from being exposed, and Choices (C) and (D) don't provide the same level of protection.
7. **D.** There may be more, smaller amounts of contaminant on the gurney than you can see. Choices (A) and (C) suggest methods that aren't recommended for destroying bloodborne pathogens. Sterilizing the unit, Choice (B), requires high heat or submersion in a chemical bath, neither of which is practical.
8. **C.** Your partner is exhibiting signs of stress, which are showing up in his treatment of his patients. Although you may need to speak to a supervisor at some point, Choice (B), it may be helpful for your partner to debrief with you first. Ignoring the situation, Choice (A), may subject your patients to unnecessary harm. Be careful not to make an assumption that the marriage is the main issue, as in Choice (D); it may be work-related.
9. **B.** The weight of the patient is too much for two rescuers to carry safely, even with a stair chair, Choice (A). Family members may not be trained to assist in a safe manner, eliminating Choice (C). A gurney, as Choice (D) suggests, is likely to worsen the situation by adding additional weight and bulk to the carry.
10. **A.** Driving with lights and siren is risky. Minimize the danger by slowing your forward speed before entering the intersection, Choice (A), rather than speeding up, Choice (B), or proceeding at your current speed, Choice (C). Using your airhorn, Choice (D), is less likely to be helpful because many drivers will not be able to hear it clearly, especially if they're coming across the intersection.
11. **B.** A medical helicopter can reduce the amount of time it takes to transport a critical trauma patient to a trauma center — if it's dispatched appropriately. Given the scenario, the best situation is to have the helicopter very close by as you begin evaluation of the patient, thereby reducing any delay of the transport. Choice (C) will cause delay; Choice (A) will add delay between the two hospitals; and Choice (D) will likely take well over an hour to implement.

12. **C.** Your safety is paramount. Despite your best intentions, you are of no use if you are injured or killed at an incident. Given the choices, the best action is to stop your vehicle a safe distance away from the incident, Choice (C). This action allows you to size up the scene and request additional resources. You should also deny entry to other personnel and bystanders if possible.

13. **A.** The patient is critically injured. Time is of the essence in managing her condition; rapid extrication is appropriate. Using a short backboard or vest device, Choice (B), delays extrication. She needs to be ventilated; supplemental oxygen, Choice (C), is not sufficient. An AED, Choice (D), isn't indicated at this time.

14. **C.** EMTs should have simple hand tools available and should know how to use them properly. You don't know if or when the owner of the car will be found, making Choice (A) impractical, and a rescue squad, Choice (B), may take time to reach the scene. Covering the car with a tarp, Choice (D), won't shield the car from the ambient air temperature.

15. **D.** START triage begins with separating patients who can ambulate from those who can't. In the second group, you should first confirm that the patient is breathing. If not, apply a jaw thrust. If he still isn't breathing, as in Choice (B), triage "expectant" or black.

    If the patient is breathing, count respirations. If the rate is greater than 30 or less than 10, triage "immediate" or red.

    If the respiratory rate is in between, check for a radial pulse. If there isn't one, as in Choice (D), triage "immediate" or red.

    If there is a radial pulse, check the patient's level of consciousness. If alert, as in Choices (A) and (C), triage "delayed" or yellow.

16. **A.** The first unit personnel assume the roles of incident commander, Choice (B), and triage, Choice (D). The second unit personnel assume treatment and transport. Subsequent units report to the staging area for further orders, Choice (C).

17. **B.** The hot zone, Choice (A), is the area immediately around the incident and is most contaminated. Patients are extricated to the warm zone, Choice (B), so decontamination can be done by those who are trained and equipped to work in this area. Decontaminated patients are then transferred to the cold zone, Choice (C), where care by EMS generally begins. There is no such thing as a washdown zone, Choice (D).

18. **C.** DNR does *not* mean "do not treat." Until you can determine the level of intervention that is authorized on the form, you are obligated to provide appropriate care (unless the patient is alert and able to tell you otherwise).

19. **D.** A patient must provide written permission for a healthcare provider or organization to release private health information. You cannot release this information to law enforcement, Choice (A), or even family, Choice (B). While the recording of the scene may be legal, it does not provide any basis for you to break confidentiality, Choice (C).

20. **B.** Although it would be nice of you to help clean up the apartment, Choice (A), the more significant issue is that she may be unable to care for herself. It's possible that she has family that is neglecting her needs; filing a report will begin an investigation to determine whether other issues are involved. There is no criminal element to this scenario, making Choice (C) unnecessary; you may end up transporting to an emergency department, but not a specialized nursing facility, Choice (D).

Part IV

Putting Your Knowledge into Practice

Five Tips for Answering Multiple-Choice Questions

- Be sure to pick the *best* answer, as there may be more than one correct answer.
- Read the question stem carefully. Try to answer the question without looking at the choices, and then see which of the choices best fits your response.
- If none of the choices seems to answer the question, play detective. Eliminate any answer that is clearly incorrect. Better to make an educated guess between two choices than three or four.
- If you get stuck between two choices, silently read the stem and each choice as if it were one sentence. One may sound more correct than the other.
- Above all, don't panic. If you get lost in the question, step back and take a moment to reread the stem. It's possible that you may have missed an important piece of information or misinterpreted part of the question.

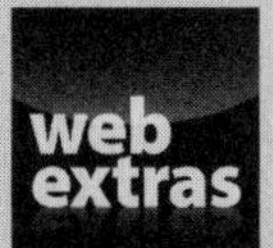

Get the scoop on getting and maintaining your EMT certification, elements of the EMT computer exam, and more on the Cheat Sheet at `www.dummies.com/extras/emtexam`.

In this part . . .

- See where you stand by taking two full-length practice exams, each composed of 120 multiple-choice questions. Don't cheat yourself; take these exams as if they were the real thing — no distractions and no stopping for breaks.
- Review the answers after you're done. Take note of any areas that seem to be weak spots for you, and review your notes, textbook, and the material in this book before taking another practice test.

Chapter 15

Practice Exam 1

Here is your first opportunity to evaluate your study efforts. Whether you just finished reviewing Chapters 9 through 14 (which cover the main areas of the EMT exam) or you're taking this exam first, try to take this practice exam under real-world conditions:

- Find a quiet place to take the exam. You can't be distracted or interrupted during this time — let people know that you need to be left alone.
- Turn off your cellphone, computer, music player, and television.
- Don't use any study aids, such as your notes or textbook.
- Don't eat or drink anything during the exam.
- Set a timer for 2.5 hours. Try to complete the exam during that time frame.

Note: Although this practice exam is on good old-fashioned paper, you'll take your actual exam on a computer at a testing center. You may want to refer to Chapter 5 for tips on taking a computer adaptive exam.

Try to follow these test-taking tips:

- Begin the exam with the first question and answer it before going to the next question.
- Answer the questions in order. Don't skip around.
- Don't look at the answers until you're completely done with the exam.
- Don't go back to change an answer. You won't be permitted to do that during your real exam.

The answers to this practice exam are in Chapter 16.

You can find an additional practice exam online at `learn.dummies.com`; get the scoop on how to access it in the Introduction. Consider taking it after you finish reviewing this exam (as well as Practice Exam 2 in Chapter 17) and studying the areas you missed. This way, you can see whether your test-taking abilities improve.

Answer Sheet for Practice Exam 1

1 (A) (B) (C) (D)
2 (A) (B) (C) (D)
3 (A) (B) (C) (D)
4 (A) (B) (C) (D)
5 (A) (B) (C) (D)
6 (A) (B) (C) (D)
7 (A) (B) (C) (D)
8 (A) (B) (C) (D)
9 (A) (B) (C) (D)
10 (A) (B) (C) (D)
11 (A) (B) (C) (D)
12 (A) (B) (C) (D)
13 (A) (B) (C) (D)
14 (A) (B) (C) (D)
15 (A) (B) (C) (D)
16 (A) (B) (C) (D)
17 (A) (B) (C) (D)
18 (A) (B) (C) (D)
19 (A) (B) (C) (D)
20 (A) (B) (C) (D)
21 (A) (B) (C) (D)
22 (A) (B) (C) (D)
23 (A) (B) (C) (D)
24 (A) (B) (C) (D)
25 (A) (B) (C) (D)
26 (A) (B) (C) (D)
27 (A) (B) (C) (D)
28 (A) (B) (C) (D)
29 (A) (B) (C) (D)
30 (A) (B) (C) (D)
31 (A) (B) (C) (D)
32 (A) (B) (C) (D)
33 (A) (B) (C) (D)
34 (A) (B) (C) (D)
35 (A) (B) (C) (D)
36 (A) (B) (C) (D)
37 (A) (B) (C) (D)
38 (A) (B) (C) (D)
39 (A) (B) (C) (D)
40 (A) (B) (C) (D)
41 (A) (B) (C) (D)
42 (A) (B) (C) (D)
43 (A) (B) (C) (D)
44 (A) (B) (C) (D)
45 (A) (B) (C) (D)
46 (A) (B) (C) (D)
47 (A) (B) (C) (D)
48 (A) (B) (C) (D)
49 (A) (B) (C) (D)
50 (A) (B) (C) (D)
51 (A) (B) (C) (D)
52 (A) (B) (C) (D)
53 (A) (B) (C) (D)
54 (A) (B) (C) (D)
55 (A) (B) (C) (D)
56 (A) (B) (C) (D)
57 (A) (B) (C) (D)
58 (A) (B) (C) (D)
59 (A) (B) (C) (D)
60 (A) (B) (C) (D)
61 (A) (B) (C) (D)
62 (A) (B) (C) (D)
63 (A) (B) (C) (D)
64 (A) (B) (C) (D)
65 (A) (B) (C) (D)
66 (A) (B) (C) (D)
67 (A) (B) (C) (D)
68 (A) (B) (C) (D)
69 (A) (B) (C) (D)
70 (A) (B) (C) (D)
71 (A) (B) (C) (D)
72 (A) (B) (C) (D)
73 (A) (B) (C) (D)
74 (A) (B) (C) (D)
75 (A) (B) (C) (D)
76 (A) (B) (C) (D)
77 (A) (B) (C) (D)
78 (A) (B) (C) (D)
79 (A) (B) (C) (D)
80 (A) (B) (C) (D)
81 (A) (B) (C) (D)
82 (A) (B) (C) (D)
83 (A) (B) (C) (D)
84 (A) (B) (C) (D)
85 (A) (B) (C) (D)
86 (A) (B) (C) (D)
87 (A) (B) (C) (D)
88 (A) (B) (C) (D)
89 (A) (B) (C) (D)
90 (A) (B) (C) (D)
91 (A) (B) (C) (D)
92 (A) (B) (C) (D)
93 (A) (B) (C) (D)
94 (A) (B) (C) (D)
95 (A) (B) (C) (D)
96 (A) (B) (C) (D)
97 (A) (B) (C) (D)
98 (A) (B) (C) (D)
99 (A) (B) (C) (D)
100 (A) (B) (C) (D)
101 (A) (B) (C) (D)
102 (A) (B) (C) (D)
103 (A) (B) (C) (D)
104 (A) (B) (C) (D)
105 (A) (B) (C) (D)
106 (A) (B) (C) (D)
107 (A) (B) (C) (D)
108 (A) (B) (C) (D)
109 (A) (B) (C) (D)
110 (A) (B) (C) (D)
111 (A) (B) (C) (D)
112 (A) (B) (C) (D)
113 (A) (B) (C) (D)
114 (A) (B) (C) (D)
115 (A) (B) (C) (D)
116 (A) (B) (C) (D)
117 (A) (B) (C) (D)
118 (A) (B) (C) (D)
119 (A) (B) (C) (D)
120 (A) (B) (C) (D)

Questions

Time: 2.5 hours

Directions: Choose the best answer to each question. Mark the corresponding oval on the answer sheet.

1. An 8-month-old infant is unresponsive. The patient is apneic, with a rapid brachial pulse. There is no trauma. The best way to open the airway is to

   (A) perform a head-tilt, chin-lift.

   (B) place a pad under the shoulders to achieve a neutral position.

   (C) perform a jaw thrust.

   (D) hyperflex the head.

2. Your patient presents with bright red blood spurting from a stab wound to her bicep. You should immediately

   (A) apply a tourniquet proximal to the wound.

   (B) apply direct pressure to the wound.

   (C) elevate the arm.

   (D) apply in-line cervical spine immobilization.

3. A patient presents conscious and alert with profuse bleeding from his nose. You should

   (A) apply a warm pack to his nose.

   (B) lay him supine and apply a cold pack to his nose.

   (C) lean him forward and pinch the nostrils together.

   (D) pack his nose with gauze.

4. The medical term for coughing up blood is

   (A) hematemesis.

   (B) hemoptysis.

   (C) epistaxis.

   (D) anaphylaxis.

5. Which of the following wounds is the result of capillary bleeding within the dermis?

   (A) Contusion

   (B) Laceration

   (C) Hematoma

   (D) Abrasion

6. Caring for an amputated hand includes

   (A) flushing the hand with sterile saline to clean it.

   (B) placing the hand directly on ice.

   (C) transporting the hand separate from the patient.

   (D) keeping the hand warm.

7. When treating a patient with an abdominal evisceration, placing her hips and knees in a flexed position will

   (A) help with pain relief.

   (B) decrease abdominal muscle tension.

   (C) slow bleeding.

   (D) help prevent infection.

8. Your patient presents with decorticate posturing after being hit in the head with a bat. Your physical exam reveals a fixed and dilated right pupil. His heart rate is 52 beats per minute, his respiratory rate is 6 breaths per minute with erratic tidal volume, and his blood pressure is 188/92 mm Hg. Your first step is to

   (A) perform full spinal immobilization.

   (B) ventilate the patient 20 times per minute with a bag-valve mask.

   (C) administer oxygen via a nonrebreather mask.

   (D) apply a cervical collar.

9. A patient presents with a stab wound to the neck. It is not bleeding. You should
   (A) apply a three-sided occlusive dressing.
   (B) dress and bandage the wound with gauze.
   (C) apply a four-sided occlusive dressing.
   (D) use a hemostatic agent.

10. A football player wearing a helmet and shoulder pads presents supine on the ground after being tackled. He is alert and complaining only of neck pain. You should remove
    (A) the helmet but leave the shoulder pads on.
    (B) the helmet and shoulder pads.
    (C) the helmet face mask but leave the helmet and shoulder pads on.
    (D) neither the helmet nor the face mask.

11. Which of the following findings would best help you differentiate a tension pneumothorax from a cardiac tamponade?
    (A) Jugular venous distention
    (B) Narrowed pulse pressure
    (C) Hypotension
    (D) Tachycardia

12. Your patient presents supine on the roadway and unconscious after being struck by a car. You note that he has a flail segment on his left lateral chest and has rapid respirations with a shallow tidal volume. He is wearing a medical alert bracelet that identifies him as a diabetic. You should immediately administer
    (A) continuous positive airway pressure (CPAP).
    (B) oxygen via a bag-valve mask.
    (C) oxygen via a nonrebreather mask.
    (D) oral glucose.

13. Your patient presents supine on the ground with a sucking chest wound after being stabbed with a knife. You note that his respiratory rate is 30 breaths per minute with shallow tidal volume. You should immediately
    (A) administer oxygen via a nonrebreather mask.
    (B) cover the chest wound with a gloved hand.
    (C) obtain a full set of vital signs.
    (D) apply a cervical collar.

14. A patient is in respiratory failure after being shot in the right anterior chest. An occlusive dressing has been placed over the wound. While ventilating the patient with a bag-valve mask, you note that ventilating the patient is becoming increasingly difficult. You also note that the patient is developing jugular venous distention, increasing tachycardia, and worsening hypotension. You should immediately
    (A) suction the airway.
    (B) begin hyperventilating the patient.
    (C) lift the occlusive dressing.
    (D) remove the oropharyngeal airway.

15. Your patient presents with pain and tenderness over his lower right anterior rib cage after being kicked repeatedly during an assault. His lung sounds are clear and equal bilaterally. His blood pressure is 92/40 mm Hg, his heart rate is 102 beats per minute, his respiratory rate is 18 breaths per minute with good tidal volume, and his pulse oximetry is 93 percent on room air. He has most likely suffered an injury to his
    (A) lung.
    (B) spleen.
    (C) kidney.
    (D) liver.

16. A 32-year-old female presents complaining of dark blood in her urine after being punched in the abdomen and back during a domestic dispute. She has most likely sustained an injury to her

(A) uterus.

(B) liver.

(C) spleen.

(D) kidney.

17. A 22-year-old male presents conscious and alert, supine on the ground, after driving a dirt bike into a fence at a high rate of speed. You note that his shirt is torn open and that he has suffered an abdominal evisceration. You should immediately

(A) have your partner stabilize the patient's cervical spine.

(B) expose the patient's abdomen.

(C) cover the eviscerated organs with moist gauze.

(D) administer oxygen.

18. Your patient presents with fractures to her right femur and tibia/fibula on her right leg after falling off a second-story balcony. Her heart rate is 94, her blood pressure is 128/78 mm Hg, her respiratory rate is 14 breaths per minute with good tidal volume, and her pulse oximetry is 97 percent on room air. You should

(A) assist ventilations with a bag-valve mask.

(B) apply the pneumatic antishock garment (PASG).

(C) apply a traction splint.

(D) transport immediately.

19. Your patient presents with an angulated fracture of her lower leg. There is no pedal pulse and her foot is cold. You should immediately

(A) attempt to realign the leg.

(B) splint the leg as found.

(C) apply a traction splint.

(D) perform full spinal immobilization.

20. A man has been assaulted. He is ambulatory, anxious, and disoriented. You note that he is self-splinting an obviously fractured left humerus; he has a weak and rapid radial pulse; and his skin is cool, pale, and diaphoretic. Your priority is to

(A) manually stabilize the injured arm.

(B) assess for other injuries.

(C) splint the humerus with a sling and swathe.

(D) apply a cold pack to the injury site.

21. Your patient is conscious and alert with difficulty breathing secondary to an exacerbation of COPD. His respiratory rate is 22, with a prolonged expiratory phase and pursed-lip breathing A pulse oximeter registers 84 percent. You should

(A) withhold oxygen.

(B) initiate CPAP.

(C) assist ventilations with a bag-valve mask.

(D) administer oxygen via blow-by mask.

22. Administering excessive tidal volume with a bag-valve-mask device can result in

(A) decreased preload.

(B) hypertension.

(C) increased cardiac output.

(D) decreased minute volume.

23. Which of the following best indicates that a patient is in respiratory failure?

(A) Intercostal retractions

(B) Difficulty breathing

(C) Stridor

(D) Shallow tidal volume

24. Your patient presents with labored respirations, peripheral cyanosis, and altered mental status. You should immediately

(A) suction the airway.

(B) determine a pulse rate.

(C) administer oxygen via a nonrebreather mask.

(D) assist ventilations with a bag-valve mask.

25. Your patient presents unconscious with slow, shallow, and snoring respirations and an intact gag reflex. You should immediately

(A) insert an oropharyngeal airway.

(B) insert a nasopharyngeal airway.

(C) suction the airway.

(D) ventilate with a bag-valve mask.

26. A woman is injured after dousing a barbeque with lighter fluid. She is awake and alert, and has burns to her face and chest. You can hear audible stridor when she breathes. You should first

(A) cover the burns with a sterile burn sheet.

(B) administer oxygen via a nonrebreather mask.

(C) insert a nasopharyngeal airway.

(D) suction the airway.

27. Your patient presents with slow, shallow, and gurgling respirations. You should immediately

(A) insert a nasopharyngeal airway.

(B) suction his airway.

(C) listen to lung sounds.

(D) ventilate with a bag-valve mask.

28. Your patient is unconscious and is breathing 4 times a minute. She gags after you insert an oropharyngeal airway. You should immediately

(A) hold it in place.

(B) ventilate with a bag mask.

(C) remove the oropharyngeal airway.

(D) insert a nasopharyngeal airway.

29. Which of the following terms best describes a patient who has an adequate tidal volume and respiratory rate but is using her accessory muscles and is diaphoretic?

(A) Respiratory distress

(B) Respiratory failure

(C) Respiratory arrest

(D) Apneic

30. You are ventilating a patient in respiratory failure with a bag-valve mask when you notice that his abdomen is becoming distended. You should

(A) increase tidal volume.

(B) increase the oxygen concentration.

(C) decrease the ventilation pressure.

(D) decrease the ventilatory rate.

31. A 34-year-old male presents supine on the ground after falling 30 feet off a roof. Your primary assessment reveals that he is not breathing and has a slow, regular, and strong radial pulse. You should immediately

(A) administer ventilations with a bag-valve-mask device.

(B) perform full spinal immobilization.

(C) instruct your partner to manually stabilize the patient's cervical spine.

(D) insert an oropharyngeal airway.

32. You are ventilating a patient with a bag-valve mask. An oropharyngeal airway is in place, and you are performing a head-tilt, chin-lift. You notice that ventilating is becoming harder. You should

(A) lay the patient on her left side.

(B) perform another head-tilt, chin-lift.

(C) suction the airway.

(D) increase the oxygen flow rate.

33. For which of the following patients would a nonrebreather mask be most appropriate?

(A) Conscious patient breathing 30 times a minute; breathing is shallow

(B) Patient breathing 4 times a minute with adequate tidal volume

(C) Unconscious patient breathing 12 times a minute with adequate tidal volume

(D) Altered patient actively vomiting and breathing 20 times a minute

34. A patient presents with agonal breathing. While ventilating this patient with a bag-valve mask, you should

(A) give one breath every 5 seconds.

(B) match his respiratory rate and "assist" ventilations.

(C) give each breath over 2 seconds.

(D) administer enough tidal volume to raise the chest 3 inches.

35. Your patient presents standing in a kitchen with stridorous respirations. A bystander reports that he is choking on a piece of meat. You should

(A) encourage the patient to cough.

(B) perform abdominal thrusts.

(C) administer back blows.

(D) perform a blind finger sweep.

36. A patient has rapid, shallow respirations and speaks with a hoarse voice after being trapped in a house fire. You should

(A) suction the airway.

(B) obtain a set of vital signs.

(C) administer oxygen via a nonrebreather mask.

(D) assist ventilations with a bag-valve mask.

37. A 65-year-old female describes waking up from sleep because she says, "I felt like I was being smothered while I was lying down." Lung auscultation reveals rales (crackles) to the bases bilaterally. Based on this information, she is most likely suffering from

(A) acute pulmonary edema.

(B) pneumonia.

(C) emphysema.

(D) pulmonary embolism.

38. A patient presents conscious and alert with a respiratory rate of 22 breaths per minute. You auscultate crackles up to the middle lobes of both lungs, and her skin is clammy with peripheral cyanosis. She has a medical history of asthma and left-sided heart failure. The best way to correct the patient's underlying problem is to

(A) administer continuous positive airway pressure (CPAP).

(B) initiate bag-valve-mask ventilation.

(C) administer oxygen via a nonrebreather mask.

(D) assist the patient with her metered-dose inhaler.

39. Why is it important to not overventilate a patient suffering from respiratory failure secondary to asthma?

(A) Decreased tidal volume can result in increased intrathoracic pressure.

(B) Air trapping can result in decreased preload.

(C) Increased intrathoracic pressure can create a hemothorax.

(D) Decreased cardiac output can result in hypertension.

40. Your patient complains of substernal chest pain radiating to his left shoulder and jaw. He has a history of angina and has his prescribed nitroglycerin with him. You should first

(A) assist him with his nitroglycerin.

(B) obtain a blood pressure.

(C) have him walk to the ambulance and transport immediately.

(D) perform a full secondary assessment.

41. A 62-year-old male complains of substernal chest pain radiating to his jaw. His pulse is 100, his respirations are 16 per minute with adequate tidal volume, his pulse oximetry equals 96 percent on room air, and his blood pressure is 88/40 mm Hg. He is allergic to aspirin. You should

(A) assist him with his prescribed nitroglycerin.

(B) administer oxygen.

(C) administer 320 milligrams of baby aspirin.

(D) transport him to a hospital.

42. Your patient presents with an acute onset of tearing pain located between his shoulder blades. His skin is cool, pale, and diaphoretic. His vital signs are as follows: pulse of 96 per minute, respirations of 18 per minute, a blood pressure of 140/90 mm Hg, and a pulse oximetry reading of 93 percent. You should first

(A) administer oxygen.

(B) assist him with his nitroglycerin.

(C) administer 160 milligrams of baby aspirin.

(D) transport him to a hospital.

43. The patient is complaining of chest pain and difficulty breathing. His breathing is labored. You should immediately

(A) administer oxygen.

(B) assist him with his nitroglycerin.

(C) take a set of vital signs.

(D) listen to lung sounds.

44. You and your partner witness a patient suffer cardiac arrest. You should immediately

(A) administer two breaths with a bag-valve mask and begin chest compressions.

(B) place the patient in the recovery position and check for a pulse.

(C) place the AED on the patient and analyze the heart rhythm.

(D) begin chest compressions and place the AED on the patient.

45. While placing the AED pads on a patient's chest, you note that a medication patch is covering the area where you're supposed to place the pad. You should

(A) remove the patch and wipe away any remaining medication.

(B) place the AED pad 3 inches away from the medication patch.

(C) continue CPR and not apply the AED.

(D) place the AED pad over the medication patch.

46. You and your partner are performing two-rescuer CPR and have just defibrillated a patient with an AED. You should immediately

(A) resume chest compressions.

(B) wait for the AED to tell you to resume CPR.

(C) check for a pulse.

(D) analyze the heart rhythm.

47. A 4-year-old is in cardiac arrest. You don't have pediatric AED/defibrillation pads with you. You should

(A) use adult defibrillation pads.

(B) not attach the AED to the patient.

(C) immediately begin transport to the emergency department.

(D) cut the adult pads to child size.

48. Which of the following cardiac rhythms will an AED not defibrillate?

(A) Ventricular fibrillation (VF)

(B) Ventricular tachycardia (VT) without a pulse

(C) Ventricular tachycardia (VT) with a pulse

(D) Pulseless electrical activity (PEA)

49. Failure of which of the following organ systems most often results in cardiac arrest in the pediatric population?

(A) Renal

(B) Neurological

(C) Respiratory

(D) Endocrine

50. You have just witnessed an adult patient go into cardiac arrest. You are alone. You should immediately

(A) listen to lung sounds.

(B) begin chest compressions.

(C) administer two breaths with a bag-valve mask.

(D) place the AED on the patient and analyze the heart rhythm.

51. You are performing single-rescuer CPR on an adult. You should

(A) take 1 second to deliver each ventilation.

(B) use a 15:2 compression to ventilation ratio.

(C) compress the chest at least 60 times per minute.

(D) use a joule attenuator device.

52. You and your partner are performing CPR on a patient in cardiac arrest. You perform defibrillation and continue chest compressions. Thirty seconds later you note that the patient is moving his arms. You should immediately

(A) stop compressions and assess for a pulse and breathing.

(B) complete your current cycle of compressions and ventilations.

(C) prepare for transport to a hospital.

(D) analyze the cardiac rhythm with the AED.

53. You and your partner are performing CPR on a cardiac arrest patient. You administer a defibrillation and complete five cycles of CPR. Your patient is now breathing and has a pulse. The AED is telling you to "push the analyze button." You should

(A) push the analyze button.

(B) continue CPR.

(C) turn the AED off.

(D) remove the defibrillation pads from the patient.

54. Which of the following best describes why an acute myocardial infarction (AMI) can result in a drop in blood pressure?

(A) Cardiac output increases during an AMI.

(B) Death of heart muscle results in a decrease in stroke volume.

(C) AMI results in peripheral vasodilation.

(D) AMI results in stimulation of baroreceptors in the aorta.

55. A 55-year-old male presents awake and alert, complaining of a sudden, severe headache. It's located directly behind his right eye and began while he was mowing his lawn. His heart rate is 72, his blood pressure is 180/120 mm Hg, and his respiratory rate is 12 breaths per minute with adequate tidal volume. He sees his physician every year, denies any past medical history, and takes no medications. His hypertension is most likely secondary to

(A) increased intracranial pressure.

(B) chronic hypertension.

(C) acute myocardial infarction.

(D) heat stroke.

56. Syncope most often is due to

(A) increased intracranial pressure.

(B) a temporary lack of blood flow to the brain.

(C) a heart attack or stroke.

(D) medication overdose.

57. You are assessing a patient with an altered mental status who you believe is postictal. Which of the following most strongly suggests that the patient had a seizure?

(A) Cold, dry skin and bradycardia

(B) Bilateral pinpoint (2-millimeter) pupils

(C) Bowel and bladder incontinence

(D) Bradycardia and hypotension

58. A 62-year-old Type 2 diabetic living in a nursing home has a four-day history of declining mental status. Staff reports that the patient has been increasingly thirsty and urinating more often. He is most likely suffering from

(A) hypoglycemia.

(B) diabetic ketoacidosis (DKA).

(C) stroke.

(D) septic shock.

59. A syncopal episode is most likely to occur when the patient is in which position?

(A) Supine

(B) Kneeling

(C) Sitting

(D) Standing

60. Your patient presents sitting on a park bench conscious and alert, though confused to person, place, and time. You should

(A) administer oral glucose.

(B) provide manual cervical spine stabilization.

(C) obtain a set of vital signs.

(D) assess her breathing.

61. Signs of hypoglycemia include

(A) cool, pale, and diaphoretic skin.

(B) anxiety and decreased respirations.

(C) tachycardia and hypotension.

(D) abdominal pain and nausea.

62. Your patient appears confused but is able to follow directions. His wife states that he is a diabetic and "may have taken too much insulin." His vital signs include a pulse rate of 102 beats per minute, a respiratory rate of 14 breaths per minute with adequate tidal volume, and a blood pressure of 128/90 mm Hg. You should first

(A) administer oxygen.

(B) administer oral glucose.

(C) inquire more into his past medical history.

(D) hold cervical spine stabilization.

63. Your patient complains of a rapid onset of fever, fatigue, and sore throat with difficulty swallowing. You note that he is sitting forward, drooling, and has inspiratory stridor. His lung sounds are clear. Based on this information, he is most likely suffering from

(A) asthma.

(B) acute pulmonary edema.

(C) pneumonia.

(D) epiglottitis.

64. Which of the following infectious diseases is spread through airborne droplets?

(A) Tuberculosis

(B) Hepatitis C

(C) Hepatitis B

(D) Human immunodeficiency virus (HIV)

65. The single most effective way to prevent the spread of infection is to

(A) wear gloves.

(B) wash your hands.

(C) avoid touching patients.

(D) be current with your vaccinations.

66. Medical control orders you to stop performing CPR on a terminally ill cancer patient. A distraught family member screams, "Do your job and save my mother!" You should

(A) resume CPR and transport the patient.

(B) immediately call the police.

(C) allow the family member to grieve.

(D) promptly leave the scene.

67. A 68-year-old male presents in bed with vomit on his face, in full cardiac arrest. You decide not to resuscitate. The patient's wife asks if she can "say goodbye to him." You should

(A) not allow the wife to view the patient.

(B) clean the patient's face and allow the wife to see him.

(C) allow the wife to visit her husband.

(D) contact medical control for permission.

68. You are treating a conscious, alert, and oriented 64-year-old male for a suspected heart attack. He refuses transport to the hospital. You should

(A) explain that once you start treatment you cannot stop.

(B) physically force the patient to go to the emergency department.

(C) have the patient's wife take the patient to his personal physician.

(D) inform the patient of the risks of not seeking medical attention.

69. A patient with a broken leg refuses to be transported to the hospital. He appears to be heavily intoxicated, and you determine that he is alert to person but not to place or time and doesn't remember how he broke his leg. You should

(A) ask a police officer to arrest the patient.

(B) have the patient sign a refusal form.

(C) have the patient's girlfriend sign a refusal form.

(D) transport the patient under the concept of implied consent.

70. A 2-month-old infant presents in his crib, pulseless with agonal respirations. You should immediately

(A) note the physical appearance of the patient and his position in the crib.

(B) declare the room a crime scene and leave the infant in place.

(C) ask the parents whether the patient has a cardiac history.

(D) leave the patient as found and call the police.

71. Your patient presents with signs and symptoms consistent with ischemic stroke. Of the following, which would be the most critical information to relay to the receiving facility?

(A) Secondary exam findings

(B) The patient's medication list

(C) The Glasgow coma scale score

(D) The time of onset of stroke symptoms

72. A 44-year-old male complains of a sudden onset of "the worst headache of my life." Which of the following is the most likely cause of this headache?

(A) Transient ischemic attack

(B) Cerebral embolism

(C) Ischemic stroke

(D) Hemorrhagic stroke

73. Which of the following is a common sign of ischemic stroke?

(A) Equal strength in both arms

(B) Projectile vomiting

(C) Slurred speech

(D) Tachycardia

74. Which of the following emergencies may present with stroke-like symptoms?

(A) Hyperglycemia

(B) Hypoglycemia

(C) Myocardial infarction

(D) Pulmonary embolism

75. The most immediate threat to life in a patient with a ruptured appendix is

(A) respiratory arrest.

(B) cardiac arrest.

(C) sepsis.

(D) hypovolemic shock.

76. A 40-year-old female has been vomiting for 24 hours and describes her emesis as being dark in color, with a coffee ground–like texture. This finding is most indicative of

(A) intestinal obstruction.

(B) esophageal varices.

(C) upper gastrointestinal bleeding.

(D) lower gastrointestinal bleeding.

77. Your patient is a 52-year-old male with a history of alcoholism. He is vomiting large amounts of bright red blood. The most likely cause of this is

(A) pancreatitis.

(B) abdominal aortic aneurysm.

(C) esophageal varices.

(D) ulcers.

78. Your patient presents with hallucinations, anxiety, and paranoia after ingesting an unknown drug. When communicating with the patient, you should

(A) search the patient for more of the drug he ingested.

(B) sit next to him, place your hand on his shoulder, and talk calmly.

(C) repeat simple and specific statements to ensure that you are understood.

(D) allow him to talk, but do not ask questions.

79. A 64-year-old female presents with an acute onset of altered mental status. She has a heart rate of 32, a blood pressure reading of 70/30 mm Hg, and respirations of 16 per minute with normal tidal volume. You suspect an accidental medication overdose. She has most likely overdosed on

(A) a beta blocker.

(B) insulin.

(C) nitroglycerin.

(D) aspirin.

80. Which of the following patients would you most expect to be experiencing delirium tremens?

(A) A 16-year-old male who ingested alcohol for the first time

(B) A 24-year-old college student who drank heavily last night

(C) A 62-year-old alcoholic who has not had a drink in three days

(D) A 42-year-old male who quit drinking "cold turkey" three years ago and hasn't had a drink since

81. You arrive on the scene of a motor vehicle crash (MVC) and find a tanker truck lying on its side, leaking an unknown fluid. You note numerous bystanders trying to assist the injured driver. You should first

(A) call for additional resources.

(B) move to a safe area uphill and upwind from the incident.

(C) instruct the bystanders to move away from the tanker truck.

(D) perform an assessment on the injured driver of the tanker truck.

82. You arrive on-scene to find your patient frantically struggling to remain above water in a deep channel about 5 feet from a dock. You should

(A) remove heavy clothing and enter the water to rescue him.

(B) stay in your ambulance and call for a water rescue team.

(C) stand on the dock and extend an object for the patient to grab.

(D) use a nearby canoe to paddle out to the patient.

83. When driving in emergency mode with lights and sirens, you should always pass cars

(A) after they come to a full and complete stop.

(B) on the right.

(C) on the left.

(D) at a speed that's no greater than 25 miles per hour.

84. Your partner asks you to clean an oropharyngeal airway (OPA) that was used on a patient during a cardiac arrest. You should

(A) wipe the OPA off with a towel.

(B) clean the OPA with a disinfectant agent.

(C) wash the OPA in hot, soapy water.

(D) clean the OPA in cold, sterile water.

85. After a call, you note that there is blood on the bench seat of your ambulance. You should

(A) wipe the blood up with a towel.

(B) clean the bench with a bleach and water solution.

(C) wash the blood off with hot, soapy water.

(D) take the ambulance out of service.

86. Malaria results in which of the following conditions in the blood?

(A) Hypoxia

(B) Anemia

(C) Clotting

(D) Dehydration

87. Hematuria is defined as the presence of

(A) blood in the urine.

(B) blood in the stool.

(C) bile in the vomit.

(D) waste products in the urine.

88. Dialysis is the process of

(A) removing blood from the urine.

(B) exchanging gases across a synthetic membrane.

(C) removing water and waste products from the blood.

(D) preventing seizures in a patient with kidney failure.

89. A patient with chronic renal failure complains of dyspnea with exertion. You auscultate crackles at the bases of both lungs and note pedal edema. He has a pulse rate of 112/minute and irregular, a blood pressure of 172/100 mm Hg, and a respiratory rate of 20/minute and deep. The pulse oximeter records 90 percent. You should

(A) administer oxygen via a nonrebreather mask at 15 liters per minute (LPM).

(B) lay the patient supine.

(C) apply an AED.

(D) administer 324 milligrams of chewable aspirin.

90. A 22-year-old female has vaginal bleeding and complains of severe abdominal cramping. She reports that she has not had her menstrual cycle in four months. Which of the following is the most likely cause of these signs and symptoms?

(A) Pelvic inflammatory disease

(B) Endometritis

(C) Ovarian cyst

(D) Spontaneous abortion

91. Your patient presents complaining of lower quadrant abdominal pain and vaginal bleeding. She shows you a pad soaked with about 50 milliliters of blood. Her heart rate is 82 and regular, her respiratory rate is 14 and nonlabored, and her blood pressure is 124/88 mm Hg. You should

(A) pack her vagina with gauze to control the bleeding.

(B) administer oxygen via a nonrebreather mask.

(C) control the bleeding with direct pressure.

(D) place a pad over the vagina to absorb any blood.

92. You are transporting a 32-week-pregnant female to the emergency department for a possible sprained ankle. After lying comfortably on your stretcher for the first 5 minutes, she develops dizziness and feels like she is going to faint. You should

(A) roll her onto her left side.

(B) take her blood pressure.

(C) attach an AED.

(D) palpate her abdomen.

93. A female patient presents with vaginal bleeding. You should

(A) open the vagina and inspect the vaginal canal.

(B) have the patient insert a tampon.

(C) place a sanitary pad over the vaginal opening.

(D) discard any used sanitary pads prior to transport.

94. You are approached by a journalist and asked whether you transported Jane Doe to the emergency department. You should

(A) give the journalist any information he needs.

(B) confirm that you did transport the patient, but not give any additional information.

(C) inform the journalist that you cannot talk about any patients you care for.

(D) direct the journalist to the emergency department staff.

95. You are performing CPR on an elderly patient. The patient's son arrives and announces that the patient has a DNR. You should

(A) stop CPR.

(B) stop CPR and ask to see the DNR.

(C) continue CPR and ask to see the DNR.

(D) continue CPR and inform the son that once you start you cannot stop.

96. A conscious 6-month-old is moving around, turning blue, and not making any sounds or moving any air. You should

(A) check her pulse.

(B) deliver abdominal thrusts.

(C) perform five back blows (slaps).

(D) administer 30 chest compressions.

97. Which of the following results in bradycardia in the pediatric patient?

(A) Fear

(B) Fever

(C) Hypoxia

(D) Hypovolemia

98. A 6-month-old male with no medical history has a two-day history of low-grade fever, tachypnea, and wheezing. Auscultation of lung sounds reveals inspiratory and expiratory wheezes to all lobes bilaterally. This is most consistent with

(A) asthma.

(B) pneumonia.

(C) croup.

(D) bronchiolitis.

99. Compared to an adult, a child's liver and spleen are more susceptible to injury from blunt force trauma because the

(A) liver and spleen are less protected by the rib cage.

(B) abdominal wall has a thicker layer of fat.

(C) thorax is more pliable.

(D) abdominal organs are more fragile.

100. An infant has suffered full thickness burns to her entire head and neck. What is the estimated total body surface area (TBSA) burned?

(A) 9 percent

(B) 12 percent

(C) 18 percent

(D) 22 percent

101. A 6-year-old female presents with a laceration to her bicep that is spurting blood. You should immediately

(A) apply direct pressure.

(B) elevate her arm.

(C) apply a tourniquet.

(D) administer oxygen.

102. A 12-year-old male presents with a gunshot wound to the chest. You should immediately

(A) fully expose the patient and look for other wounds.

(B) cover the wound with an occlusive dressing.

(C) administer oxygen via a nonrebreather mask.

(D) perform full spinal immobilization.

103. You are presented with a 2-year-old who appears limp and sleepy and doesn't respond to painful stimulus. The father describes a 24-hour history of vomiting and diarrhea with limited fluid intake. What condition do you suspect?

(A) Compensated cardiogenic shock

(B) Decompensating hypovolemic shock

(C) Compensated hypovolemic shock

(D) Irreversible distributive shock

104. A 12-year-old, insulin-dependent diabetic presents with a three-day history of abdominal pain, nausea, and vomiting. Your exam reveals warm, dry skin and poor skin turgor. You also note a fruity odor on the patient's breath. She is most likely suffering from

(A) hypoglycemia.

(B) diabetic ketoacidosis (DKA).

(C) epiglottitis.

(D) septic shock.

105. An 8-year-old patient has ingested a medication unfamiliar to you. On-scene, your best source of information regarding the medication itself is

(A) the Internet.

(B) the patient's family.

(C) the patient's physician.

(D) poison control.

106. Which of the following skin signs is most characteristic of hypovolemic shock?

(A) Pale, cool, diaphoretic skin

(B) Warm, flushed, dry skin

(C) Diaphoretic, red, hot skin

(D) Mottled, warm, dry skin

107. An indication for the application of the pneumatic anti-shock garment (PASG) is

(A) cardiopulmonary arrest.

(B) an impaled object in the abdomen.

(C) penetrating thoracic trauma.

(D) a pelvic fracture with hypotension.

108. A 12-month-old female presents supine in bed having a generalized seizure. There is vomit around her mouth and she is peripherally cyanotic. You note that her respirations are rapid and shallow. You should

(A) insert an oropharyngeal airway.

(B) ventilate with a bag-valve mask.

(C) inspect her airway.

(D) administer blow-by oxygen.

109. A 3-year-old male presents lethargic and irritable. His mother states that he developed a fever of 102 degrees Fahrenheit over the past 2 hours. As such, he is at high risk of

(A) dehydration.

(B) hypertension.

(C) febrile seizure.

(D) bradycardia.

110. Your patient has numerous cuts to his inside forearms and wrists. You should be concerned that the patient

(A) may have attempted suicide.

(B) is the victim of abuse.

(C) has been involved in a fight.

(D) is an IV drug abuser.

111. You have determined that a patient is a suicide risk and requires transport to the hospital. He refuses transport and says, "I'm not going without a fight." You should

(A) allow the patient to leave the room and your sight.

(B) contact medical control for advice.

(C) request that law enforcement be dispatched to the scene.

(D) notify your supervisor.

112. Your patient presents with hallucinations and violent behavior. You restrain him to the stretcher by his wrists and ankles. While en route to the hospital he calms down noticeably, apologizes for his behavior, and asks you to remove the restraints. You should

(A) remove all the restraints.

(B) not remove the restraints.

(C) remove the ankle restraints but not the wrists.

(D) remove the wrist restraints and reevaluate the situation.

113. A 31-year-old female presents with urticaria and a rash on her forearm after being stung by a bee. She has a history of being allergic to nuts and carries an epinephrine autoinjector, which she produces. You should immediately

(A) assess her pulse and blood pressure.

(B) listen to lung sounds.

(C) have her use her epinephrine autoinjector.

(D) transport to a hospital.

114. Your patient presents with altered mental status, difficulty breathing, hypotension, and tachycardia after being stung by a bee. He is allergic to bees and carries an epinephrine autoinjector. You should immediately

(A) administer oxygen.

(B) have the patient use his epinephrine autoinjector.

(C) determine the blood pressure.

(D) administer oral glucose.

115. Which of the following is an indication for the use of an epinephrine autoinjector?

(A) Tachycardia

(B) Itching

(C) Hypotension

(D) Hives

116. Your EMT certification is due to expire in six months. Who is responsible for ensuring that you have met all of your recertification requirements?

(A) Your physician medical director

(B) Your supervisor

(C) You

(D) The local EMS regulatory agency

117. What is the most immediate benefit of continuing education?

(A) Improved patient outcomes

(B) Increased knowledge base

(C) Increased wages and benefits

(D) Better relationships with other healthcare professionals

118. Completing a patient care report completely and accurately

(A) keeps you from getting sued.

(B) prevents employee discipline.

(C) provides information to those responsible for the patient's care.

(D) assures full reimbursement in billing.

119. Your medical director asks you to assist in an audit to determine how often EMTs use oropharyngeal airways and how often they are successful. This is an example of

(A) off-line medical direction.

(B) standing orders.

(C) medical oversight.

(D) continuous quality improvement.

120. Which of the following is *not* a role or responsibility of the EMT?

(A) Serving as a patient advocate

(B) Providing administrative support

(C) Maintaining vehicle and equipment readiness

(D) Providing follow-up medical care

Chapter 16

Practice Exam 1: Answers and Explanations

Score your practice exam from Chapter 15 with these answers. As you go through the answer explanations, try the following:

- **See whether there are any broad areas of weakness.** For example, suppose you find that you answer quite a few of the cardiology questions incorrectly. This discovery should push you to review your course notes, go over the textbook chapters related to cardiology, and take another look at Chapter 10.
- **Think about how you felt during the practice exam.** Don't worry if you felt panicked or stressed while you took the exam. It's better to feel these emotions now and work through them before you take the real exam. Read Chapter 7 for tips on how to reduce your stress during exams.
- **You can score your effort, but don't take the result blindly.** There are 120 questions on the exam. Count up the number of questions you got right, divide that by 120, and multiply the result by 100; this will be your percent score. Keep in mind that the NREMT exam doesn't simply go by one overall score; you have to pass all content areas in order to pass. If you find that you did well overall but poorly in one content area, beware of being overconfident. Make sure to review the content area where you didn't do so well.

Answers and Explanations

1. **B.** When compared to an adult's upper airway, the pediatric upper airway is smaller and more easily blocked by hyperextension or flexion, Choices (A) and (D). Keeping the airway in a neutral position minimizes the possibility of blockage. Because trauma isn't noted, a jaw thrust, Choice (C), isn't necessary. (Content area: Airway, Respiration, and Ventilation)
2. **B.** The correct sequence of treatment for an uncontrolled arterial hemorrhage to an extremity is to first provide direct pressure over the injury site; then apply a tourniquet if direct pressure doesn't stop the hemorrhage. Elevating the arm, Choice (C), has not been demonstrated to help control bleeding, and there is no information to indicate a spinal cord injury, Choice (D). (Content area: Trauma)
3. **C.** Pinching the nostrils provides some direct pressure to control bleeding, and having him lean forward helps keep the airway clear of blood. Applying a warm pack, Choice (A), has no benefit and may actually make the bleeding worse. Laying him supine, Choice (B), makes it difficult for him to keep his airway clear, and you never pack the nose with gauze, Choice (D). (Content area: Trauma)
4. **B.** Coughing up blood is *hemoptysis,* Choice (B). *Hematemesis,* Choice (A), describes the vomiting of blood. *Epistaxis,* Choice (C), describes bleeding that originates in the nose or nasal cavity. *Anaphylaxis,* Choice (D), is a severe allergic reaction. (Content area: Trauma)

5. **A.** A *contusion,* or bruise, Choice (A), is the result of capillary bleeding within the dermis. A *laceration,* Choice (B), is a jagged tear or cut through the skin. A *hematoma,* Choice (C), is a localized collection of blood outside of the blood vessels. An *abrasion,* Choice (D), is the result of the scraping off of the skin. (Content area: Trauma)

6. **A.** You should clean an amputated hand by flushing it with sterile saline. Choice (B) doesn't mention placing the hand in a protective bag or other material so that it doesn't rest directly on the ice, so it's not a good choice. Choices (C) and (D) aren't routine care for amputation. (Content area: Trauma)

7. **B.** Placing the knees and hips in a flexed position helps decrease the tension of the abdominal muscles and lower the intraabdominal pressure, preventing further evisceration of intraabdominal organs and tissue. (Content area: Trauma)

8. **B.** The patient is showing signs of brain herniation, the treatment of which is hyperventilation with a bag-valve mask, Choice (B). Application of a cervical collar, Choice (D), and spinal immobilization, Choice (A), will be performed at some point but not prior to ventilation. Choice (C) is incorrect because the patient's breathing is inadequate. (Content area: Trauma)

9. **C.** A four-sided occlusive dressing, Choice (C), is used to prevent air from entering a damaged vein or artery, resulting in an air embolus. A three-sided occlusive dressing, Choice (A), is used with a penetrating chest injury. Gauze, Choice (B), doesn't create an airtight seal. Choice (D) is contraindicated because there's no active bleeding. (Content area: Trauma)

10. **C.** A stable patient with isolated neck or back pain who presents in shoulder pads and a football helmet should be immobilized to a long spine board with the shoulder pads and helmet left on. This allows for an in-line positioning of the cervical, thoracic, and lumbar spine. The face mask should be removed from the helmet to allow access to the airway. (Content area: Trauma)

11. **B.** A narrowed pulse pressure, Choice (B), is a clinical exam finding associated with cardiac tamponade but not tension pneumothorax. Choices (A), (C), and (D) are clinical exam findings shared by both injuries. (Content area: Trauma)

12. **B.** Two observations indicate use of a bag-valve mask in this patient: His breathing is inadequate, and he has a flail segment. Choice (A) is incorrect because CPAP is contraindicated both in unconscious patients and patients with trauma. Choice (C) is incorrect because a nonrebreather mask should not be used in patients with inadequate breathing. Choice (D) is incorrect because the patient is unconscious, a contraindication for the use of oral glucose. (Content area: Trauma)

13. **B.** All open wounds to the chest should be first covered with a gloved hand and then covered with an occlusive dressing. Choice (A) is incorrect as this patient is in respiratory failure and requires assisted ventilation with a bag-valve mask. Choices (C) and (D) are both actions that may be taken with this patient, but not before identifying and treating any immediate threats to life found in the primary exam. (Content area: Trauma)

14. **C.** The patient is exhibiting signs consistent with a developing tension pneumothorax. The occlusive dressing should be lifted in an attempt to allow for the release of pressure in the chest. Suctioning, Choice (A), is not required as there's no evidence of fluid in the airway. There are no indications for Choices (B) or (D). (Content area: Trauma)

15. **D.** This patient is showing signs of decompensated shock, most likely the result of significant blood loss from the blunt force trauma he received. The liver is predominately located in the right upper quadrant and is partially protected by the lower right portion of the rib cage. When injured, it bleeds significantly and leads to hemorrhagic shock. The lung, Choice (A), is another likely site for blood loss in trauma, but lung sounds are clear and equal bilaterally, indicating that a significant amount of blood in the patient's thorax isn't present. The spleen, Choice (B), and the kidney, Choice (C), are located in the upper left quadrant and retroperitoneal spaces, respectively, making them less likely to be injured in this scenario. (Content area: Trauma)

16. **D.** Blood in this patient's urine suggests that there is an injury somewhere in her urinary system. The kidney, Choice (D), is the only organ listed that is part of the urinary system. (Content area: Trauma)

17. **A.** Choices (B), (C), and (D) are all actions that will most likely take place in this patient with an abdominal evisceration, but the mechanism of injury requires that cervical spine stabilization be maintained immediately and throughout care. (Content area: Trauma)

18. **D.** Choice (D) is the only answer that's indicated in this situation. Choice (A) is incorrect because the patient's respirations are adequate. Choice (B) isn't indicated because the patient is not in shock. Choice (C) is contraindicated in the presence of lower extremity fractures. (Content area: Trauma)

19. **A.** Any angulated fracture that results in a distal loss of perfusion should be realigned. Splinting the leg as found, Choice (B), should occur only after an attempt at realignment has failed. A traction splint, Choice (C), is contraindicated in lower extremity fractures. There is no indication for cervical spine immobilization, Choice (D). (Content area: Trauma)

20. **B.** The patient's primary exam findings suggest that he may be in shock, making the identification of life-threatening injuries a priority. A full rapid trauma exam should be performed. Choices (A), (C), and (D) may all be performed during care of this patient, but only after assessing for other injuries. (Content area: Trauma)

21. **B.** CPAP, Choice (B), is the best treatment option for this patient experiencing an exacerbation of his COPD because it will decrease the work of his breathing. EMTs should not withhold oxygen, Choice (A), in patients with difficulty breathing, even if there is a history of COPD. Choice (D) will not be sufficient for the patient who is having difficulty ventilating. Choice (C) is not indicated because the patient is not in respiratory failure. (Content area: Airway, Respiration, and Ventilation)

22. **A.** Too much tidal volume results in an increase in intrathoracic pressure, which puts pressure against the great blood vessels in the thorax, thereby decreasing preload. As a result, cardiac output falls and causes hypotension, making Choices (C) and (B), respectively, incorrect. Too much tidal volume doesn't result in a decrease in minute volume, Choice (D). (Content area: Airway, Respiration, and Ventilation)

23. **D.** Respiratory failure is characterized by inadequate rate and/or tidal volume. Choices (A), (B), and (C) are all signs characteristic of respiratory distress. (Content area: Airway, Respiration, and Ventilation)

24. **D.** This patient is in respiratory failure, requiring bag-valve-mask ventilation (Choice D) and making Choice (C) an incorrect response. Choice (A) isn't indicated as there's no evidence of fluid in the airway. A pulse rate, Choice (B), should be determined eventually, but not before you take care of issues with the airway and breathing. (Content area: Airway, Respiration, and Ventilation)

25. **B.** The patient's tongue must be removed as an airway obstruction, and the presence of a gag reflex makes Choice (B) better than Choice (A). Choice (D) should be performed, but only after a basic life support (BLS) airway adjunct has been inserted. Choice (C) isn't indicated because there's no evidence of fluid in the airway. (Content area: Airway, Respiration, and Ventilation)

26. **B.** The administration of oxygen is indicated in a patient with airway burns and stridor. Choice (A) may be performed, but only after the administration of oxygen. Choices (C) and (D) are not indicated. (Content area: Airway, Respiration, and Ventilation)

27. **B.** The patient's airway should be cleared of fluid with suctioning, Choice (B), prior to administering ventilation with a bag-valve mask, Choice (D), and listening to lung sounds, Choice (C). Use of a nasopharyngeal airway, Choice (A), may be appropriate, but the suctioning is a priority in this case. (Content area: Airway, Respiration, and Ventilation)

28. **C.** An oropharyngeal airway should immediately be removed if a patient gags after it is inserted. Next, Choices (D) and then (B) should be performed in sequence. You should never do Choice (A) because the patient will likely vomit, worsening the patency of the airway. (Content area: Airway, Respiration, and Ventilation)

29. **A.** Respiratory distress is present when a patient is exhibiting signs of increased work of breathing. Respiratory failure, Choice (B), is present when respiratory rate or tidal volume is inadequate. Respiratory arrest, Choice (C), is present when a patient is not breathing, or is apneic, Choice (D). (Content area: Airway, Respiration, and Ventilation)

30. **C.** Ventilation with a bag-valve-mask device should be provided with an airway pressure that's as low as possible in order to prevent gastric distention. None of the other choices would result in decreased gastric distention. (Content area: Airway, Respiration, and Ventilation)

31. **C.** As this is a trauma patient, cervical spine stabilization, Choice (C), should be performed immediately. After that, Choices (D), (A), and (B) should be performed, in that order. (Content area: Airway, Respiration, and Ventilation)

32. **B.** If airway or ventilation problems occur while performing bag-valve-mask ventilations, the procedure should be started from the beginning, making Choice (B) the best answer. (Content area: Airway, Respiration, and Ventilation)

33. **C.** Patients with inadequate breathing, as in Choices (A) and (B), should be ventilated with a bag-valve mask. Patients who are vomiting, Choice (D), should have oxygen administered via blow-by or nasal cannula, because vomit can become trapped in a nonrebreather mask, increasing the risk of aspiration. (Content area: Airway, Respiration, and Ventilation)

34. **A.** Patients with agonal breathing have an inadequate respiratory rate, making Choice (B) a poor choice. Ventilations should be administered over 1 second, not 2 seconds as in Choice (C). Raising the chest 3 inches with each breath, Choice (D), can only occur when too much tidal volume is administered and should be avoided. (Content area: Airway, Respiration, and Ventilation)

35. **A.** A choking patient with stridorous respirations is breathing and has only a partial airway obstruction. Abdominal thrusts, Choice (B), are only performed on adults with complete foreign body airway obstructions. Back blows, Choice (C), are only performed on infants, and blind finger sweeps, Choice (D), should be avoided in all patients. (Content area: Airway, Respiration, and Ventilation)

36. **D.** The patient's ventilations are inadequate, making Choice (D) the correct one. There's no indication for the need to suction, Choice (A), and a nonrebreather mask, Choice (C), is contraindicated in patients with inadequate breathing. A set of vital signs, Choice (B), should be obtained after taking care of issues found in the primary exam. (Content area: Airway, Respiration, and Ventilation)

37. **A.** The presence of rales (crackles) rules out Choices (C) and (D). The fact that the patient is sitting up and has difficulty lying flat is more suggestive of acute pulmonary edema, Choice (A), than it is of pneumonia, Choice (B). (Content area: Airway, Respiration, and Ventilation)

38. **A.** CPAP will decrease the work of breathing and drive the edema in and around the alveoli back into the pulmonary capillaries by providing a constant airway pressure. A bag-valve-mask device, Choice (B), or a nonrebreather mask, Choice (C), won't provide this. The patient isn't experiencing bronchospasm, making Choice (D) incorrect. (Content area: Airway, Respiration, and Ventilation)

39. **B.** Air trapping results in increased intrathoracic pressure, which in turn results in decreased preload, decreased stroke volume, decreased cardiac output, and decreased blood pressure. Choices (A), (C), and (D) are simply incorrect. (Content area: Airway, Respiration, and Ventilation)

40. **B.** This patient is experiencing pain characteristic of acute coronary syndrome and you should obtain his blood pressure, Choice (B), prior to the administration of nitroglycerin, Choice (A). A secondary assessment, Choice (D), can be performed after treating the chest pain. The patient should not be allowed to walk to the ambulance, Choice (C). (Content area: Cardiology and Resuscitation)

41. **D.** The patient's low blood pressure is a contraindication for the administration of nitroglycerin, Choice (A), and his allergy is a contraindication for the administration of aspirin, Choice (C). His chest pain is characteristic of acute coronary syndrome (ACS), so his pulse oximetry of 96 percent and lack of any pulmonary complications rule out the use of oxygen, Choice (B), in accordance with American Heart Association (AHA) guidelines for ACS. (Content area: Cardiology and Resuscitation)

42. **A.** The patient's pain is characteristic of aortic dissection, rendering Choices (B) and (C) incorrect. You should administer oxygen, Choice (A), prior to transporting the patient to the hospital, Choice (D). (Content area: Cardiology and Resuscitation)

43. **A.** The patient's breathing is labored, indicating the need for the administration of oxygen, Choice (A). Choices (B), (C), and (D) may indeed all be performed on this patient, but after the administration of oxygen. (Content area: Cardiology and Resuscitation)

44. **D.** As this is a witnessed arrest, the patient should be placed on the AED and defibrillated immediately. Because two rescuers are present, one should provide chest compressions while the other applies and operates the AED. (Content area: Cardiology and Resuscitation)

45. **A.** Placing the AED pad over the medication patch, Choice (D), may result in poor pad contact or patient burns. Not applying the AED, Choice (C), is not in the patient's best interest. Placing the AED pad in an area other than the appropriate one, Choice (B), may result in inadequate defibrillation energy levels reaching the heart tissue. (Content area: Cardiology and Resuscitation)

46. **A.** Though some units may do so, there is no need to wait for the AED to tell you to resume CPR, Choice (B). You should only check for a pulse, Choice (C), if signs of life are apparent; you should analyze the heart rhythm, Choice (D), at the end of five cycles of CPR, not at the start. (Content area: Cardiology and Resuscitation)

47. **A.** Even if only adult pads are present, a pediatric patient should have the AED applied and the cardiac rhythm analyzed, making Choices (B) and (C) incorrect. Adult pads should never be cut, Choice (D), to "fit" a pediatric or infant patient. (Content area: Cardiology and Resuscitation)

48. **D.** Choices (A), (B), and (C) are all cardiac rhythms that an AED will identify and shock. Remember that an AED cannot detect a pulse, which is why you shouldn't apply an AED to a patient who is breathing and has a pulse. (Content area: Cardiology and Resuscitation)

49. **C.** The pediatric population is particularly sensitive to hypoxia, and cardiac arrest is often the result of respiratory impairment and hypoxia. (Content area: Cardiology and Resuscitation)

50. **D.** If you witness a cardiac arrest, you should immediately apply the AED and analyze the cardiac rhythm. In the case of one rescuer, AED application supersedes all other treatments, including chest compressions. (Content area: Cardiology and Resuscitation)

51. **A.** The correct compression to ventilation ratio in single-rescuer CPR is 30:2, making Choice (B) incorrect. The proper rate of chest compressions is at least 100 per minute, and a joule attenuator device is used in children, not adults, making Choices (C) and (D) incorrect. (Content area: Cardiology and Resuscitation)

52. **A.** If a patient in cardiac arrest shows signs of life, stop CPR and perform a primary assessment immediately. (Content area: Cardiology and Resuscitation)

53. **C.** The analyze button should not be pushed, Choice (A), because cardiac dysrhythmias can result in a pulse and perfusing rhythm that the AED identifies as "shockable." The AED pads should not be removed, Choice (D), because the patient may go back into cardiac arrest and require the continued use of the AED. CPR, Choice (B), is not required as the patient has a pulse. (Content area: Cardiology and Resuscitation)

54. **B.** A decrease in stroke volume results in decreases in cardiac output and blood pressure. Choices (A), (C), and (D) are all false statements. (Content area: Cardiology and Resuscitation)

55. **A.** The patient's symptoms are consistent with a hemorrhagic stroke and increased intracranial pressure, and the hypertension is the result of his body trying to keep the brain perfused. Chronic hypertension, Choice (B), is unlikely as he sees his physician yearly and has no history of hypertension. His signs and symptoms are not characteristic of acute myocardial infarction, Choice (C), or heat stroke, Choice (D). (Content area: Cardiology and Resuscitation)

56. **B.** Choices (C) and (D) can cause the issue, but there are other causes as well. As such, syncope is usually an event that is transient and not long-lasting. Choice (A) is not a common cause of syncope. (Content area: Medical and Obstetrics/Gynecology)

57. **C.** In addition to incontinence, patients often present with tachycardia, pupillary dilation, warm and diaphoretic skin, and normotension or mild hypertension. These symptoms render Choices (A), (B), and (D) incorrect. (Content area: Medical and Obstetrics/Gynecology)

58. **B.** Hypoglycemia, Choice (A), is associated with a rapid decrease in mental status and does not result in increased thirst and increased urine output. The signs present are also inconsistent with stroke, Choice (C), or septic shock, Choice (D). (Content area: Medical and Obstetrics/Gynecology)

59. **D.** A decrease in perfusion to the brain is most likely to occur when a patient is standing. The other body positions are less likely to cause a sudden loss of blood pressure. (Content area: Medical and Obstetrics/Gynecology)

60. **D.** Performing a primary assessment is always a priority in every patient. You may administer oral glucose, Choice (A), and obtain a set of vital signs, Choice (C), but not until completion of the primary assessment. There's no indication that cervical spine stabilization, Choice (B), is necessary. (Content area: Medical and Obstetrics/Gynecology)

61. **A.** Hypoglycemia results in the release of epinephrine, resulting in signs such as cool, pale, and diaphoretic skin; tachycardia and possibly mild hypertension; and other signs associated with sympathetic nervous system activation. As such, Choices (B) and (C) are incorrect. Abdominal pain and nausea, Choice (D), are symptoms associated with hyperglycemia, not hypoglycemia. (Content area: Medical and Obstetrics/Gynecology)

62. **A.** You should administer oxygen, Choice (A), to all patients with altered mental status until the cause is determined. You may administer oral glucose, Choice (B), and obtain a past medical history, Choice (C), but not until after the administration of oxygen. There's no indication that cervical spine stabilization, Choice (D), is necessary. (Content area: Medical and Obstetrics/Gynecology)

63. **D.** Clear lung sounds are enough to rule out Choices (A), (B), and (C). (Content area: Medical and Obstetrics/Gynecology)

64. **A.** Choices (B), (C), and (D) are all transmitted by contact with infected blood and/or other body fluids. (Content area: Medical and Obstetrics/Gynecology)

65. **B.** It's well established that hand washing is the most effective way to prevent the spread of infectious disease! (Content area: Medical and Obstetrics/Gynecology)

66. **C.** Choice (A) is incorrect because medical control has authorized you to withhold any further intervention. There's no indication of a scene safety issue, so you don't need to summon the police, Choice (B), nor is leaving the scene immediately necessary, Choice (D). (Content area: EMS Operations)

67. **B.** Choice (C) doesn't mention cleaning the patient prior to letting the wife view him, making Choice (B) the better answer. There's no reason to prevent the wife from seeing her husband, Choice (A), nor to contact medical control for permission, Choice (D). (Content area: EMS Operations)

68. **D.** Although you desire to treat this patient, he has the right to refuse your medical care, as long as he is alert, oriented, not under the influence of drugs or alcohol, and an adult. In this situation, physically forcing a patient to be transported against his will, Choice (B), is considered a form of kidnapping. Although the wife may end up taking the patient to see his personal physician, Choice (C), doing so is of limited help to the patient, who may require significant testing and treatment at a hospital. Treatment may be refused by a patient at any time, so Choice (A) is not accurate. (Content area: EMS Operations)

69. **D.** This person is not in a position to make a reasonable decision about his care, so the concept of implied consent applies. Therefore, the patient cannot sign a refusal form, Choice (B), nor does the girlfriend have any legal right to sign for the patient, Choice (C). No crime is described in the scenario, so asking a police officer to arrest the patient, Choice (A), is inappropriate. (Content area: EMS Operations)

70. **A.** The infant will have to be removed from his crib for assessment and resuscitation, so noting specifics about the scene will assist in your documentation later. You will certainly ask about a past medical history, Choice (C), but only after removing the patient from the crib and beginning treatment. The presence of agonal respirations suggests a recent cardiac arrest and the need for resuscitation, making Choices (B) and (D) incorrect. (Content area: Cardiology and Resuscitation)

71. **D.** The time of onset of symptoms, Choice (D), is crucial information for determining whether the patient is a candidate for fibrinolytic therapy. The other choices, while important, are not as valuable in determining the next step in the patient's medical treatment. (Content area: Cardiology and Resuscitation)

72. **D.** Hemorrhagic stroke is the only choice that is characterized by acute onset of a severe headache. (Content area: Cardiology and Resuscitation)

73. **C.** Projectile vomiting, Choice (B), is a sign more associated with increased cranial pressure following a hemorrhagic stroke. A patient may have equal strength in both arms, Choice (A), in certain strokes, but this characteristic isn't common. Tachycardia, Choice (D), does not commonly occur. (Content area: Cardiology and Resuscitation)

74. **B.** Hypoglycemia is known as a "stroke mimicker," and patients can present with neurological findings such as hemipalegia, slurred speech, or facial droop. (Content area: Cardiology and Resuscitation)

75. **D.** Hypovolemic shock, Choice (D), may eventually lead to respiratory and cardiac arrest, Choices (A) and (B). Sepsis, Choice (C), is a complication associated with a ruptured appendix, but it isn't as immediate a threat as hypovolemic shock. (Content area: Medical and Obstetrics/Gynecology)

76. **C.** Lower gastrointestinal bleeding, Choice (D), doesn't often result in the vomiting of blood or coffee ground–like emesis. Esophageal varices, Choice (B), result in the vomiting of bright red blood. Intestinal obstruction, Choice (A), does not typically result in gastrointestinal bleeding. (Content area: Medical and Obstetrics/Gynecology)

77. **C.** Pancreatitis, Choice (A), does not result in the vomiting of blood, nor does a ruptured abdominal aortic aneurysm, Choice (B). An ulcer, Choice (D), may result in the vomiting of some blood, but not copious amounts of bright red blood. (Content area: Medical and Obstetrics/Gynecology)

78. **C.** Choices (A) and (B) are both aggressive behaviors that violate the patient's personal space and could lead to violence. Choice (D) would hinder you in your assessment. (Content area: Medical and Obstetrics/Gynecology)

79. **A.** A beta blocker is designed to reduce blood pressure by reducing heart rate and the strength of contractions. Too much of a beta blocker causes the heart to slow down too much and blood pressure to fall dramatically. An insulin overdose, Choice (B), causes blood sugar levels to fall, but that doesn't usually result in bradycardia. Nitroglycerin, Choice (C), can cause hypotension, but the rate is usually faster in order to compensate. An aspirin overdose, Choice (D), does not cause bradycardia. (Content area: Medical and Obstetrics/Gynecology)

80. **C.** Ingesting alcohol for the first time, Choice (A), doesn't result in addiction, a condition needed for withdrawal. Delirium tremens start approximately 72 hours after an alcoholic's last drink, as in Choice (C), ruling out Choice (B). The patient in Choice (D) would not experience delirium tremens as he is no longer addicted to alcohol. (Content area: Medical and Obstetrics/Gynecology)

81. **B.** The actions in Choices (A), (C), and (D) should all be taken, but the safety of the rescuers is the first concern. (Content area: EMS Operations)

82. **C.** You should never enter the water, as in Choices (A) and (D), unless you're properly trained and doing so is part of your job. Likewise, doing nothing while sitting in your ambulance, Choice (B), isn't appropriate, either. (Content area: EMS Operations)

83. **C.** Drivers are told to pull to the right when they hear sirens or see an emergency vehicle with its lights on, clearing a lane to pass safely on the left. (Content area: EMS Operations)

84. **B.** A disinfectant agent should be used to clean any equipment that has come into contact with bodily fluids. (Content area: EMS Operations)

85. **B.** Wiping the blood with a towel alone, Choice (A), may not get all the blood. There's no need to take the unit out of service, Choice (D). Hot, soapy water, Choice (C), may work but is inconvenient. A 10 parts water to 1 part bleach mixture can be safely saved in a spray bottle, which can be stored in the ambulance. (Content area: EMS Operations)

86. **B.** Malaria results in the destruction and misshaping of red blood cells, reducing the total amount of red blood cells and producing anemia, Choice (B). It does not cause any of the other conditions. (Content area: Medical and Obstetrics/Gynecology)

87. **A.** The medical term *-uria* should remind you of *urine.* Blood in the stool, Choice (B), is termed *hematochezia*. Choices (C) and (D) are not definitions of hematuria. (Content area: Medical and Obstetrics/Gynecology)

88. **C.** Patients with kidney failure require dialysis to remove waste products from their blood. Although dialysis may prevent serious medical conditions such as seizures from occurring in a patient with kidney failure, that is not its definition. (Content area: Medical and Obstetrics/Gynecology)

89. **A.** The patient should not be laid supine, Choice (B), because he has pulmonary edema and would experience worsening dyspnea. An AED should not be applied, Choice (C), as the patient has a pulse. Aspirin, Choice (D), is not indicated in this case. (Content area: Medical and Obstetrics/Gynecology)

90. **D.** The lack of menses for four months strongly suggests that the patient was pregnant, making Choice (D) the best answer. In addition, spontaneous abortion is the choice that's most likely to result in vaginal hemorrhage. (Content area: Medical and Obstetrics/Gynecology)

91. **D.** The vagina should never be packed with material, Choice (A), in an effort to stop bleeding. There's no indication for the administration of oxygen, Choice (B), as the patient is stable. Direct pressure, Choice (C), doesn't control vaginal bleeding, which typically originates not in the vagina but higher up in the female reproductive anatomy. (Content area: Medical and Obstetrics/Gynecology)

92. **A.** The patient is experiencing supine hypotensive syndrome. Rolling her onto her left side, Choice (A), moves the gravid uterus off of the vena cava. You will assess her blood pressure, Choice (B), but treating her first is more important. There are no indications for an AED, Choice (C), and palpating her abdomen, Choice (D), is not critical at this point. (Content area: Medical and Obstetrics/Gynecology)

93. **C.** You should never open and inspect the vagina, Choice (A), nor should you insert a tampon into it, Choice (B). Blood-soaked sanitary pads should be transported to the emergency department for evaluation, not discarded as Choice (D) suggests. (Content area: Medical and Obstetrics/Gynecology)

94. **C.** Choices (A) and (B) are in direct violation of the Health Insurance Portability and Accountability Act (HIPAA), and Choice (D) can be seen as a tacit agreement that indeed the crew did transport a particular patient to the emergency department. The best reply is one that neither confirms nor denies that you know anything about any patient. (Content area: Airway, Respiration, and Ventilation)

95. **C.** CPR should be performed until a valid DNR is produced. The other choices are not appropriate for this situation. (Content area: Airway, Respiration, and Ventilation)

96. **C.** Five chest compressions should follow the back slaps, not 30, Choice (D), and then the airway should be observed for the foreign object. If seen, it should be removed with a finger sweep. Abdominal thrusts, Choice (B), should never be performed on a 6-month-old. A pulse check, Choice (A), should not be performed until the airway is cleared. (Content area: Airway, Respiration, and Ventilation)

97. **C.** Hypoxia is the most common cause of pediatric bradycardia and should be immediately corrected when identified. Choices (A), (B), and (D) are all expected to result in tachycardia. (Content area: Airway, Respiration, and Ventilation)

98. **D.** Signs and symptoms of bronchiolitis closely mimic those of asthma, Choice (A), but children less than 1 year of age are generally said to have bronchiolitis, not asthma. Croup, Choice (C), is a viral infection characterized by a barking cough and clear lung sounds, and pneumonia, Choice (B), isn't expected to result in wheezing to all lung fields. (Content area: Airway, Respiration, and Ventilation)

99. **A.** Choices (B) and (C) are true, but they don't relate to the question. Choice (D) is not a true statement. (Content area: Trauma)

100. **C.** According to the rule of nines, the infant head and neck are approximately 18 percent of the total body surface area. (Content area: Trauma)

101. **A.** Treatment for an arterial hemorrhage consists of applying direct pressure, Choice (A), and then applying a tourniquet, Choice (C), if the bleeding doesn't stop. Oxygen should be administered, Choice (D), after the bleeding has been controlled. Elevation, Choice (B), is no longer recommended as part of the treatment for arterial hemorrhage. (Content area: Trauma)

102. **B.** Choices (A), (C), and (D) should all be performed in this case, but only after Choice (B). (Content area: Trauma)

103. **B.** Prolonged vomiting and diarrhea can lead to hypovolemic shock. The patient is not responding appropriately, meaning the brain is not being perfused well. This condition indicates the decompensating phase of shock, where blood pressure is falling. (Content area: Medical and Obstetrics/Gynecology)

104. **B.** Hypoglycemia, Choice (A), is characterized by an acute change of mental status and cool, pale, diaphoretic skin. Epiglottitis, Choice (C), is characterized by rapid onset of sore throat, pain with swallowing, and drooling. Septic shock, Choice (D), is unlikely in this case. (Content area: Medical and Obstetrics/Gynecology)

105. **D.** Poison control is the best resource for information about poisonings and toxicological emergencies. The patient's family, Choice (B), and physician, Choice (C), may know the names of the medications but not exactly what they do or how to treat them in case of accidental ingestion. Although Choice (A) may be helpful, you will need to determine whether the information you review is accurate. (Content area: Medical and Obstetrics/Gynecology)

106. **A.** Hypovolemic shock results in epinephrine release that results in tachycardia and cool, pale, diaphoretic skin. (Content area: Trauma)

107. **D.** The pneumatic anti-shock garment (PASG) is not indicated for use in cardiopulmonary arrest, Choice (A). Choice (C) is actually considered a contraindication because the pressure resulting from the PASG's use may worsen bleeding in the chest. You could make an argument for just inflating the leg compartments in Choice (B), but that, too, may result in more bleeding around the impaled abdominal object. (Content area: Trauma)

108. **C.** The patient has vomit around her mouth, so it's important to ensure that the airway is clear. An oropharyngeal airway, Choice (A), should not be used in a seizing patient, as it may become an airway obstruction. Ventilation, Choice (B), and administration of blow-by oxygen, Choice (D), are possible options, but only after the airway is assessed. (Content area: Medical and Obstetrics/Gynecology)

109. **C.** Febrile seizures most often occur when a fever develops rapidly. Dehydration, Choice (A), may be an issue if the fever persists. Choices (B) and (D) are not commonly associated with fever. (Content area: Medical and Obstetrics/Gynecology)

110. **A.** Wounds on the inside of the forearms and wrists are not characteristic of abuse, Choice (B), or the defensive or offensive wounds suffered in a fight, Choice (C). Wounds from IV drug use, Choice (D), are typically puncture wounds. (Content area: Medical and Obstetrics/Gynecology)

111. **C.** Unobserved, as in Choice (A), the patient could harm himself, leave the scene, or obtain a weapon. Contacting medical control, Choice (B), isn't likely to help. Notifying your supervisor, Choice (D), may be helpful, but law enforcement has the tools and techniques necessary to help you safely restrain the patient if necessary. (Content area: Medical and Obstetrics/Gynecology)

112. **B.** Once a patient has been restrained, he should not be unrestrained unless a safety issue is present. Choices (A), (C), and (D) reduce the safety of the situation for the patient and for you. (Content area: Medical and Obstetrics/Gynecology)

113. **B.** Auscultating lung sounds early is important as they may reveal a compromise to the airway and breathing. You will perform Choices (A) and (D), but not until after listening to lung sounds during the primary assessment. The use of an epinephrine autoinjector, Choice (C), is not indicated. (Content area: Medical and Obstetrics/Gynecology)

114. **B.** Choices (A) and (C) should be performed, but only after the patient has self-administered his epinephrine autoinjector, which will correct the underlying problem. The administration of oral glucose, Choice (D), is not indicated here. (Content area: Medical and Obstetrics/Gynecology)

115. **C.** An epinephrine autoinjector is used when the patient is experiencing anaphylaxis. Choices (A), (B), and (D) are all characteristic of a simple allergic reaction. (Content area: Medical and Obstetrics/Gynecology)

116. **C.** Each individual EMT is responsible for keeping his or her certification current and valid. (Content area: EMS Operations)

117. **B.** Your education doesn't stop after completion of an original education program. Increasing your knowledge base improves your ability to care for your patients, which may lead to better patient outcomes, Choice (A). Answers (C) and (D) may also happen, but are not direct results of continuing education. (Content area: EMS Operations)

118. **C.** Contrary to Choice (A), someone can always sue you for perceived poor care, but having a well-documented report helps shield you from legal harm. Choice (B) is too simplistic; you can be disciplined for a variety of reasons other than documentation. Alas, even the best documentation doesn't always result in full financial reimbursement, as Choice (D) would have you believe. (Content area: EMS Operations)

119. **D.** Choices (A) and (B) both refer to the concept of having protocols that do not require the EMT to contact a medical control physician for orders. Medical oversight, Choice (C), is the concept of physician leadership in EMS practice and decision-making. (Content area: EMS Operations)

120. **D.** Choices (A), (B), and (C) are all responsibilities of the EMT. (Content area: EMS Operations)

Answer Key

1. **B**	2. **B**	3. **C**
4. **B**	5. **A**	6. **A**
7. **B**	8. **B**	9. **C**
10. **C**	11. **B**	12. **B**
13. **B**	14. **C**	15. **D**
16. **D**	17. **A**	18. **D**
19. **A**	20. **B**	21. **B**
22. **A**	23. **D**	24. **D**
25. **B**	26. **B**	27. **B**
28. **C**	29. **A**	30. **C**
31. **C**	32. **B**	33. **C**
34. **A**	35. **A**	36. **D**
37. **A**	38. **A**	39. **B**
40. **B**	41. **D**	42. **A**
43. **A**	44. **D**	45. **A**
46. **A**	47. **A**	48. **D**
49. **C**	50. **D**	51. **A**
52. **A**	53. **C**	54. **B**
55. **A**	56. **B**	57. **C**
58. **B**	59. **D**	60. **D**
61. **A**	62. **A**	63. **D**
64. **A**	65. **B**	66. **C**
67. **B**	68. **D**	69. **D**
70. **A**	71. **D**	72. **D**
73. **C**	74. **B**	75. **D**
76. **C**	77. **C**	78. **C**
79. **A**	80. **C**	81. **B**

82. **C**
83. **C**
84. **B**
85. **B**
86. **B**
87. **A**
88. **C**
89. **A**
90. **D**
91. **D**
92. **A**
93. **C**
94. **C**
95. **C**
96. **C**
97. **C**
98. **D**
99. **A**
100. **C**
101. **A**
102. **B**
103. **B**
104. **B**
105. **D**
106. **A**
107. **D**
108. **C**
109. **C**
110. **A**
111. **C**
112. **B**
113. **B**
114. **B**
115. **C**
116. **C**
117. **B**
118. **C**
119. **D**
120. **D**

Chapter 17

Practice Exam 2

Here is a second opportunity to evaluate your study efforts. As I explain at the start of Practice Exam 1 in Chapter 15, try to take this practice exam under real-world conditions:

- Find a quiet place to take the exam. You can't be distracted or interrupted during this time — let people know that you need to be left alone.
- Turn off your cellphone, computer, music player, and television.
- Don't use any study aids, such as your notes or textbook.
- Don't eat or drink anything during the exam.
- Set a timer for 2.5 hours. Try to complete the exam during that time frame.

Note: Although this practice exam is on good old-fashioned paper, you'll take your actual exam on a computer at a testing center. You may want to refer to Chapter 5 for tips on taking a computer adaptive exam.

Try to follow these test-taking tips:

- Begin the exam with the first question and answer it before going to the next question.
- Answer the questions in order. Don't skip around.
- Don't look at the answers until you're completely done with the exam.
- Don't go back to change an answer. You won't be permitted to do that during your real exam.

The answers to this practice exam are in Chapter 18.

You can find an additional practice exam online at `learn.dummies.com`; get the scoop on how to access it in the Introduction. Consider taking it after you finish reviewing this exam (as well as Practice Exam 1 in Chapter 15) and studying the areas you missed. This way, you can see whether your test-taking abilities improve.

Answer Sheet for Practice Exam 2

1 (A) (B) (C) (D)
2 (A) (B) (C) (D)
3 (A) (B) (C) (D)
4 (A) (B) (C) (D)
5 (A) (B) (C) (D)
6 (A) (B) (C) (D)
7 (A) (B) (C) (D)
8 (A) (B) (C) (D)
9 (A) (B) (C) (D)
10 (A) (B) (C) (D)
11 (A) (B) (C) (D)
12 (A) (B) (C) (D)
13 (A) (B) (C) (D)
14 (A) (B) (C) (D)
15 (A) (B) (C) (D)
16 (A) (B) (C) (D)
17 (A) (B) (C) (D)
18 (A) (B) (C) (D)
19 (A) (B) (C) (D)
20 (A) (B) (C) (D)
21 (A) (B) (C) (D)
22 (A) (B) (C) (D)
23 (A) (B) (C) (D)
24 (A) (B) (C) (D)
25 (A) (B) (C) (D)
26 (A) (B) (C) (D)
27 (A) (B) (C) (D)
28 (A) (B) (C) (D)
29 (A) (B) (C) (D)
30 (A) (B) (C) (D)
31 (A) (B) (C) (D)
32 (A) (B) (C) (D)
33 (A) (B) (C) (D)
34 (A) (B) (C) (D)
35 (A) (B) (C) (D)
36 (A) (B) (C) (D)
37 (A) (B) (C) (D)
38 (A) (B) (C) (D)
39 (A) (B) (C) (D)
40 (A) (B) (C) (D)
41 (A) (B) (C) (D)
42 (A) (B) (C) (D)
43 (A) (B) (C) (D)
44 (A) (B) (C) (D)
45 (A) (B) (C) (D)
46 (A) (B) (C) (D)
47 (A) (B) (C) (D)
48 (A) (B) (C) (D)
49 (A) (B) (C) (D)
50 (A) (B) (C) (D)
51 (A) (B) (C) (D)
52 (A) (B) (C) (D)
53 (A) (B) (C) (D)
54 (A) (B) (C) (D)
55 (A) (B) (C) (D)
56 (A) (B) (C) (D)
57 (A) (B) (C) (D)
58 (A) (B) (C) (D)
59 (A) (B) (C) (D)
60 (A) (B) (C) (D)
61 (A) (B) (C) (D)
62 (A) (B) (C) (D)
63 (A) (B) (C) (D)
64 (A) (B) (C) (D)
65 (A) (B) (C) (D)
66 (A) (B) (C) (D)
67 (A) (B) (C) (D)
68 (A) (B) (C) (D)
69 (A) (B) (C) (D)
70 (A) (B) (C) (D)
71 (A) (B) (C) (D)
72 (A) (B) (C) (D)
73 (A) (B) (C) (D)
74 (A) (B) (C) (D)
75 (A) (B) (C) (D)
76 (A) (B) (C) (D)
77 (A) (B) (C) (D)
78 (A) (B) (C) (D)
79 (A) (B) (C) (D)
80 (A) (B) (C) (D)
81 (A) (B) (C) (D)
82 (A) (B) (C) (D)
83 (A) (B) (C) (D)
84 (A) (B) (C) (D)
85 (A) (B) (C) (D)
86 (A) (B) (C) (D)
87 (A) (B) (C) (D)
88 (A) (B) (C) (D)
89 (A) (B) (C) (D)
90 (A) (B) (C) (D)
91 (A) (B) (C) (D)
92 (A) (B) (C) (D)
93 (A) (B) (C) (D)
94 (A) (B) (C) (D)
95 (A) (B) (C) (D)
96 (A) (B) (C) (D)
97 (A) (B) (C) (D)
98 (A) (B) (C) (D)
99 (A) (B) (C) (D)
100 (A) (B) (C) (D)
101 (A) (B) (C) (D)
102 (A) (B) (C) (D)
103 (A) (B) (C) (D)
104 (A) (B) (C) (D)
105 (A) (B) (C) (D)
106 (A) (B) (C) (D)
107 (A) (B) (C) (D)
108 (A) (B) (C) (D)
109 (A) (B) (C) (D)
110 (A) (B) (C) (D)
111 (A) (B) (C) (D)
112 (A) (B) (C) (D)
113 (A) (B) (C) (D)
114 (A) (B) (C) (D)
115 (A) (B) (C) (D)
116 (A) (B) (C) (D)
117 (A) (B) (C) (D)
118 (A) (B) (C) (D)
119 (A) (B) (C) (D)
120 (A) (B) (C) (D)

Questions

Time: 2.5 hours

Directions: Choose the best answer to each question. Mark the corresponding oval on the answer sheet.

1. Your patient is fully immobilized on a backboard when he starts to vomit into his airway. You should
   (A) suction the airway with a portable suction unit.
   (B) ventilate the patient with 100 percent oxygen.
   (C) unstrap the patient and roll him on his side.
   (D) roll the backboard, and the patient, on its side.

2. You are assessing the airway of a patient you are about to ventilate with a bag-valve mask. She has dentures, which are firmly in place. You should
   (A) remove the upper denture.
   (B) remove the lower denture.
   (C) remove both the upper and lower dentures.
   (D) leave the dentures in place.

3. A 7-year-old presents conscious with a partial foreign body airway obstruction. She suddenly becomes unresponsive. You should
   (A) administer 30 chest compressions.
   (B) perform five back blows (slaps).
   (C) check a pulse.
   (D) deliver abdominal thrusts.

4. A 12-year-old male presents in respiratory arrest after falling off a second-floor balcony. You note a large contusion to his forehead, and he has a heart rate of 62. You should first
   (A) determine his blood pressure.
   (B) perform full spinal immobilization.
   (C) ventilate with a bag-valve mask.
   (D) administer chest compressions.

5. Your patient presents with altered mental status, an oxygen saturation level (SpO_2) of 71 percent on room air, and labored, shallow breathing at a rate of 24 times a minute. You should
   (A) take cervical spine precautions and administer high-flow oxygen.
   (B) give one breath every 5 seconds with a continuous positive airway pressure (CPAP) unit.
   (C) match his respiratory rate and assist ventilations with a bag-valve mask.
   (D) administer oral glucose with a tongue depressor, and administer low-flow oxygen.

6. You are ventilating an unconscious, apneic patient experiencing a severe asthma attack. Your rate is 20 breaths per minute and oxygen is flowing at 15 liters per minute (LPM). You note that his chest is increasingly distended, and it's getting harder to ventilate. You should
   (A) decrease the oxygen flow rate to 5 LPM.
   (B) decrease the ventilation rate to 12 per minute.
   (C) suction the airway.
   (D) assist the patient with administration of his metered-dose inhaler.

7. Which of the following is the best indicator that ventilation with a bag-valve mask is correcting hypoxia?
   (A) Normal chest rise and fall
   (B) Ventilation rate of 12 per minute
   (C) Increasing SpO_2 (oxygen saturation level)
   (D) Pulse of 88/minute and regular

8. A 22-year-old female with a history of asthma presents with dyspnea. She is alert, her respiratory rate is 20 and deep, and her skin is cool and moist with peripheral cyanosis. You auscultate wheezes in all lung fields. She has her prescribed albuterol metered-dose inhaler. You should first

(A) administer oxygen via nasal cannula.

(B) assist the patient with her metered-dose inhaler.

(C) administer oxygen via a nonrebreather mask.

(D) cover her with a blanket.

9. A 34-year-old female presents conscious and alert, complaining of difficulty breathing. You note a respiratory rate of 22 per minute with deep tidal volume, and her skin is cool, pale, and diaphoretic. You should immediately

(A) insert an oropharyngeal airway.

(B) suction her airway.

(C) assist ventilations with a bag-valve mask.

(D) administer oxygen via a nonrebreather mask.

10. A 64-year-old female with a history of congestive heart failure has a sudden onset of shortness of breath. She is alert, with rapid and deep respirations and cool, pale, and diaphoretic skin. You auscultate rales (crackles) bilaterally. You should

(A) administer continuous positive airway pressure (CPAP).

(B) administer oxygen via nasal cannula.

(C) administer oxygen via a nonrebreather mask.

(D) determine the patient's blood pressure.

11. Which of the following clinical exam findings would best indicate that your patient is in respiratory distress and not respiratory failure?

(A) Shallow tidal volume

(B) Respiratory rate of 4 breaths per minute

(C) Absent respirations

(D) Respiratory rate of 16 breaths per minute

12. A 34-year-old female presents with an acute onset of dyspnea and right-sided chest pain that worsens when she takes a deep breath. She has a history of asthma and gave birth to her first child four days ago. Lung sounds are clear and equal bilaterally. Her skin is cool, pale, and diaphoretic, and there is jugular venous distention. You should first

(A) obtain a complete set of vital signs.

(B) administer oxygen via a nonrebreather mask.

(C) assist the patient with her albuterol metered-dose inhaler.

(D) inspect for vaginal hemorrhage.

13. An 8-year-old male is slumped in a chair, responsive to pain only. His mother describes an acute onset of his asthma that was unrelieved with his metered-dose inhaler. He has a shallow respiratory rate of 8 breaths per minute, a brachial pulse of 64, and wheezes to all lung fields. You should first

(A) start CPR.

(B) assist with his metered-dose inhaler.

(C) administer bag-valve mask ventilations.

(D) lay the patient supine and pad behind his shoulders.

14. A 72-year-old female with a history of chronic obstructive pulmonary disease (COPD) presents unconscious and apneic with a strong and rapid radial pulse. Her family describes a 4-hour history of increasingly difficult breathing, unrelieved with her home nebulizer and metered-dose inhalers. You should immediately

(A) administer continuous positive airway pressure (CPAP).

(B) ventilate the patient with a bag-valve mask.

(C) assist the patient with her albuterol metered-dose inhaler.

(D) insert an oropharyngeal airway.

15. You are ventilating a patient who is apneic. Which of the following errors will most likely result in gastric distension?

(A) Ventilating too fast

(B) Ventilating too hard

(C) Ventilating too slow

(D) Ventilating too shallow

16. A 23-year-old male presents with stridor and difficulty breathing after being stung by a bee. He is breathing 28 times a minute, he has a heart rate of 108, and his blood pressure is 110/70 mm Hg. You should first

(A) ventilate with a bag-valve mask.

(B) insert an oropharyngeal airway.

(C) listen to lung sounds.

(D) administer his epinephrine auto-injector.

17. Your patient presents alert to pain only after being pulled out of a house fire by firefighters. You hear audible stridor; his respiratory rate is 18 breaths per minute with good tidal volume. There is a strong, rapid radial pulse, and his skin is warm and dry. The patient's most immediate threat to life is

(A) an airway obstruction.

(B) hypovolemic shock.

(C) increased intracranial pressure.

(D) decreased perfusion.

18. A patient presents sitting on the edge of his bed, leaning forward, and drooling, with inspiratory stridor. He is alert, his respiratory rate is 20 breaths per minute with visible chest rise and fall, and his skin is hot, dry, and pale. You should

(A) manually inspect the airway.

(B) assist ventilations with a bag-valve mask.

(C) insert an oropharyngeal airway.

(D) administer oxygen via a nonrebreather mask.

19. Administration of which of the following medications will result in bronchodilation?

(A) Alpha-1 antagonist

(B) Alpha-2 agonist

(C) Beta-1 antagonist

(D) Beta-2 agonist

20. Bronchospasm, bronchial edema, and increased mucus production in the lower airways best describe the pathophysiology of

(A) asthma.

(B) pneumonia.

(C) chronic bronchitis.

(D) emphysema.

21. A patient presents with a left-sided spontaneous pneumothorax. Which of the following would best suggest that a tension pneumothorax was developing?

(A) Decreased lung sounds on the left

(B) Jugular venous distention

(C) Hypertension

(D) SpO_2 (oxygen saturation level) = 98 percent on room air

22. A 4-year-old male presents complaining of a sore throat. His parents describe a three-day progression of fever, malaise, and respiratory distress. You note slight intercostal retraction, tachycardia, tachypnea, and a loud cough. Lung sounds are clear. This is most consistent with

(A) asthma.

(B) epiglottitis.

(C) croup.

(D) pneumonia.

23. A 10-year-old asthmatic female presents with altered mental status, head-bobbing, and peripheral cyanosis. She is breathing 60 times per minute. There are inspiratory and expiratory wheezes in all lung fields, and her capillary refill is 5 seconds. You should first

(A) assist ventilations with a bag-valve mask.

(B) administer humidified oxygen via a nonrebreather mask.

(C) place the patient in a sitting position.

(D) ask the mother whether she has used her metered-dose inhaler.

24. An infant has suffered full thickness burns to the entirety of both of her legs. What is the estimated total body surface area (TBSA) burned?

(A) 14 percent

(B) 18 percent

(C) 27 percent

(D) 36 percent

25. You are ventilating an apneic 6-year-old trauma patient at 20 breaths per minute. There is a weak radial pulse of 52 beats per minute. You should

(A) increase the ventilation rate to 40 breaths per minute.

(B) start chest compressions.

(C) perform full spinal immobilization.

(D) administer oral glucose.

26. Your patient is an 8-month-old found pulseless and apneic in her crib by her parents. Rigor mortis is present. The patient has no medical history. The mother states, "She was absolutely fine when we put her to bed last night. How can this happen?" The best reply is

(A) "I have no idea."

(B) "I think this may be sudden infant death syndrome (SIDS)."

(C) "It was most likely a breathing problem that killed your child."

(D) "Have you called a funeral home yet?"

27. The appropriate compression-to-ventilation ratio in two-rescuer CPR on a child is

(A) 30:1

(B) 30:2

(C) 15:1

(D) 15:2

28. You are caring for a 4-year-old female with severe head trauma after a fall from a significant height. The patient's mother asks you, "Is my daughter seriously injured?" The best reply is

(A) "No, she is not seriously injured."

(B) "I do not know how badly she is injured."

(C) "The doctor at the hospital will be better able to talk with you about this."

(D) "Yes, your daughter is seriously injured, and we are doing everything we can for her."

29. A 2-year-old male presents sitting in his mother's lap, with an injured arm after a fall. You should

(A) take off his shirt to expose the arm and keep it off during transport.

(B) perform your assessment with the child in the mother's lap.

(C) touch the patient as much as possible to allow him to get familiar with you.

(D) place a nonrebreather mask over his face to keep him calm.

30. Why does a child's rib cage not protect the intrathoracic organs as effectively as an adult's?

(A) The respiratory rate is faster.

(B) The ribs are more pliable.

(C) There is smaller circulating blood volume.

(D) The ribs are more horizontal.

31. A 4-year-old patient presents supine on a kitchen floor. You determine that he is pulseless and apneic. You and your partner should immediately

(A) begin CPR at a ratio of 15 compressions to 2 breaths.

(B) ventilate the patient once every 5 seconds.

(C) begin CPR, compressing the chest at least 1 inch.

(D) attach an automated external defibrillator (AED) and analyze the heart rhythm.

32. A 7-year-old male complains of neck pain after a fall off his bicycle. You see no obvious injury, and you find no neurological deficits. His heart rate is 82, his respiratory rate is 16 with good tidal volume, and his blood pressure is 112/70 mm Hg. You should

(A) administer high-flow oxygen via a nonrebreather mask.

(B) pad behind his shoulders when placing him on a long spine board.

(C) transport the patient to a trauma center.

(D) call for a paramedic unit to care for the patient.

33. You are assessing a 13-month-old child and determine the need for spinal immobilization. You do not have a cervical collar that fits the patient. You should

(A) use the smallest sized adult collar you have.

(B) use a towel or other padding as an improvised cervical collar.

(C) immobilize the child without cervical spine protection.

(D) hold manual cervical spine stabilization throughout transport.

34. A 42-year-old male has a sudden onset of sharp, knife-like pain that is located between his shoulder blades. His right radial pulse is weaker than his left. He is most likely suffering from a(n)

(A) heart attack.

(B) pulmonary embolism.

(C) aortic dissection.

(D) muscle strain.

35. A 62-year-old male with a history of heart attack complains of crushing, substernal chest pain that radiates to his neck. He is allergic to aspirin and has his prescribed nitroglycerin. You should first

(A) administer aspirin.

(B) assist the patient with his nitroglycerin.

(C) obtain a blood pressure.

(D) administer continuous positive airway pressure (CPAP).

36. A 56-year-old female presents lying in bed complaining of chest pain and dyspnea. Her leg is in a cast. She has a history of angina and is an insulin-dependent diabetic. She has clear and equal lung sounds bilaterally. Her vital signs are a heart rate of 102, a respiratory rate of 18 breaths per minute, and a blood pressure of 102/60 mm Hg. Pulse oximetry indicates 90 percent saturation. You should first administer

(A) oral glucose.

(B) supplemental oxygen.

(C) the patient's nitroglycerin.

(D) aspirin.

37. An elderly male is unconscious, responding to painful stimuli with groaning. His family reports that he complained of a sudden onset of chest discomfort and nausea, and then lost consciousness. You note a weak carotid pulse of 92 and a respiratory rate of 12 breaths per minute. His skin is cool and diaphoretic, with peripheral cyanosis. You should first

(A) administer aspirin.

(B) assist the patient with his nitroglycerin.

(C) administer oxygen.

(D) determine his vital signs.

38. You and your partner are caring for an elderly patient with chest pain when he suddenly becomes unresponsive. He is not breathing and has no pulse. Your next, most immediate steps are to

(A) suction the airway and provide supplemental oxygen.

(B) open the airway and ventilate the patient with a bag-valve mask.

(C) begin chest compressions while attaching automated external defibrillator (AED) pads to the patient's chest.

(D) provide two ventilations, and then begin chest compressions.

39. You have just defibrillated a patient who was in cardiac arrest. He is coughing, and you hear gurgling as he attempts to breathe. You should

(A) insert an oropharyngeal airway.

(B) check for the presence of a pulse.

(C) place him in the recovery position.

(D) push the "analyze" button on the automated external defibrillator (AED).

40. A 68-year-old male states that his "heart is beating really fast." He has a weak, irregular radial pulse of 190 and a respiratory rate of 12 breaths per minute with adequate tidal volume. He has a history of atrial fibrillation and heart attack. He takes an aspirin a day and has been prescribed nitroglycerin. You should

(A) administer oxygen.

(B) assist the patient with his nitroglycerin.

(C) administer aspirin.

(D) determine his blood pressure.

41. First responders have placed an automated external defibrillator (AED) on a patient who is conscious and complaining of palpitations and chest pain. The AED has analyzed the cardiac rhythm and is beginning to charge. You should

(A) allow the AED to charge and deliver a shock.

(B) take the defibrillation pads off the patient.

(C) turn off the AED.

(D) check the patient's pulse.

42. During a cardiac arrest, a paramedic has inserted an endotracheal tube into the patient's trachea. When ventilating the patient through the tube, you should

(A) use a 30:2 compression-to-ventilation ratio.

(B) squeeze the bag once every 6–8 seconds.

(C) disconnect the bag-valve mask from oxygen.

(D) administer twice the tidal volume you were delivering without an endotracheal tube.

43. You have just defibrillated a cardiac arrest patient, and after 2 minutes of CPR, he is now breathing and you find a carotid pulse. You are attempting to obtain his blood pressure when you note that he stops breathing. You should

(A) begin chest compressions.

(B) ventilate the patient with a bag-valve mask.

(C) analyze the cardiac rhythm with an automated external defibrillator (AED).

(D) check for a pulse.

44. Your patient is sitting and complains of chest pain and dizziness. He has a history of diabetes, hypertension, and angina. His skin is cool, pale, and diaphoretic. His pulse is 102, his blood pressure is 76/34 mm Hg, and his respiratory rate is 18 breaths per minute and deep. You should

(A) assist the patient with his prescribed nitroglycerin.

(B) administer oral glucose.

(C) lay the patient supine.

(D) assist his ventilations with a bag-valve mask.

45. Your patient complains of dizziness and a headache. He has a history of angina that is treated with nitroglycerin and high blood pressure for which he has not been taking his prescribed medications. His blood pressure is 230/164 mm Hg, his heart rate is 84, and his respiratory rate is 16 breaths per minute. You should

(A) assist the patient with his nitroglycerin to lower his blood pressure.

(B) administer oxygen via nasal cannula.

(C) lay the patient in a head-down position.

(D) perform a complete secondary assessment.

46. A 23-year-old male presents conscious and alert, supine on the ground with an obvious abdominal evisceration. Bystanders tell you that he fell from a second story balcony and struck an iron fence. You should first

(A) flex the patient's hips and knees.

(B) cover the evisceration with a moist, sterile dressing.

(C) provide cervical spine stabilization.

(D) administer oxygen.

47. A patient presents with a knife impaled in his neck. There is profuse bleeding from the wound. You hear no gurgling or stridor as the patient breathes. You should

(A) remove the knife and apply direct pressure.

(B) provide direct pressure to the wound around the knife.

(C) apply direct pressure to the knife.

(D) cover the wound with a four-sided occlusive dressing.

48. Your patient is supine on the sidewalk. As you approach, you observe an open wound to the anterior chest wall. You should first

(A) administer oxygen.

(B) dress and bandage the wound.

(C) apply an occlusive dressing.

(D) determine his heart rate.

49. Your patient presents unconscious with a metal rod impaled through her jaw. Her respirations are slow and shallow; she is cyanotic. Because of the rod, you can't form an adequate seal with the bag-valve mask. You should

(A) administer oxygen via a nonrebreather mask.

(B) administer oxygen via blow-by.

(C) remove the object.

(D) call advanced life support (ALS) to perform a surgical airway.

50. Your patient presents unconscious with a gunshot wound to the thigh just above the knee. The wound is spurting bright red blood. You can't control the bleeding with direct pressure. You should

(A) perform full spinal immobilization and transport.

(B) elevate the patient's leg.

(C) apply a pressure bandage.

(D) apply a tourniquet.

51. Where should you apply a tourniquet to a wound located on the wrist?

(A) Just proximal to the injury

(B) Directly on the hand

(C) Directly over the wound

(D) On the bicep, just proximal to the elbow

52. Which of the following is an example of a closed soft tissue injury?

(A) Laceration

(B) Avulsion

(C) Contusion

(D) Puncture

53. Your patient presents with a screwdriver impaled through his pants, into his thigh. You should immediately

(A) expose the wound area.

(B) manually stabilize the screwdriver.

(C) use a bulky dressing to stabilize the object.

(D) remove the object.

54. Your patient is unconscious after being struck by a car. His breathing is slow and shallow, and you hear snoring. You feel crepitus when you palpate his pelvis and both femurs. His pulse rate is 126, and his blood pressure is 82/56 mm Hg. Which of the following treatments is indicated?

(A) Application of a tourniquet

(B) Application of a pneumatic antishock garment (PASG)

(C) Oxygen via a nonrebreather mask

(D) Use of a traction splint

55. Human bites are of particular concern because

(A) bleeding can be difficult to control.

(B) there is a high risk of infection.

(C) crush injuries are common.

(D) bones are often fractured.

56. A patient is ejected from his vehicle during a high-speed rollover crash. There is blood in his airway and he has gurgling respirations that are slow and shallow. You note paradoxical movement on the right anterior chest wall, an unstable pelvis, and an open femur fracture. You should first

(A) stabilize the flail segment.

(B) ventilate with a bag-valve mask.

(C) suction the airway.

(D) manually stabilize the pelvis and femur.

57. Your patient was kicked repeatedly in the chest and head during an assault. As you approach, you see him lying on the ground, moaning, with paradoxical motion of the chest. His breathing is rapid and deep. You should first

(A) wrap a bandage around his chest.

(B) have your partner hold cervical spine stabilization.

(C) obtain a set of vital signs.

(D) administer oxygen.

58. A 20-year-old male is sitting on a sidewalk, leaning against a wall. There is an open stab wound to his chest, which makes a loud, gurgling noise as he breathes. He tells you that he is having trouble breathing. You should first

(A) suction his airway.

(B) insert a nasopharyngeal airway.

(C) assist his ventilations with a bag-valve mask.

(D) cover the wound with your gloved hand.

59. A 32-year-old male has a stab wound to his right lateral chest at the 4th intercostal space. There is jugular venous distention, and lung sounds are absent over the right side. His heart rate is 118, and his blood pressure is 60 by palpation. You suspect which of the following injuries?

(A) Simple pneumothorax

(B) Pericardial tamponade

(C) Tension pneumothorax

(D) Flail chest

60. Your patient was slashed across her abdomen with a razor knife. You see an open wound with protruding intestines. You should first

(A) provide cervical spine stabilization.

(B) cover the injury with a moist gauze dressing.

(C) apply direct pressure over the injury.

(D) cover the injury with a three-sided occlusive dressing.

61. A 25-year-old male has multiple stab wounds to his lower right abdominal quadrant. There is little bleeding you can see. Lung sounds are clear and equal bilaterally. His skin is cool, pale, and diaphoretic. His blood pressure is 60/40 mm Hg and his heart rate is 112. You should

(A) apply direct pressure over the injury site.

(B) cover the stab wounds with occlusive dressings.

(C) apply moist dressings to the wounds.

(D) treat for shock.

62. Your patient presents with a fractured pelvis. He has a blood pressure of 132/84 mm Hg and a heart rate of 108. You should

(A) apply and inflate the pneumatic anti-shock garment (PASG).

(B) apply a traction splint.

(C) wrap the pelvis with a sheet.

(D) splint with a sling and swathe.

63. You try to realign a severely angulated lower leg injury but meet significant resistance. You should

(A) force the leg into realignment.

(B) increase the amount of force you are providing.

(C) splint the leg in the position found.

(D) have the patient straighten her leg.

64. Your patient is walking around, anxious and disoriented, after an assault. You note that he has an obviously fractured left humerus, a weak and rapid radial pulse, and his skin is cool, pale, and diaphoretic. You should first

(A) assess for other injuries.

(B) manually stabilize the injured arm.

(C) splint the humerus with a sling and swathe.

(D) manually stabilize the cervical spine.

65. Which of the following exam findings indicates the greatest potential for harm in a patient with a head injury?

(A) Retrograde amnesia

(B) High blood pressure

(C) Ringing in the ears

(D) Nausea

66. Your patient has severe eye pain after being struck in the face with a bat. Your exam reveals a ruptured globe in his right eye. Proper care of this injury includes

(A) irrigating the eye for 20 minutes.

(B) placing an eye shield over both eyes.

(C) applying a cold pack over the injury site.

(D) applying direct pressure to the ruptured globe.

67. Which nervous system mechanism is responsible for bradycardia and hypotension associated with neurogenic shock?

(A) Interruption of the sympathetic nervous system

(B) Increased sympathetic nervous system activation

(C) Increased parasympathetic nervous system activation

(D) Paralysis of motor neurons

68. You find a patient having a grand mal seizure in a cluttered living room. Bystanders have placed a bite block in her mouth. You should first

(A) remove hazards from the area.

(B) administer oxygen.

(C) remove the bite block.

(D) place her in the recovery position.

69. Which of the following would most likely indicate that your patient has suffered a stroke?

(A) Sudden onset left-sided weakness

(B) Altered mental status

(C) A blood pressure of 184/120 mm Hg

(D) Headache

70. A patient who has experienced a syncopal episode will most often

(A) experience a postictal period afterward.

(B) remain unconscious for a long period of time.

(C) regain consciousness after being positioned supine.

(D) present with tachycardia and hypertension.

71. Your patient is alert, with right-sided arm and leg weakness and slurred speech. Family members state that the symptoms began 12 hours ago. He has a blood pressure of 182/118 mm Hg, a heart rate of 82, and is breathing 12 times a minute. Treatment should include

(A) transport to a stroke center.

(B) oxygen via nasal cannula.

(C) laying supine with his feet elevated.

(D) administration of oral glucose.

72. Your patient presents responsive to pain by withdrawing, and muttering incomprehensible sounds. His Glasgow Coma Scale score is

(A) 6

(B) 7

(C) 8

(D) 9

73. A 4-year-old female presents in bed, postictal, after a grand mal seizure. Her mother states that she "spiked a high fever this afternoon." Her skin is hot and dry to the touch. You should

(A) apply ice packs to cool her off.

(B) immerse her in cold water to cool her off.

(C) provide supplemental oxygen.

(D) apply a cervical collar.

74. Your patient has difficulty breathing. He has a history of renal failure and receives dialysis three times a week. Which of the following questions will give you the most information regarding his condition?

(A) "Have you missed your scheduled dialysis treatments?"

(B) "What medications are you taking?"

(C) "Do you have any allergies to medications?"

(D) "Have you vomited?"

75. Your patient has a history of renal failure and has missed his past two scheduled dialysis treatments. Which of the following exam findings would you most expect?

(A) Pulmonary edema

(B) Hypotension

(C) Cloudy urine

(D) Facial droop

76. Your patient presents complaining of cloudy, foul-smelling urine, pain with urination, and left flank pain. Which of the following is the most likely cause of these symptoms?

(A) Kidney stones

(B) Peritonitis

(C) Urinary tract infection

(D) Kidney failure

77. Which of the following statements is correct with regard to evaluating female patients with abdominal pain?

(A) You should determine the exact cause of the patient's pain.

(B) You should administer oxygen each time.

(C) You don't have to evaluate sexual history if the patient is over 60 years old.

(D) You should evaluate the patient's defecation and urination habits.

78. Which of the following questions would be *least* helpful in determining the cause of a patient's vaginal bleeding?

(A) "When was your last menstrual period?"

(B) "Are you having difficulty breathing?"

(C) "Could you be pregnant?"

(D) "Have you had any surgeries?"

79. After three days of diffuse abdominal pain, a 21-year-old patient states that the pain is now located in her lower right quadrant. This is most consistent with

(A) appendicitis.

(B) intestinal obstruction.

(C) gastroenteritis.

(D) cholecystitis.

80. The presence of bright red blood in the feces is called

(A) hematemesis.

(B) melena.

(C) varices.

(D) hematochezia.

81. Which of the following assessment procedures would best confirm your suspicion of an abdominal aortic aneurysm?

(A) Palpate the abdomen for rebound tenderness.

(B) Perform deep palpation of the abdomen.

(C) Perform the Markle test.

(D) Assess pedal pulses.

82. A 32-year-old female has sharp abdominal pain. She is eight weeks pregnant. She has a history of cocaine addiction and pelvic inflammatory disease. There is pain with palpation to her lower right quadrant. The most likely cause of her pain is a(n)

(A) miscarriage.

(B) ectopic pregnancy.

(C) abruptio placentae.

(D) placenta previa.

83. While transporting a patient with a vaginal hemorrhage, you note that the sanitary napkin that was placed over her vagina has become soaked with blood. Your best next step would be to

(A) discard the soaked napkin.

(B) pack the vagina with a new napkin.

(C) place another napkin directly on top of the first one.

(D) remove the first napkin and place a new napkin over the vaginal opening.

84. Hypotension associated with anaphylaxis occurs because of

(A) bradycardia.

(B) increased capillary permeability.

(C) bronchodilation.

(D) increased peripheral vascular resistance.

85. Your patient presents with a rash on both hands after being exposed to poison oak. She has an allergy to peanuts and has her epinephrine autoinjector. You should

(A) administer oxygen.

(B) administer her epinephrine autoinjector.

(C) have the patient self-administer diphenhydramine (Benadryl).

(D) listen to her lung sounds.

86. A 22-year-old male is unconscious after being stung by a bee. He has a weak radial pulse, and his skin is cool, pale, and diaphoretic. You auscultate wheezes in both lung fields. Which of the following would most likely correct the underlying problem?

(A) Administration of the patient's prescribed metered-dose inhaler

(B) Ventilation with a bag-valve-mask device

(C) Oxygen administration

(D) Administration of the patient's prescribed epinephrine autoinjector

87. The most effective way of preventing the spread of infectious disease is to

(A) use sterile techniques when possible.

(B) wash your hands.

(C) require immunizations for all infectious disease.

(D) properly dispose of all contaminated linens.

88. Your patient presents with a history of fever, night sweats, and malaise. You note that he is coughing up spots of blood. You should

(A) administer oxygen.

(B) obtain a full set of vital signs.

(C) listen to his lungs.

(D) put on a HEPA mask.

89. Which of the following infectious diseases is transmittable by coming in contact with an infected person's blood?

(A) Croup

(B) Hepatitis

(C) Tuberculosis

(D) Influenza

90. A 6-month-old male has a two-day history of low-grade fever, tachypnea, and wheezing. Auscultation of lung sounds reveals inspiratory and expiratory wheezes to all lobes bilaterally. You suspect that the patient has

(A) epiglottitis.

(B) pneumonia.

(C) croup.

(D) bronchiolitis.

91. Your patient is confused but is able to follow directions. His wife states that he "may have taken too much insulin." His pulse rate is 102 per minute, and his blood pressure is 128/90 mm Hg. He is breathing 14 times per minute with noticeable chest rise and fall. Your next step is to

(A) administer oxygen via a nonrebreather mask.

(B) administer oral glucose.

(C) inquire more into his past medical history.

(D) hold cervical spine stabilization.

92. A 12-year-old Type 1 diabetic female is unresponsive. There is gurgling in her airway. A parent says her blood sugar level is low. You should first

(A) administer oral glucose.

(B) obtain a set of vital signs.

(C) suction her airway.

(D) insert a nasopharyngeal airway.

93. A 62-year-old Type 2 diabetic is in a nursing home. Staff reports that the patient has had a four-day history of declining mental status, with increased thirst and urine output over the same time period. He is most likely suffering from

(A) hypoglycemia.

(B) hyperglycemia.

(C) pneumonia.

(D) septic shock.

94. Which of the following occurs as blood glucose levels fall below about 70 mg/dL?

(A) Type 2 diabetes develops.

(B) Glucagon secretion increases.

(C) Insulin secretion increases.

(D) Hyperglycemia develops.

95. A 34-year-old female complains of chest tightness and difficulty breathing. She states that she has a history of anxiety disorder but has been noncompliant with her medications. She is breathing 30 times per minute. You should

(A) advise her to take her medications.

(B) administer oxygen.

(C) have the patient breathe into a paper bag.

(D) withhold oxygen.

96. Your patient presents with extreme agitation and anxiety after methamphetamine ingestion. He becomes increasingly combative and threatening as you attempt to provide care. He is most likely suffering from

(A) agitated delirium.

(B) bipolar disorder.

(C) depression.

(D) a panic attack.

97. Depression is considered a disorder when it

(A) results in feelings of sadness in the patient.

(B) produces physiologic symptoms such as weakness.

(C) persists for more than three days.

(D) interferes with normal daily activity.

98. Your patient presents severely agitated, paranoid, and hyper-alert. His pupils are dilated bilaterally, and his skin is warm and diaphoretic. His heart rate is 104, and his blood pressure is 148/100 mm Hg. His respiratory rate is 22 breaths per minute with normal tidal volume. Which of the following drugs has he most likely been using?

(A) Marijuana

(B) Methamphetamine

(C) Heroin

(D) Barbiturates

99. A 24-year-old college student is unconscious in bed. There is a strong odor of alcohol on his breath, and his skin is cool, pale, and diaphoretic. His heart rate is 114, and his blood pressure is 126/90 mm Hg. He is breathing 14 times per minute with normal tidal volume. You should

(A) position the patient left lateral recumbent.

(B) ventilate with a bag-valve mask.

(C) administer oral glucose.

(D) request police assistance.

100. Of the following actions, which should you do first for a patient who has overdosed on an unknown medication?

(A) Identify the medication.

(B) Administer an antidote to the medication.

(C) Administer oxygen.

(D) Maintain a patent airway.

101. Your patient is sitting on a living room couch, confused and lethargic after inhaling glue fumes. Vital signs are a regular heart rate of 88, blood pressure of 128/90 mm Hg, a respiratory rate of 18 breaths per minute, and an oxygen saturation level of 98 percent. You should

(A) administer activated charcoal.

(B) administer oxygen via a nonrebreather mask.

(C) decontaminate the patient by removing his clothes.

(D) transport the patient to a facility with a hyperbaric chamber.

102. Which of the following conditions is most likely to result in acute anemia?

(A) Sickle cell disease

(B) Liver disease

(C) Stroke

(D) Heart attack

103. Which of the following statements best describes how to drive an ambulance with due regard?

(A) Disregard traffic laws under any condition.

(B) Obey all traffic laws and regulations.

(C) Drive aggressively in order to assure safety.

(D) Disregard certain traffic laws based upon the driving environment.

104. When driving in emergency mode, you should

(A) brake quickly.

(B) anticipate the actions of other drivers.

(C) pass other vehicles on the right.

(D) use your siren only when necessary.

105. While inspecting your vehicle, you notice that the siren is not operating properly. You should

(A) fill out the appropriate paperwork and begin your shift with the ambulance.

(B) take the ambulance out of service until the siren can be fixed.

(C) attempt to fix the siren yourself.

(D) put yourself in service and use the horn as a warning device.

106. How often should you check your medical equipment?

(A) Before every shift

(B) Weekly

(C) Monthly

(D) Bimonthly

107. You are caring for a patient who is suffering from a heart attack. You will most likely transport her to a(n)

(A) stroke center.

(B) pediatric center.

(C) cardiac center.

(D) obstetrical center.

108. Which of the following traits will *best* allow you to effectively communicate with patients and their families?

(A) Good judgment

(B) Ability to listen

(C) Resourcefulness

(D) Leadership ability

109. You and your partner find a gasoline tanker truck on fire and lying on its side. The driver is unconscious and trapped in the cab, and bystanders are attempting to free him. You should

(A) move a safe distance away.

(B) tell the bystanders how to extricate the patient.

(C) attempt to free the driver from the wreckage yourself.

(D) use a fire extinguisher to put out the fire.

110. Which of the following items would be the most appropriate to increase rescuer visibility while working on a roadway?

(A) Full turnout gear

(B) Flashlights

(C) Hazardous materials protective suit

(D) Class 3 safety vest

111. After a call, you note that there is vomit on your uniform pants. You should

(A) wipe the vomit off with a wet towel.

(B) clean your pants with a disinfectant agent.

(C) wash your pants in hot, soapy water.

(D) sterilize your pants with steam.

112. You are performing CPR on a patient in cardiac arrest. His wife asks you, "Is my husband dead?" Of the following, which is the best answer?

(A) "The doctor at the emergency department will be able to tell you."

(B) "No, your husband is not dead."

(C) "Could you please step away and let us work?"

(D) "Your husband's heart has stopped beating, and he is not breathing."

113. You have just received permission from medical control to stop CPR on a terminally ill cancer patient. You had moved him from his bedroom floor, and he is naked. The family asks if they can view the deceased's body. You should

(A) not allow the family to view the patient.

(B) return the patient to his bed.

(C) cover the patient up to his chest with a blanket.

(D) allow the family to view the patient as is.

114. While you're transporting a terminally ill patient from her doctor's office to her home, she states, "You know, I regret that I never traveled to Europe." This statement suggests that the patient is in which of the following stages of grief?

(A) Anger

(B) Bargaining

(C) Depression

(D) Acceptance

115. Your system's physician medical director discontinues the use of pneumatic anti-shock garments (PASG) in trauma after reading numerous studies that show increased mortality with their use. This is an example of the use of

(A) evidence-based medicine.

(B) on-line medical direction.

(C) off-line medical direction.

(D) quality improvement.

116. A man who claims to be the father of an 8-year-old patient that you transported earlier requests information regarding the incident. You should

(A) provide the person with any information he requires.

(B) establish that the person is the patient's legal guardian.

(C) refer the person to the emergency department that provided care.

(D) inform the father that you are not permitted to release patient information.

117. You are treating a conscious, alert, and oriented 64-year-old male for a suspected heart attack. He refuses transport to the hospital. You should

(A) explain to the patient that once you start treatment you can't stop.

(B) force the patient to go to the emergency department.

(C) have the patient's wife take the patient to his personal physician.

(D) inform the patient of the risks of not seeking medical attention.

118. Your patient presents with an acute onset of right-sided weakness and slurred speech. The symptoms go away during transport. The patient has most likely suffered a

(A) syncopal episode.

(B) seizure.

(C) stroke.

(D) transient ischemic attack.

119. Your patient presents conscious and alert with a sudden onset of slurred speech and facial droop. His heart rate is 100, his blood pressure is 210/120 mm Hg, his respirations are 12 per minute with good tidal volume, and his pulse oximetry is 98 percent on room air. You should

(A) withhold oxygen.

(B) transport to a stroke center.

(C) ventilate with a bag-valve-mask device.

(D) administer aspirin.

120. Which of the following would best indicate that you should not begin resuscitative efforts in a cardiac arrest?

(A) Absence of a pulse

(B) No pupil response

(C) Rigor mortis

(D) Unresponsiveness

Chapter 18

Practice Exam 2: Answers and Explanations

Score your practice exam from Chapter 17 with these answers. As you go through the answer explanations, try the following:

- **See whether there are any broad areas of weakness.** For example, suppose you find that you answer quite a few of the cardiology questions incorrectly. This discovery should push you to review your course notes, go over the textbook chapters related to cardiology, and take another look at Chapter 10.
- **Think about how you felt during the practice exam.** Don't worry if you felt panicked or stressed while you took the exam. It's better to feel these emotions now and work through them before you take the real exam. Read Chapter 7 for tips on how to reduce your stress during exams.
- **You can score your effort, but don't take the result blindly.** There are 120 questions on the exam. Count up the number of questions you got right, divide that by 120, and multiply the result by 100; this will be your percent score. Keep in mind that the NREMT exam doesn't simply go by one overall score; you have to pass all content areas in order to pass. If you find that you did well overall but poorly in one content area, beware of being overconfident. Make sure to review the content area where you didn't do so well.

Answers and Explanations

1. **D.** The most immediate way to clear the airway is to roll the patient, on the backboard, onto his side. Ventilation, Choice (B), isn't indicated in this situation, and unstrapping the patient from the backboard, Choice (C), is unnecessary because the board actually helps you roll the patient while still maintaining spinal precautions. Suctioning with a portable suction unit, Choice (A), may seem like a good idea, but it's not as effective at clearing the airway of copious amounts of large, chunky stomach contents. (Content area: Airway, Respiration, and Ventilation)
2. **D.** Leaving the dentures in place creates a firm surface to press the bag-valve mask against, helping to create a better mask seal. (Content area: Airway, Respiration, and Ventilation)
3. **A.** Abdominal thrusts, Choice (D), are not used in pediatric patients with a foreign body airway obstruction because you may harm relatively unprotected organs. Back blows, Choice (B), should not be performed on a 7-year-old because they delay chest compressions. A pulse should not be checked, as Choice (C) suggests, until the foreign body airway obstruction has been removed. (Content area: Airway, Respiration, and Ventilation)
4. **C.** Chest compressions, Choice (D), are not indicated in a pediatric patient with a heart rate of 62. Blood pressure determination, Choice (A), and full spinal immobilization, Choice (B), will both be performed, but not until after ventilations have been provided. (Content area: Airway, Respiration, and Ventilation)

5. **C.** Cervical spine precautions, Choice (A), are not necessary as there is no indication of cervical spine injury. Choice (B) would be correct if the patient were in respiratory arrest. Oral glucose, Choice (D), may be indicated, but the patient's hypoxia should be corrected first because the chances of harm are far greater from a lack of oxygen. (Content area: Airway, Respiration, and Ventilation)

6. **B.** Decreasing the oxygen flow rate, Choice (A), or suctioning the airway, Choice (C), won't decrease the air trapping that is happening in this patient with bronchospasm. The patient is unconscious and in respiratory arrest, both of which are contraindications for assisting with his metered-dose inhaler, Choice (D). (Content area: Airway, Respiration, and Ventilation)

7. **C.** None of the other choices are indications that hypoxia is being corrected. Choices (A) and (B) are both indications that ventilations are adequate, but oxygen levels in the bloodstream are not. (Content area: Airway, Respiration, and Ventilation)

8. **B.** Assisting the patient with the administration of her bronchodilator will correct the underlying problem (bronchospasm) better than will the administration of oxygen, Choices (A) and (C), or keeping the patient warm, Choice (D). (Content area: Airway, Respiration, and Ventilation)

9. **D.** Choices (A), (B), and (C) are not indicated because there is no gurgling, snoring, or inadequate ventilation, respectively. (Content area: Airway, Respiration, and Ventilation)

10. **A.** CPAP will help push the fluid in the patient's lungs across the alveolar-capillary membrane as well as deliver oxygen. It will better correct the underlying problem (pulmonary edema) than will the administration of oxygen alone, Choices (B) and (C). Blood pressure should be determined, Choice (D), but only after the patient's airway, breathing, and circulatory issues (ABCs) have been managed. (Content area: Airway, Respiration, and Ventilation)

11. **D.** A patient in respiratory distress has an adequate respiratory rate and tidal volume, making Choice (D) the correct answer. (Content area: Airway, Respiration, and Ventilation)

12. **B.** The patient is most likely suffering from a pulmonary embolism. The patient is not experiencing bronchospasm, ruling out Choice (C) as an answer. You'll definitely obtain vital signs, Choice (A), later in your patient assessment and may even attempt to determine whether the patient has any vaginal bleeding, Choice (D). But first you should administer oxygen, Choice (B), because potential hypoxia presents a greater challenge at this point. (Content area: Airway, Respiration, and Ventilation)

13. **D.** Prior to administering ventilations with a bag-valve mask, Choice (C), you need to lay the patient supine and pad behind his shoulders, Choice (D), to open his airway. CPR, Choice (A), isn't indicated as his heart rate is above 60, and his decreased level of consciousness is a contraindication to assisting with his metered-dose inhaler, Choice (B). (Content area: Airway, Respiration, and Ventilation)

14. **D.** You should insert an oropharyngeal airway, Choice (D), before ventilating a patient with a bag-valve mask, Choice (B). CPAP, Choice (A), and use of a metered-dose inhaler, Choice (C), are both contraindicated in this patient who is apneic. (Content area: Airway, Respiration, and Ventilation)

15. **B.** Hyperventilation, Choice (A), may contribute to gastric insufflation, but ventilating at a high airway pressure, Choice (B), is more likely to result in gastric insufflation. Choices (C) and (D) aren't likely to produce enough pressure to create gastric distension. (Content area: Airway, Respiration, and Ventilation)

16. **D.** Choices (A) and (C) will be done with this patient, but epinephrine should be administered first as it will correct the underlying, developing upper-airway problem. The use of an oropharyngeal airway, Choice (B), is not indicated. (Content area: Airway, Respiration, and Ventilation)

17. **A.** There are no indications that the patient is experiencing hypovolemic shock, Choice (B), or increased intracranial pressure, Choice (C). His decreased level of consciousness may be the result of decreased perfusion to his brain, Choice (D), but his stridor, Choice (A), is definitely the result of a partially occluded airway, which may continue to swell and totally occlude. (Content area: Airway, Respiration, and Ventilation)

18. **D.** Avoid doing anything that could potentially irritate soft tissues of the posterior mouth and throat, causing them to swell and completely occlude the airway. This includes inspecting the airway, Choice (A), and inserting an oropharyngeal airway, Choice (C). The patient is breathing, which makes Choice (B) unnecessary. (Content area: Airway, Respiration, and Ventilation)
19. **D.** An alpha-1 antagonist, Choice (A), and an alpha-2 agonist, Choice (B), both result in an elevated blood pressure. A beta-1 antagonist, Choice (C), results in bradycardia. (Content area: Airway, Respiration, and Ventilation)
20. **A.** Pneumonia, Choice (B), is an infection in the lung; chronic bronchitis, Choice (C), results in increased mucus production and edema of the bronchi and bronchioles; and emphysema, Choice (D), is characterized by destruction of the alveolar walls, loss of lung tissue elasticity, and air trapping. (Content area: Airway, Respiration, and Ventilation)
21. **B.** Decreased lung sounds on the left side, Choice (A), are expected in this patient, so they don't assist in determining that a tension pneumothorax is developing. You'd expect hypotension and developing hypoxia with a tension pneumothorax, not hypertension, Choice (C), and a normal pulse oximetry, Choice (D). (Content area: Airway, Respiration, and Ventilation)
22. **C.** Asthma, Choice (A), presents with wheezing in the lungs, and pneumonia, Choice (D), has rales (crackles) or rhonchi or possibly wheezing. Epiglottitis, Choice (B), has a faster progression, a higher fever, and possibly drooling. (Content area: Airway, Respiration, and Ventilation)
23. **A.** The patient is in respiratory failure, making the use of a nonrebreather mask, Choice (B), a poor choice compared to the use of a bag-valve mask, Choice (A). As such, the patient should be placed in the supine position, not in a sitting position, Choice (C). Knowing whether the patient has used her metered-dose inhaler, Choice (D), is not as important as improving the patient's inadequate ventilations at this point. (Content area: Airway, Respiration, and Ventilation)
24. **C.** When estimating the total body surface area burned in an infant patient, using the rule of nines, each leg is worth 13.5 percent. (Content area: Trauma)
25. **B.** When ventilating a pediatric, infant, or neonate patient, chest compressions should be started if the heart rate drops below 60 beats per minute. The 40-per-minute rate indicated by Choice (A) is too high of a ventilation rate for this age group, and there is no need to perform spinal immobilization, Choice (C), at this time when there are issues with the ABCs that must be corrected. Oral glucose, Choice (D), is not indicated in this patient. (Content area: Cardiology and Resuscitation)
26. **A.** Trying to determine and report the exact cause of death, as in Choices (B) and (C), is beyond the scope of an EMT on a scene. Choice (D) is a subject that may be discussed at some point with the family, but Choice (A) most directly answers the question that was asked. (Content area: EMS Operations)
27. **D.** Per the American Heart Association, the appropriate compression-to-ventilation ratio in two-rescuer CPR on a child is 15:2. (Content area: Cardiology and Resuscitation)
28. **D.** Choice (D) is a true statement and does not artificially raise expectations. Choices (A) and (B) are not truthful, and Choice (C) is evasive, so they are not good choices. (Content area: EMS Operations)
29. **B.** The stem indicates that the patient is not critical, so keeping him close to his parent is appropriate. A young child is likely to become increasingly distressed if any of the actions described in Choices (A), (C), or (D) are performed. (Content area: Trauma)
30. **B.** The ribs of a child are more pliable, allowing for greater flex and movement and energy transfer to the underlying intrathoracic organs. (Content area: Trauma)

31. **A.** CPR should be started immediately, prior to attaching the AED, Choice (D). Chest compressions should be at least 4 centimeters (1.5 inches) in the infant, making Choice (C) incorrect. Choice (B) doesn't address the cardiac arrest. (Content area: Cardiology and Resuscitation)

32. **B.** Padding behind the patient's shoulders helps to place his cervical spine in the desired neutral, in-line position. There are no findings that suggest the need for oxygen administration, Choice (A), nor the need for a paramedic and ALS-level care or evaluation, Choice (D). In addition to a lack of clinical exam findings, there is no mechanism of injury or other contributing factors that suggest the need for transport to a trauma center, Choice (C). (Content area: Trauma)

33. **B.** An inappropriately sized adult collar, as Choice (A) suggests, should not be used, and full spinal immobilization should not be performed without stabilization of the cervical spine, as Choice (C) indicates. Holding manual cervical spine stabilization throughout transport, Choice (D), is an option but may not be as reliable as Choice (B). (Content area: EMS Operations)

34. **C.** A heart attack, Choice (A), pulmonary embolism, Choice (B), or muscle strain, Choice (D), isn't likely to change the quality of the radial pulse on one side only. (Content area: Cardiology and Resuscitation)

35. **C.** Aspirin, Choice (A), is contraindicated because of the patient's allergy, and you should not assist the patient with his nitroglycerin, Choice (B), until you're sure that his blood pressure is adequate. CPAP, Choice (D), is not indicated in this patient. (Content area: Cardiology and Resuscitation)

36. **B.** Oral glucose, Choice (A), is not indicated, as the patient does not have an altered mental status. Nitroglycerin, Choice (C), and aspirin, Choice (D), may be indicated if the patient is experiencing cardiac chest pain, but the clinical exam findings and the patient's broken leg suggest that a pulmonary embolism may be the source of her signs and symptoms. A good idea would be to administer oxygen, Choice (B), and ask more questions regarding the patient's signs and symptoms. (Content area: Cardiology and Resuscitation)

37. **C.** The patient is alert to pain only, so his decreased level of consciousness is a contraindication for the administration of aspirin or nitroglycerin, Choices (A) and (B). You will determine his vital signs, Choice (D), but only after administering oxygen, Choice (C), to correct any possible hypoxia. (Content area: Cardiology and Resuscitation)

38. **C.** This is a witnessed cardiac arrest and requires immediate defibrillation. There is no information indicating a blocked airway, as Choice (A) indicates. Ventilations are less of a priority than are high-quality chest compressions and defibrillation, making Choices (B) and (D) incorrect. (Content area: Cardiology and Resuscitation)

39. **C.** An oropharyngeal airway, Choice (A), is not indicated in this patient, as there's no evidence that his tongue is acting as an airway obstruction. You don't need to check for the presence of a pulse, Choice (B), or have the AED analyze the patient's cardiac rhythm, Choice (D), because the patient is showing signs of life. (Content area: Cardiology and Resuscitation)

40. **A.** The patient is having an episode of tachydysrhythmia (fast heart rate) and has no chest discomfort, making Choices (B) and (C) ineffective. You will determine his blood pressure, Choice (D), at some point, but it's not as important as administering oxygen, Choice (A), to treat his complaint of dizziness. (Content area: Cardiology and Resuscitation)

41. **C.** Defibrillation, Choice (A), is contraindicated in conscious patients. Simply taking the defibrillation pads off the patient, Choice (B), won't correct the fact that you'll have a fully charged AED, creating a safety hazard. The patient is conscious and alert, so there is no need to check for a pulse, Choice (D). (Content area: Cardiology and Resuscitation)

42. **B.** With an endotracheal tube in place, you don't need to interrupt compressions when ventilating, as in Choice (A). There is no need to disconnect the bag-valve mask from oxygen, Choice (C). Administering twice the tidal volume, Choice (D), may injure the patient. (Content area: Cardiology and Resuscitation)
43. **D.** The goal for a witnessed cardiac arrest is immediate defibrillation, Choice (C), but you must first confirm that the patient doesn't have a pulse, Choice (D). Choices (A) and (B) both delay checking for a pulse. (Content area: Cardiology and Resuscitation)
44. **C.** The patient's low blood pressure is a contraindication for nitroglycerin use, Choice (A). He doesn't have an altered mental status, so oral glucose, Choice (B), is also not indicated. His respiratory effort is adequate, so assisted ventilations with a bag-valve mask, Choice (D) are not indicated. (Content area: Cardiology and Resuscitation)
45. **B.** Nitroglycerin, Choice (A), should not be used to lower the blood pressure of a hypertensive patient in the field. Laying the patient in a head-down position, Choice (C), will likely worsen his headache. You will perform a complete secondary assessment, Choice (D), but only after administering oxygen, Choice (B). (Content area: Cardiology and Resuscitation)
46. **C.** Both Choices (A) and (B) are part of routine care for an abdominal evisceration, but should be performed after you first hold cervical spine stabilization, Choice (C), and then administer oxygen if needed, Choice (D), as these are greater concerns. (Content area: Trauma)
47. **B.** An impaled object should not be removed, Choice (A), unless it interferes with airway control and/or ventilation, which isn't the case here. Direct pressure to the knife, Choice (C), may result in a worse injury, and covering the knife with an occlusive dressing, Choice (D), is impractical. (Content area: Trauma)
48. **C.** A normal dressing and bandage, Choice (B), is inappropriate for a sucking chest wound. You need to determine the patient's heart rate and administer oxygen, Choices (D) and (A), after correcting the life-threatening injury you've already identified. (Content area: Trauma)
49. **C.** The patient is in respiratory failure, making Choices (A) and (B) incorrect. Calling for ALS support, Choice (D), is necessary, but first the patient's airway needs to be controlled and she needs to be ventilated immediately. (Content area: Trauma)
50. **D.** Arterial bleeding that is uncontrolled with direct pressure requires the immediate application of a tourniquet, Choice (D), not elevation, Choice (B), or the application of a pressure dressing, Choice (C). If full spinal immobilization, Choice (A), is going to be performed, it should be done after bleeding has been controlled. (Content area: Trauma)
51. **A.** Applying the tourniquet directly on the hand, Choice (B), wouldn't stop the bleeding nor would placing it directly over the wound, Choice (C). Placing it proximal to the elbow, Choice (D), would cut off perfusion to much of the arm unnecessarily. (Content area: Trauma)
52. **C.** Lacerations, avulsions, and punctures, Choices (A), (B), and (D), are all examples of open wounds. (Content area: Trauma)
53. **B.** Choice (D) is incorrect because impaled objects are left in place unless they are interfering with airway control and/or ventilation, or CPR. Choices (A) and (C) are both procedures that will be performed, but only after the impaled object is manually stabilized to prevent further injury, Choice (B). (Content area: Trauma)
54. **B.** There is no evidence of uncontrolled external arterial bleeding, so there's no need for a tourniquet, Choice (A). The patient is in respiratory failure, which requires a bag-valve mask, not a nonrebreather mask, Choice (C). The fractured pelvis is a contraindication for the use of a traction splint, Choice (D). (Content area: Trauma)
55. **B.** Bleeding from a human bite injury is not any harder to control than in any other soft tissue injury, and crush injuries are not common, making Choices (A) and (C) incorrect. Fractures, Choice (D), are not common findings with human bites. (Content area: Trauma)

56. **C.** Choices (A), (B), and (D) are all procedures that will be performed, but the airway should be controlled first. Otherwise, the patient will succumb quickly. (Content area: Trauma)

57. **B.** A circumferential bandage, Choice (A), should not be applied around the chest as it may restrict breathing. You'll administer oxygen and obtain vital signs as Choices (C) and (D) suggest, but cervical spine stabilization, Choice (B), should be performed first because of the mechanism of injury. (Content area: Trauma)

58. **D.** There is no gurgling from his airway, so suction, Choice (A), isn't needed. The patient is able to keep his airway open, so a nasopharyngeal airway, Choice (B), is unnecessary. Breathing is adequate, so assisted ventilations, Choice (C), are not needed. (Content area: Trauma)

59. **C.** A simple pneumothorax, Choice (A), doesn't cause jugular venous distension. The mechanism of injury (MOI) is not likely to injure the heart, as Choice (B) suggests. There's no paradoxical chest wall movement or other evidence of broken ribs, so a flail chest, Choice (D), is unlikely. (Content area: Trauma)

60. **B.** The mechanism of injury does not indicate the need for cervical spine stabilization, Choice (A). Direct pressure, Choice (C), is not applied to an abdominal evisceration unless there is bleeding, and a four-sided occlusive dressing is used to seal the injury, not a three-sided one as Choice (D) indicates. (Content area: Trauma)

61. **D.** Direct pressure, Choice (A), is not applied to an abdominal stab wound. The use of occlusive dressings, Choice (B), or moist dressings, Choice (C), is not indicated unless an evisceration is evident. (Content area: Trauma)

62. **C.** The patient is not hypotensive, so application of the PASG, Choice (A), isn't indicated. A traction splint, Choice (B), is contraindicated in the presence of a pelvic fracture. A sling and swathe, Choice (D), isn't adequate to splint a pelvic fracture. (Content area: Trauma)

63. **C.** Forcing the leg into realignment, increasing the amount of force, or having the patient straighten her leg, Choices (A), (B), and (D), respectively, could all result in a worsening of the injury. (Content area: Trauma)

64. **D.** The patient is confused, so manually stabilizing the spine is necessary until you have fully evaluated the patient. You can treat the minor injuries, as Choices (A), (B), and (C) indicate, after the major problems are managed. (Content area: Trauma)

65. **B.** High blood pressure may be part of Cushing's reflex, a potentially lethal condition that signals increased cranial pressure from a brain injury. The other findings are important, but are not critical. (Content area: Trauma)

66. **B.** There's no need to irrigate a ruptured globe, as Choice (A) suggests. Applying a cold pack, Choice (C), and applying direct pressure to the ruptured globe, Choice (D), should be avoided, as should any treatment that applies pressure to the globe. (Content area: Trauma)

67. **A.** Increased sympathetic nervous system activation, Choice (B), increases heart rate and blood pressure. Parasympathetic nervous system activity is not increased as Choice (C) suggests in neurogenic shock, just unopposed. Paralysis of the motor neurons, Choice (D), doesn't result in neurogenic shock. (Content area: Trauma)

68. **C.** The bite block is a potential airway foreign body and should be removed immediately, as Choice (C) indicates. Choices (A), (B), and (C) are potential treatment options, but only after taking care of the possible airway issue. (Content area: Medical and Obstetrics/Gynecology)

69. **A.** Altered mental status, a blood pressure of 184/120 mm Hg, and a headache, Choices (B), (C), and (D), *may* accompany a stroke, but don't always. New onset left-sided weakness, Choice (A), is the most indicative of stroke, explaining why it's a component of the Cincinnati Stroke Scale. (Content area: Medical and Obstetrics/Gynecology)

70. **C.** A postictal period, Choice (A), isn't expected with a syncopal episode, nor does the patient remain unconscious for an extended period of time, Choice (B). You can expect a patient to present with tachycardia and hypotension, but not hypertension, Choice (D). (Content area: Medical and Obstetrics/Gynecology)

71. **B.** The patient's symptoms are 12 hours old, excluding him from reperfusion therapy. Transport to a stroke center, Choice (A), is not essential. Laying supine with the feet elevated, Choice (C), is not a treatment for stroke. Oral glucose, Choice (D), isn't indicated because there's no indication of altered mental status. (Content area: Medical and Obstetrics/Gynecology)

72. **C.** Responsive to pain (2) by withdrawing (4) and muttering incomprehensible sounds (2) results in a Glasgow Coma Scale score of 8. (Content area: Medical and Obstetrics/Gynecology)

73. **C.** Cooling the patient off, as Choices (A) and (B) suggest, is not part of the prehospital care for fever. Applying a cervical collar, Choice (D), isn't necessary because there's no mechanism of injury that would indicate the potential for spinal trauma. (Content area: Medical and Obstetrics/Gynecology)

74. **A.** Missing or delaying dialysis treatments causes the patient to retain fluid and waste, which may cause breathing difficulty due to pulmonary edema. Choices (B), (C), and (D) are all questions that should be asked, but Choice (A) best helps you determine the underlying problem. (Content area: Medical and Obstetrics/Gynecology)

75. **A.** You would expect hypertension, not hypotension, Choice (B), with a missed dialysis treatment. Cloudy urine and facial droop, Choices (C) and (D), are not signs associated with renal failure. (Content area: Medical and Obstetrics/Gynecology)

76. **C.** Peritonitis, Choice (B), causes diffuse abdominal pain and is not associated with changes in urine condition. Kidney stones, Choice (A), may cause pain in the left flank but not the foul smell. Signs of kidney failure, Choice (D), are low amounts of urine and fluid overload, such as pulmonary edema and swelling in the feet and hands. (Content area: Medical and Obstetrics/Gynecology)

77. **D.** The gastrointestinal tract is often a cause of abdominal pain; Choice (D) is related to that system. You don't need to pinpoint the exact cause of the discomfort, as Choice (A) suggests. Oxygen may not be necessary unless the patient is potentially hypoxic, Choice (B). Although the patient may not be able to become pregnant at the age of 60, she may be sexually active and be exposed to genital-urinary infections, so Choice (C) is incorrect. (Content area: Medical and Obstetrics/Gynecology)

78. **B.** The questions in Choices (A), (C), and (D) are all directed at identifying the etiology of vaginal bleeding. (Content area: Medical and Obstetrics/Gynecology)

79. **A.** The pain characteristic of intestinal obstruction, Choice (B), and gastroenteritis, Choice (C), may be diffuse but does not tend to isolate in the lower right quadrant. The pain characteristic of cholecystitis, Choice (D), tends to be located in the upper right quadrant. (Content area: Medical and Obstetrics/Gynecology)

80. **D.** Hematemesis, Choice (A), is blood in vomit. Melena, Choice (B), is a dark, tarry stool that occurs secondary to an upper gastrointestinal hemorrhage. Varices, Choice (D), are abnormally distended vessels. (Content area: Medical and Obstetrics/Gynecology)

81. **D.** If you suspect an abdominal aortic aneurysm (AAA), you should avoid palpating the abdomen, as Choices (A) and (B) suggest. The Markle test, Choice (C), is used to assess for peritoneal irritation. An AAA may cause pedal pulse strength to decrease as the blood pressure to the legs decreases. (Content area: Medical and Obstetrics/Gynecology)

82. **B.** A miscarriage, Choice (A), would most likely cause central pain in the lower quadrants and be associated with vaginal bleeding. Abruptio placentae and placenta previa, Choices (C) and (D), are both obstetrical emergencies that occur in the third trimester, not the first. (Content area: Medical and Obstetrics/Gynecology)

83. **D.** Packing the vagina with a napkin, Choice (B), is never indicated. Placing a second napkin over a blood-soaked one, Choice (C), is not effective. Discarding the first bloody napkin, Choice (A), isn't harmful, but is not the best next step in managing this patient. (Content area: Medical and Obstetrics/Gynecology)

84. **B.** Signs associated with anaphylactic shock include tachycardia, not bradycardia, Choice (A); bronchoconstriction, not bronchodilation, Choice (C); and decreased, not increased, peripheral vascular resistance, Choice (D). (Content area: Medical and Obstetrics/Gynecology)

85. **D.** You want to know whether the patient is having a simple allergic reaction or whether anaphylaxis may be occurring. Evaluating her skin signs, taking her vital signs, and listening for wheezing in her lungs, Choice (D), helps you tell the difference between the two conditions. Because you don't yet know about the severity of the patient's condition, oxygen administration, Choice (A), and use of the patient's autoinjector, Choice (B), are not indicated at this point. You are not authorized to tell the patient about using diphenhydramine, Choice (C). (Content area: Medical and Obstetrics/Gynecology)

86. **D.** Although there is wheezing, which may lead you to Choice (A), the wheezing is likely to be from the bee sting. Bag-valve-mask ventilation, Choice (B), and oxygen administration, Choice (C), are both treatments that the patient will receive, but the administration of epinephrine will correct the vasodilation and bronchospasm characteristic of anaphylaxis. (Content area: Medical and Obstetrics/Gynecology)

87. **B.** Hand washing is the most effective way to prevent the spread of infectious disease. (Content area: Medical and Obstetrics/Gynecology)

88. **D.** You will administer oxygen, Choice (A); obtain a set of vital signs, Choice (B); and listen to the patient's lung sounds, Choice (C); but only after protecting yourself first with a HEPA mask, Choice (D). (Content area: Medical and Obstetrics/Gynecology)

89. **B.** Croup, tuberculosis, and influenza, Choices (A), (C), and (D), respectively, are spread primarily through the airborne route. (Content area: Medical and Obstetrics/Gynecology)

90. **D.** Epiglottitis, Choice (A), and croup, Choice (C), are upper airway conditions and don't result in wheezing. Wheezing may be associated with pneumonia, Choice (B), but it's unlikely that pneumonia would involve all lung fields in both lungs. (Content area: Medical and Obstetrics/Gynecology)

91. **B.** The administration of oxygen, Choice (A), and asking more questions about his medical history, Choice (C), are things that should be done, but only after administering oral glucose, Choice (B), to correct the underlying problem. Holding cervical spine stabilization, Choice (D), is unnecessary considering the information provided. (Content area: Medical and Obstetrics/Gynecology)

92. **C.** The administration of oral glucose, Choice (A), is contraindicated in this patient due to her decreased level of consciousness. You should obtain vital signs, Choice (B), after completion of the primary assessment. A nasopharyngeal airway, Choice (D), may be used, but only after suctioning the secretions from her airway, Choice (C). (Content area: Medical and Obstetrics/Gynecology)

93. **B.** Increased urination and increased thirst are not associated with hypoglycemia, Choice (A). There are no signs associated with an infection, as Choices (C) and (D) suggest, such as fever, bedsore, cough, nausea, vomiting, or diarrhea. (Content area: Medical and Obstetrics/Gynecology)

94. **B.** Type 2 diabetes, Choice (A), is associated with hyperglycemia, not hypoglycemia. Insulin secretion, Choice (C), decreases as blood glucose levels decrease. Hyperglycemia, Choice (D), is said to exist when blood glucose levels rise above 110–120 mg/dL. (Content area: Medical and Obstetrics/Gynecology)

95. **B.** Never withhold oxygen, as Choice (D) suggests, from any patient with respiratory distress. Don't have a patient with suspected hyperventilation or anxiety disorder breathe into a paper bag, Choice (C), because there's a chance that she is, in fact, hypoxic. Having the patient take her medications, Choice (A), won't help the acute emergency she is having at this time. (Content area: Medical and Obstetrics/Gynecology)

96. **A.** Exacerbations of bipolar disorder, Choice (B), don't happen immediately after ingesting drugs. Exacerbation of depression, Choice (C), is not characterized by agitation and anxiety. A panic attack, Choice (D), isn't characterized by combative and threatening behavior. (Content area: Medical and Obstetrics/Gynecology)

97. **D.** All patients with depression, regardless of whether they meet clinical criteria, feel sadness, Choice (A). Patients may have subclinical depression yet feel symptoms, Choice (B). There are no criteria for length of symptoms, Choice (C), for a clinical diagnosis of depression. (Content area: Medical and Obstetrics/Gynecology)

98. **B.** Marijuana, heroin, and barbiturates, Choices (A), (C), and (D), respectively, are all depressants and don't result in the patient presenting hyper-alert, paranoid, and agitated. (Content area: Medical and Obstetrics/Gynecology)

99. **A.** There is no indication that artificial ventilations, Choice (B), are required. Anything given orally, as in Choice (C), is contraindicated in an unconscious patient, and there is no indication of a potentially unsafe scene requiring police assistance, Choice (D). (Content area: Medical and Obstetrics/Gynecology)

100. **D.** A patent airway, Choice (D), ensures that the patient will continue to ventilate and oxygenate, Choice (C), while you evaluate the patient. Identifying the medication, Choice (A), is helpful but not as critical. Few antidotes, Choice (B), are available to the EMT. (Content area: Medical and Obstetrics/Gynecology)

101. **B.** Activated charcoal, Choice (A), is not indicated for inhaled toxins. There's no need to decontaminate the patient, Choice (C), nor is there a need to transport the patient to a hyperbaric chamber, Choice (D). (Content area: Medical and Obstetrics/Gynecology)

102. **A.** Liver disease, Choice (B), is not associated with acute anemia. Stroke, Choice (C), and heart attack, Choice (D), are not major contributors to anemia, acute or chronic. (Content area: Medical and Obstetrics/Gynecology)

103. **D.** There are times when an ambulance operator is allowed to disobey traffic laws and regulations safely when necessary, making Choice (B) incorrect. You should not drive aggressively, Choice (C), nor disregard traffic laws all the time, Choice (A). (Content area: EMS Operations)

104. **B.** Contrary to Choices (A), (C), and (D), when driving in emergency mode, you should brake in a controlled fashion, pass other vehicles on the left whenever possible, and use your siren continuously. (Content area: EMS Operations)

105. **B.** The ambulance should not be used for emergency calls with an improperly working siren as Choices (A) and (D) suggest. You should not attempt to fix the siren yourself, Choice (C); a properly trained person should inspect and repair any of the emergency warning devices on the ambulance. (Content area: EMS Operations)

106. **A.** Because you don't know what was used during prior shifts, it makes sense to check out the unit each time you begin a shift. (Content area: EMS Operations)

107. **C.** Patients suffering from a stroke should be transported to a stroke center, Choice (A); pediatric patients should be transported to a pediatric center, Choice (B); and pregnant patients should be transported to an obstetrical center, Choice (D). (Content area: EMS Operations)

108. **B.** Good judgment, resourcefulness, and leadership, Choices (A), (B), and (D), are all desired qualities in an EMT, but the ability to listen, Choice (B), is most likely to make you an effective communicator. (Content area: EMS Operations)

109. **A.** Scene safety is a major issue in this scenario. Bystanders should be told to move away, not to extricate the patient as in Choice (B), and you should not attempt a rescue, Choice (C), or try to put out the fire with an extinguisher, Choice (D). (Content area: EMS Operations)

110. **D.** Turnout gear, Choice (A), and a HAZMAT protective suit, Choice (C), are not designed for increased visibility on a roadway. Flashlights, Choice (B), provide no safety on a roadway and may actually blind oncoming traffic. (Content area: EMS Operations)

111. **C.** Wiping the vomit off with a towel, Choice (A), doesn't remove the biohazard. Using a disinfectant agent, Choice (B), or sterilizing with steam, Choice (D), are not necessary to achieve the goal of removing the contamination. (Content area: EMS Operations)

112. **D.** You should never lie about a patient's condition, as Choice (B) suggests, fail to answer a question, as in Choice (C), or be evasive when answering questions, as in Choice (A). (Content area: EMS Operations)

113. **C.** You should not deny the family viewing of the patient's body, as in Choice (A). You shouldn't move a patient, Choice (B), unless it's absolutely necessary after a resuscitation attempt has been halted. Allowing the family to observe the patient's naked body, Choice (D), may make an already difficult situation worse. (Content area: EMS Operations)

114. **C.** In the anger stage, Choice (A), patients may be outwardly angry at those around them. During bargaining, Choice (B), patients may bargain with themselves, God, or others. During the acceptance stage, Choice (D), the patient appears to have come to accept her fate. (Content area: EMS Operations)

115. **A.** On-line medical direction, Choice (B), involves directly contacting medical control for orders. Off-line medical direction, Choice (C), involves the use of protocols or standing orders to guide patient care. Quality improvement, Choice (D), is the process of continuous self-review for the purpose of identifying and correcting issues in a system. (Content area: EMS Operations)

116. **D.** No information about any patient should be released to any person who is not authorized to receive it, so Choice (A) is incorrect. You have no way of determining whether the person approaching you is actually the patient's father, making Choice (B) impossible. Referring the person to the emergency department that the patient was transported to, Choice (C), is in fact releasing private information; you're telling the person that indeed the patient was transported to an emergency department. (Content area: EMS Operations)

117. **D.** Even if you believe that a patient should get medical care at a hospital, you should not lie, as in Choice (A), in an effort to get him to seek it, nor can you force a patient who is alert and oriented to go, as Choice (B) suggests. If the patient refuses to seek medical care despite your informing him of the risks, per Choice (D), you can always try to talk the patient into seeing his personal physician, Choice (C), but this is not the best option. (Content area: EMS Operations)

118. **D.** A patient won't experience right-sided weakness and slurred speech after a syncopal episode, Choice (A), or a seizure, Choice (B). You could have considered a stroke, Choice (C), if the symptoms had not resolved on their own. (Content area: Cardiology and Resuscitation)

119. **B.** Patients with suspected stroke should not have oxygen withheld, Choice (A), or take aspirin, Choice (D), which can make the stroke worse. This patient doesn't require bag-valve-mask ventilations, Choice (C). (Content area: Cardiology and Resuscitation)

120. **C.** Choices (A), (B), and (D) may occur early in a cardiac arrest, while there is still an opportunity for a successful resuscitation. Rigor mortis, or stiffening of the muscles, occurs several hours after death occurs. (Content area: Cardiology and Resuscitation)

Answer Key

1. **D**	2. **D**	3. **A**
4. **C**	5. **C**	6. **B**
7. **C**	8. **B**	9. **D**
10. **A**	11. **D**	12. **B**
13. **D**	14. **D**	15. **B**
16. **D**	17. **A**	18. **D**
19. **D**	20. **A**	21. **B**
22. **C**	23. **A**	24. **C**
25. **B**	26. **A**	27. **D**
28. **D**	29. **B**	30. **B**
31. **A**	32. **B**	33. **B**
34. **C**	35. **C**	36. **B**
37. **C**	38. **C**	39. **C**
40. **A**	41. **C**	42. **B**
43. **D**	44. **C**	45. **B**
46. **C**	47. **B**	48. **C**
49. **C**	50. **D**	51. **A**
52. **C**	53. **B**	54. **B**
55. **B**	56. **C**	57. **B**
58. **D**	59. **C**	60. **B**
61. **D**	62. **C**	63. **C**
64. **D**	65. **B**	66. **B**
67. **A**	68. **C**	69. **A**
70. **C**	71. **B**	72. **C**
73. **C**	74. **A**	75. **A**
76. **C**	77. **D**	78. **B**
79. **A**	80. **D**	81. **D**

82. **B**	83. **D**	84. **B**
85. **D**	86. **D**	87. **B**
88. **D**	89. **B**	90. **D**
91. **B**	92. **C**	93. **B**
94. **B**	95. **B**	96. **A**
97. **D**	98. **B**	99. **A**
100. **D**	101. **B**	102. **A**
103. **D**	104. **B**	105. **B**
106. **A**	107. **C**	108. **B**
109. **A**	110. **D**	111. **C**
112. **D**	113. **C**	114. **C**
115. **A**	116. **D**	117. **D**
118. **D**	119. **B**	120. **C**

Part V
The Part of Tens

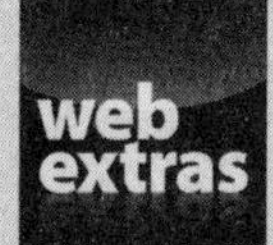

Check out a free Part of Tens list on common medical abbreviations for EMTs at `www.dummies.com/extras/emtexam`.

In this part . . .

- Discover ten handy tips for performing a better assessment more effectively. These tips include looking at the whole patient; taking care of the airway, breathing, and circulation before anything else; and more.
- Read ten tips that can improve your skills performance both on the EMT exam and in real life. Having book knowledge is one thing, but getting it from the head to the hands is another.

Chapter 19

Ten Assessment Tips for EMTs

In This Chapter

- Improving your patient assessment
- Making decisions quickly but accurately
- Correlating certain signs to certain conditions

The EMT exam evaluates your ability to assess patients quickly and formulate a treatment plan even if you don't have all the information yet. You can adopt certain assessment approaches, both in testing and with real-life patients, that can rapidly identify patterns or collections of signs that identify life-threatening situations or serious medical conditions. Here are the top ten assessment tips for you to keep in mind.

Looking at the Whole Patient

As an EMT student, it's easy to get hung up on one finding, one number, one something that makes you jump to a conclusion. For example, you may see a test question where the respiratory rate is 10. Based on this single finding, you may be tempted to choose an answer that provides supplemental oxygen using a nonrebreather mask. But if the patient is also described as being altered, with shallow respirations, a slow heart rate, and cool, cyanotic skin, a breathing rate of 10 is probably inadequate and the patient requires manual ventilation.

Look at the big picture. Pull all the findings together before making a decision. Don't get tunneled into one single finding. It's a sure-fire way to choose the wrong answer or treatment approach.

Assessing the ABCs before Anything Else

Don't get distracted by the broken bone sticking out of the skin or the really bad burns. What will kill your patient faster than anything else is compromise to the airway, breathing difficulty, or poor circulation (you guessed it: the ABCs). Whether in an exam question or on a real patient, the game of EMS is won or lost during the first minute of assessing a critical patient.

If something is affecting the ABCs, fix it before moving on. And if you find something wrong during the primary assessment, the patient becomes an immediate transport.

Deciding Whether to Oxygenate or Ventilate

The body does whatever it takes to move oxygenated blood to the brain, heart, lungs, and kidneys. Because the brain is very sensitive to oxygen levels, any drop in concentration affects it. If the patient is having trouble breathing, make sure you understand the patient's mental status before you decide whether to oxygenate or ventilate:

- **Oxygenate:** If she is alert or able to follow your commands, her body is compensating for whatever the problem is. Supplemental oxygen via a nasal cannula or a nonrebreather mask may help to relieve the respiratory distress.
- **Ventilate:** If she is altered or unresponsive, she may be in respiratory failure and decompensating. You need to ventilate with a bag-valve mask and oxygen to ensure she has adequate tidal volume to push oxygen into the bloodstream.

Determining Shock

Shock can happen any time the body's circulatory status, or *perfusion,* becomes inadequate. In general, the problem lies within the three parts of the cardiovascular system:

- **Heart problems:** Myocardial infarction, myocardial contusion, cardiac tamponade
- **Pipe problems:** Sepsis, anaphylaxis, spinal injury
- **Fluid problems:** Dehydration or major bleeding

As with breathing difficulty (see the preceding section), there are two levels of shock:

- **Compensated:** The patient is alert or follows commands, his breathing rate and pulse are elevated, his skin is pale and cool to the touch, and his blood pressure is normal or even high.
- **Decompensated:** The patient is altered or unresponsive, his breathing rate and pulse are really fast or slow, his skin is pale or cyanotic and cold or clammy to the touch, and his blood pressure is falling or low.

What's as important as recognizing shock is treating it. In either state, reducing the workload on the body while it's in shock is crucial. Lay the patient flat or on his side, provide oxygen if saturation levels are low, and maintain body temperature by keeping him covered, especially if you expose the body during assessment. If ventilations aren't adequate, use a bag-valve mask and oxygen.

Searching for the Signs of Beck's Triad

A *triad* refers to three signs that, when seen together, may point to a specific condition. Beck's triad refers to cardiac tamponade, where the space between the heart and its pericardium fills with fluid or blood, sometimes as a result of trauma or from a heart infection. This fluid compresses the heart chambers, which in turn makes it difficult for the heart to pump blood. Systolic blood pressure falls. At the same time, the pressure around the heart causes diastolic pressure to rise. The combination of falling systolic and rising diastolic is called a narrowing pulse width or pressure.

The rising pressure causes the neck veins to bulge under the skin, or jugular venous distention. The fluid surrounding the heart makes it difficult to hear lung sounds; they become more muffled. Tie all of these findings together, and you have Beck's triad: narrowing pulse width, jugular venous distension, and muffled heart sounds.

There's not much for prehospital treatment; the patient will likely want to sit up to relieve the pain that's sometimes associated with the condition. Maintain oxygen saturation levels and transport as soon as possible. At the emergency department, a physician may insert a long, slender needle into the pericardial sac and remove as much of the fluid as possible, a procedure called *pericardiocentesis.*

Checking for Cushing's Triad

When the brain is injured from trauma, it does what any other tissue does — it swells. But the skull keeps it from becoming bigger as it swells, which results in pressure building up within the brain tissue, or *intracranial pressure* (ICP). ICP reduces the amount of blood flowing to the brain. The body attempts to compensate by increasing blood pressure. Although that sounds great — more blood to the brain — it also worsens the ICP. So the body tries to compensate further by slowing down the heart rate. Nevertheless, ICP continues to rise, which begins to crush the lower part of the brain, slowing down the heart rate even more and causing the breathing rate and rhythm to change. The patient has irregular respirations, even hyperventilation, because dropping carbon dioxide levels in the bloodstream can cause blood vessels to constrict, reducing brain blood flow a little.

If you suspect your patient with altered mental status has increasing ICP, check for Cushing's triad: increasing blood pressure, decreasing heart rate, and changes in breathing patterns. You may need to manually ventilate the patient with a bag-valve mask and oxygen if the breathing rate becomes too slow or irregular. If the pupils become unequal in size or if they become dilated and fixed, you have to actually increase the ventilation rate slightly, or *hyperventilate.* This means ventilating an adult patient at 20 breaths per minute, 25 breaths per minute for a child, and 30 breaths per minute for an infant under 1 year of age.

Recognizing That Not All Wheezes Are Asthma

One common mistake EMTs make is thinking that wheezing in the lungs can only mean an asthma attack. Wheezing simply means the bronchioles are constricted. That may be because they are irritated, causing an asthma attack. But the constriction can also be due to fluid buildup around smaller bronchioles, as in congestive heart failure (CHF).

Be sure to look at the whole picture; a patient with breathing difficulty, jugular venous distension, high blood pressure, pedal edema *and* wheezing is more likely to be in CHF, not having an asthma attack.

Listing the Causes of Altered Mental Status

The brain is sensitive to blood levels of oxygen, carbon dioxide, nutrients, and waste. That's why EMTs are always assessing how alert the patient is and become concerned when mental status changes. An easy way to remember a variety of causes for altered mental status is

AEIOUTIPS. The following list shows the condition that each letter of the mnemonic stands for, along with signs and symptoms to look for:

- **A – Alcohol intoxication:** Breath odor, alcohol containers, slurred speech, staggering gait.
- **E – Epilepsy or seizure:** Bleeding tongue, incontinence, medical history, med-alert jewelry.
- **I – Insulin shock (hypoglycemia) or diabetic coma (hyperglycemia):** Insulin or diabetic medications; small syringes; evidence of the hyperglycemic "3 Polly's": polydipsia (excessive thirst), polyuria (excessive urination), and polyphasia (excessive hunger/ eating).
- **O – Overdose of medications or drugs:** Missing pills, evidence of drug abuse, needles and syringes, very constricted pupils (narcotic OD), very dilated pupils (stimulant OD).
- **U – Uremia or renal failure:** History of renal disease, worsening weakness in extremities, headache or seizures, dialysis shunt.
- **T – Trauma (brain injury):** Trauma mechanism of injury (MOI; see Chapter 12), Beck's triad (described earlier in this chapter).
- **I – Infection (sepsis):** Fever; signs of infection; history of aches, chills, cough, or poor oral intake.
- **P – Psychological (behavioral):** Psychiatric history, evidence of medication abuse or overdose.
- **S – Stroke or shock:** Look for signs of stroke using the Cincinnati Stroke Scale or another assessment tool that you learned in class; signs of shock are described earlier in this chapter.

Understanding That Not All Myocardial Infarctions Have Chest Pain as a Symptom

The classic sign of a myocardial infarction (MI) in Caucasian males is chest pain or pressure that radiates to the arm or jaw. Women or patients from other racial backgrounds may experience more of an achiness or nondescript discomfort centered between the shoulders or in the epigastrium. Older patients and patients with advanced diabetic disease may not have any complaint of chest discomfort at all and may experience unexplained shortness of breath, nausea, or sudden syncope (fainting). If you see these symptoms, first think of cardiac conditions before suspecting something else as the underlying cause.

Knowing That Crying Is a Good Sign in Pediatric Patients

No one likes to hear a child cry. But in emergency care, loud crying is a sign that the pediatric patient recognizes pain or an unknown, frightening situation. Another good sign is the pediatric patient who clings or stays close to the parent. If the child isn't responding to the environment, is quiet, or otherwise doesn't respond appropriately, you have cause for concern and should perform an assessment quickly.

Chapter 20

Ten Tips for Performing EMT Procedures

In This Chapter

- Using practical tips for better hands-on performance
- Assessing consistent documentation approaches

As much as the EMT exam is focused on your knowledge base and decision-making ability, much of the practice of the EMT is a hands-on experience. In other words, you touch patients, either with your hands or with a piece of equipment. Here are ten tips for improving your ability to do so and increasing your confidence factor.

Practice, Practice, Practice

There's a short saying that reflects the importance of practicing your skills: "Train as you work; work as you trained."

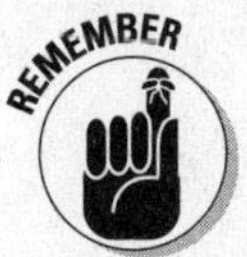

In other words, how you perform a skill in the field is based on how you learned it in school. The *only* way to get better at a skill is to practice it often, until the steps become second nature. Skills like taking a blood pressure, applying a splint, and palpating a broken bone take practice to perfect. The more times you practice, the easier the task becomes. And over time, when something unusual pops up and you have to make an adjustment, it'll be easier to do so.

Closely Evaluate Breathing

It's tempting to assume that the patient who is talking with you is breathing normally. Resist the temptation. A patient's breathing takes priority over everything else. If she is having difficulty breathing, she may have to stop talking in order to take her next breath. As the patient talks, listen for unusually short sentences or sentences that break prematurely.

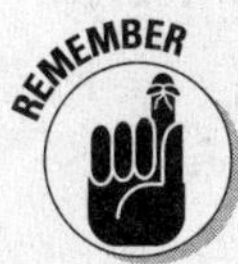

Even better, when you begin your primary assessment, take a moment to really observe the chest rising and falling. Normal breathing is hard to see; abnormal breathing may appear as being faster, shallower, or even deeper. If you see faster breathing, look for accessory muscle use in the abdomen and neck. If you see these in action, be very concerned — assume that this patient is in serious trouble until proven otherwise.

Palpate Firmly and Steadily

You have to put your hands on the patient during your examination. Hands-on assessments range from taking a patient's radial pulse to palpating the abdominal region for tenderness and masses. Many EMTs are afraid to hurt a patient during palpation and press too lightly as a result.

Palpation has to be firm enough to depress the tissue underneath the flats of your fingers. Press at a steady rate and watch the person's face for any signs of discomfort. Stop as soon as you cause pain.

You can quickly check a patient's extremities during a rapid trauma assessment by putting your hands on the opposite sides of the extremity and pushing them toward each other slightly. If there is an injury, this maneuver will cause pain.

Improve the Volume of Lung Sounds

Lung sounds are difficult to hear at first. Normal lung sounds are quiet, like a soft breeze in your ears. You can improve the volume by doing two things:

- Make sure the stethoscope is planted firmly in your ears. The tips of the stethoscope should be pointing slightly forward, in the same direction as your nose. Then place the bell of the stethoscope in between two ribs, not on top of one.
- Ask the patient to take a deep breath and exhale normally. This causes air to rush in more quickly and increases turbulence in the bronchioles, making lung sounds louder and easier to hear.

If the patient or other people on-scene are talking, ask them to stop speaking for a few seconds while you auscultate.

Immobilize the Patient's Spine at the Correct Time

When talking trauma, a common practice is to protect the patient's spinal cord after a potential injury has occurred. It used to be that EMTs would take spinal precautions based on mechanism of injury (MOI) alone (for example, a fall or car crash). Recent research has changed the practice; in addition to the MOI, a patient should have signs of a possible spinal cord injury, such as pain to the spine, tingling *(parathesia),* and/or weakness in the extremities *(paraplegia).* In these cases, you should immobilize the patient.

If there's an MOI but the patient doesn't have signs of a spinal cord injury, evaluate whether any of the following conditions exist:

- Another injury is causing so much pain that it may be distracting the patient from spine pain.
- The patient is intoxicated by alcohol or drugs.
- The patient is unable to communicate with you because of altered mental status, a language barrier, or other medical conditions.

If any of these situations exist, you need to protect the patient's spine.

Control Bleeding Immediately

In serious trauma, the patient needs every red blood cell he has to carry oxygen throughout the body. This means that you must control bleeding as soon as you detect it. When you first approach the patient, you may be tempted to avoid treating the obvious bleeding first and focus on his airway and breathing. If there is active external bleeding, place a gloved hand on the site and apply direct pressure while you evaluate the patient's airway and breathing. Better yet, direct a team member to control bleeding while you perform the primary assessment.

Keep in mind that direct pressure controls nearly all forms of external bleeding. If bleeding doesn't stop within a few seconds, you may need to apply a tourniquet.

Splint an Angulated Fracture the Way You Found It (If Possible)

Unless otherwise directed, an angulated fracture of a long bone should be splinted in the position in which you found it if a pulse can be detected distal to the fracture. If no pulse is detected, you can apply mild traction to the extremity and attempt once to align the bone's ends back to their normal position. If the pulse returns, continue to splint the injury.

If you can't find a pulse after straightening the extremity, continue to splint the injury. Be sure to let the emergency department know you had to straighten the fracture because of what you found.

Perform a Focused Physical Exam

You can't complete your assessment of the patient with a medical complaint without performing some type of focused physical assessment. For example, if the patient is complaining of chest pain, you should palpate the chest wall and auscultate lung sounds. If the patient is complaining of shortness of breath, you should listen to lung sounds, palpate for pedal edema, and observe for jugular venous distension. Each medical condition has a set of physical findings that can help you refine your suspicion of the underlying condition.

Make an Abdominal Exam More Accurate

For the patient with abdominal discomfort or some type of gastrointestinal complaint, you need to palpate the abdomen as part of the physical exam. To perform this exam accurately, have the patient lay supine on his back, with his knees bent. This relaxes the abdominal muscles, making palpation easier, and puts the organs in the right positions. The organs shift when the patient sits or stands. Use the flats of your fingers to press firmly into each quadrant and watch for any sign of discomfort.

Provide Consistent Medical Documentation

Regardless of how variable patient presentations can be, you want to document the same way each time. Consistency helps you to document completely and makes the process easier each time you do it. There are a few methods to record your findings, such as the CHART or SOAP method.

CHART stands for:

- **C – Complaint:** Why EMS was called; the patient's chief complaint
- **H – History:** The history of the present illness or injury; what happened
- **A – Assessment:** What you found during your assessment, including a SAMPLE history (signs/symptoms, allergies, medications, past medical history, last oral intake, events leading up to the complaint)
- **R – Rx or Treatment:** What care you provided during your assessment
- **T – Transport:** What happened during your care; where you transported the patient

SOAP stands for:

- **S – Subjective findings:** These include the patient's chief complaint, the history of the present illness, and the patient's past medical history including medications and allergies.
- **O – Objective findings:** These include vital signs and physical exam findings.
- **A – Assessment:** What you think is happening to the patient. You may have more than one suspicion.
- **P – Plan:** This is your treatment plan, indicating what actions you performed.

You can use either of these methods or one you create, so long as it captures a similar level of detail. Regardless of which method you use, use it all the time.

Index

• A •

• B •

• C •

• D •

• E •

• F •

• G •

• H •

• I •

• J •

• K •

• L •

• M •

• N •

• O •

• T •

• U •

• V •

• W •

About the Author

Art Hsieh, MA, NREMT-P, has been in the EMS profession since 1982 and has worked as a volunteer, line medic, educator, and chief officer in private, third-service, and fire-based EMS. He has directed both primary and EMS continuing education programs, and currently he is the Paramedic Program Director for the Public Safety Training Center at Santa Rosa Junior College in California. A past president of the National Association of EMS Educators, Art is a published textbook author and editorial columnist, and he has presented at conferences across the United States and internationally.

Dedication

The EMS family is filled with the most caring, compassionate people that I have the privilege of calling friends. Many have been my teachers and mentors. I have learned much from them and can only hope to continue to pay it forward. I am honored to be part of this family, and dedicate this work to them.

Even more important is my own family. Their love and sacrifice have allowed me to serve my profession in ways few EMS providers can imagine. To my wife, Veronica, no words can convey my deepest gratitude for your love and friendship. Thank you.

Author's Acknowledgments

To paraphrase the saying, it takes a village to raise the village Dummy.

I was surprised and honored when I was asked to create a *Dummies* book for the EMT exam. This venerable series of how-to books is well known for breaking down complex information into easier-to-understand concepts and manageable chunks. However, when I started writing the content for this book, I felt like I was the dummy!

Fortunately, the good folks at John Wiley & Sons provided me the confidence to complete this book. Erin Calligan Mooney, acquisitions editor, paved the way to get me onboard with the project. Senior project editor Georgette Beatty's expert editing, much-too-kind words, and gentle nudging of maintaining deadlines made the project much more straightforward and helped to calm my ever-present stress. Copy editor Christy Pingleton provided the extra pair of eyes in making sure what I wrote would make sense to the reader. My technical reviewer, colleague, and friend Lori Gallian had the thankless task of keeping me on the straight and narrow when keeping the facts straight. Kathryn Born's artistic hand created the perfect set of simple but effective illustrations to highlight some of the key points in the text.

EMS is a small profession; those who teach others to save lives, smaller still. I'm blessed to call many of them my colleagues and close friends. Their willingness to share their mistakes and successes has helped shape my teaching practice and continues to influence it to this day.

Publisher's Acknowledgments

Acquisitions Editor: Erin Calligan Mooney

Senior Project Editor: Georgette Beatty

Copy Editor: Christine Pingleton

Technical Editor: Lori Gallian

Art Coordinator: Alicia B. South

Project Coordinator: Sheree Montgomery

Illustrator: Kathryn Born, MA

Cover Image: ©iStock.com/lauradyoung

e & Mac

For Dummies, 6th Edition
-118-72306-7

ne For Dummies, 7th Edition
-118-69083-3

All-in-One For Dummies,
dition
-118-82210-4

Mavericks For Dummies
-118-69188-5

ging & Social Media

book For Dummies, 5th Edition
-118-63312-0

l Media Engagement For Dummies
-118-53019-1

Press For Dummies, 6th Edition
-118-79161-5

ness

Investing For Dummies,
dition
-118-37678-2

ting For Dummies, 6th Edition
)-470-90545-6

nal Finance For Dummies,
dition
-118-11785-9

Books 2014 For Dummies
-118-72005-9

Business Marketing Kit
ummies, 3rd Edition
-118-31183-7

Careers

Job Interviews For Dummies, 4th Edition
978-1-118-11290-8

Job Searching with Social Media For Dummies, 2nd Edition
978-1-118-67856-5

Personal Branding For Dummies
978-1-118-11792-7

Resumes For Dummies, 6th Edition
978-0-470-87361-8

Starting an Etsy Business For Dummies, 2nd Edition
978-1-118-59024-9

Diet & Nutrition

Belly Fat Diet For Dummies
978-1-118-34585-6

Mediterranean Diet For Dummies
978-1-118-71525-3

Nutrition For Dummies, 5th Edition
978-0-470-93231-5

Digital Photography

Digital SLR Photography All-in-One For Dummies, 2nd Edition
978-1-118-59082-9

Digital SLR Video & Filmmaking For Dummies
978-1-118-36598-4

Photoshop Elements 12 For Dummies
978-1-118-72714-0

Gardening

Herb Gardening For Dummies, 2nd Edition
978-0-470-61778-6

Gardening with Free-Range Chickens For Dummies
978-1-118-54754-0

Health

Boosting Your Immunity For Dummies
978-1-118-40200-9

Diabetes For Dummies, 4th Edition
978-1-118-29447-5

Living Paleo For Dummies
978-1-118-29405-5

Big Data

Big Data For Dummies
978-1-118-50422-2

Data Visualization For Dummies
978-1-118-50289-1

Hadoop For Dummies
978-1-118-60755-8

Language & Foreign Language

500 Spanish Verbs For Dummies
978-1-118-02382-2

English Grammar For Dummies, 2nd Edition
978-0-470-54664-2

French All-in-One For Dummies
978-1-118-22815-9

German Essentials For Dummies
978-1-118-18422-6

Italian For Dummies, 2nd Edition
978-1-118-00465-4

Math & Science

Algebra I For Dummies, 2nd Edition
978-0-470-55964-2

Available in print and e-book formats.

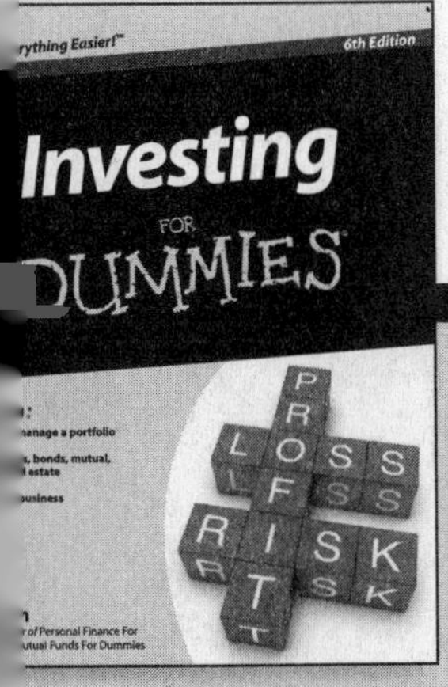

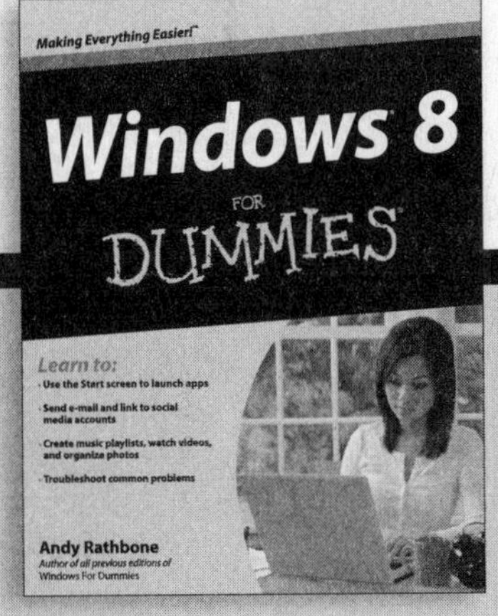

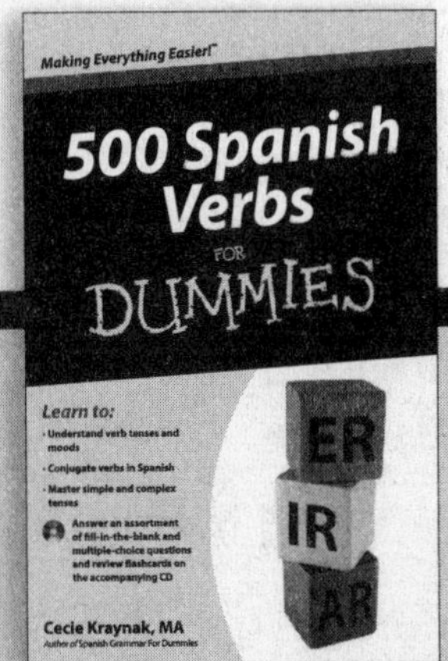

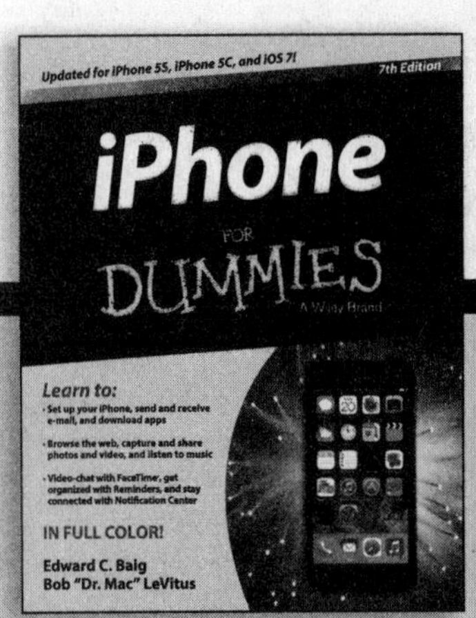

Available wherever books are sold. **For more information or to order direct visit www.dummies.com**

Anatomy and Physiology For Dummies, 2nd Edition
978-0-470-92326-9

Astronomy For Dummies, 3rd Edition
978-1-118-37697-3

Biology For Dummies, 2nd Edition
978-0-470-59875-7

Chemistry For Dummies, 2nd Edition
978-1-118-00730-3

1001 Algebra II Practice Problems For Dummies
978-1-118-44662-1

Microsoft Office

Excel 2013 For Dummies
978-1-118-51012-4

Office 2013 All-in-One For Dummies
978-1-118-51636-2

PowerPoint 2013 For Dummies
978-1-118-50253-2

Word 2013 For Dummies
978-1-118-49123-2

Music

Blues Harmonica For Dummies
978-1-118-25269-7

Guitar For Dummies, 3rd Edition
978-1-118-11554-1

iPod & iTunes For Dummies, 10th Edition
978-1-118-50864-0

Programming

Beginning Programming with C For Dummies
978-1-118-73763-7

Excel VBA Programming For Dummies, 3rd Edition
978-1-118-49037-2

Java For Dummies, 6th Edition
978-1-118-40780-6

Religion & Inspiration

The Bible For Dummies
978-0-7645-5296-0

Buddhism For Dummies, 2nd Edition
978-1-118-02379-2

Catholicism For Dummies, 2nd Edition
978-1-118-07778-8

Self-Help & Relationships

Beating Sugar Addiction For Dummies
978-1-118-54645-1

Meditation For Dummies, 3rd Edition
978-1-118-29144-3

Seniors

Laptops For Seniors For Dummies, 3rd Edition
978-1-118-71105-7

Computers For Seniors For Dummies, 3rd Edition
978-1-118-11553-4

iPad For Seniors For Dummies, 6th Edition
978-1-118-72826-0

Social Security For Dummies
978-1-118-20573-0

Smartphones & Tablets

Android Phones For Dummies, 2nd Edition
978-1-118-72030-1

Nexus Tablets For Dummies
978-1-118-77243-0

Samsung Galaxy S 4 For Dummies
978-1-118-64222-1

Samsung Galaxy Tabs For Dummies
978-1-118-77294-2

Test Prep

ACT For Dummies, 5th Edition
978-1-118-01259-8

ASVAB For Dummies, 3rd Edition
978-0-470-63760-9

GRE For Dummies, 7th Edition
978-0-470-88921-3

Officer Candidate Tests For Dummie
978-0-470-59876-4

Physician's Assistant Exam For Dum
978-1-118-11556-5

Series 7 Exam For Dummies
978-0-470-09932-2

Windows 8

Windows 8.1 All-in-One For Dummi
978-1-118-82087-2

Windows 8.1 For Dummies
978-1-118-82121-3

Windows 8.1 For Dummies, Book + Bundle
978-1-118-82107-7

Available in print and e-book formats.

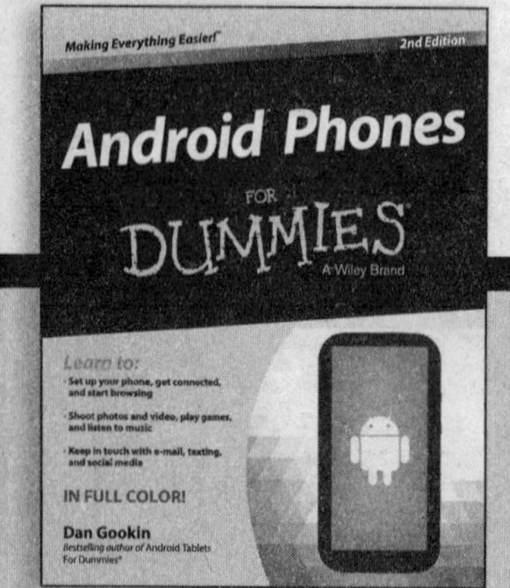

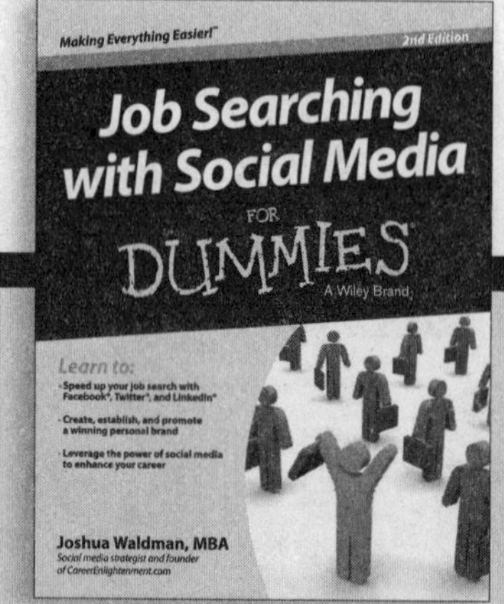

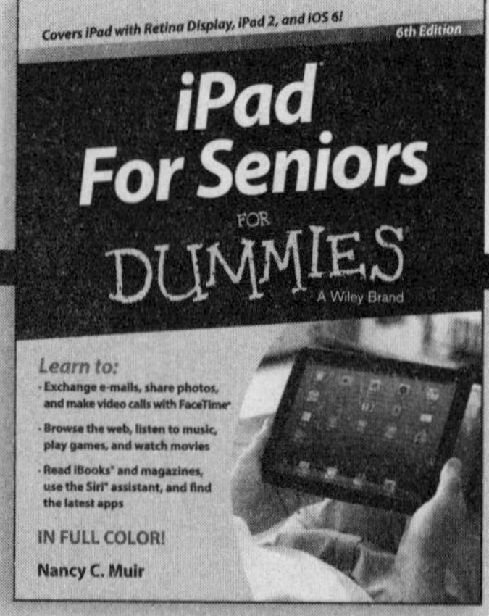

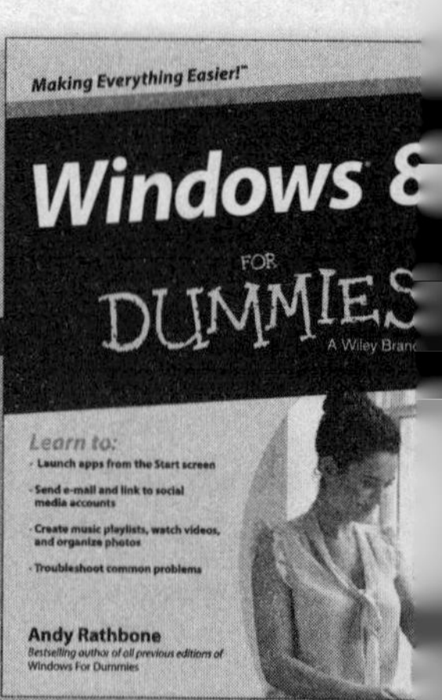

Available wherever books are sold. **For more information or to order direct visit www.dummies.com**